The Texture of Life

Purposeful Activities
in Occupational Therapy

Jim Hinojosa, PhD, OT, FAOTA
Marie-Louise Blount, AM, OT, FAOTA
Editors

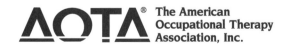

AOTA® The American
Occupational Therapy
Association, Inc.

The American Occupational Therapy Association, Inc.
4720 Montgomery Lane
PO Box 31220
Bethesda, Maryland 20824-1220

Disclaimers

This publication is designed to provide accurate and authoritative information in regard to the subject matter covered. It is sold or distributed with the understanding that the publisher is not engaged in rendering legal, accounting, or other professional service. If legal advice or other expert assistance is required, the services of a competent professional person should be sought.

—From the Declaration of Principles jointly adopted by the American Bar Association and a Committee of Publishers and Associations

It is the objective of The American Occupational Therapy Association to be a forum for free expression and interchange of ideas. The opinions expressed by the contributors to this work are their own and not necessarily those of either the editors or The American Occupational Therapy Association.

ISBN 1-56900-145-6

Printed in the United States of America.

Contents

Foreword

"Of course I know what activities are. Doesn't everyone?" This kind of response is a familiar one and not altogether unexpected. After all, each and every one of us, including those of us who practice as occupational therapists, engage in numerous diverse activities each day, every day, every week, every month, and every year of our lives. Moreover, these activities are so tightly woven into the fabric of our everyday lives that most of the time we tend to take them for granted. By common consent, we deem these activities ordinary, mundane, even commonplace.

Many years ago, Mary Reilly (1962) raised the issue of commonplaceness as she contemplated the question of whether occupational therapy is a "sufficiently vital and unique service for medicine to support and society to reward" (p. 1). She went on to say that this question in part stems from "the wide and gaping chasm which exists between the complexity of illness and commonplaceness of our treatment tools . . . (which) is, and always will be, both the pride and anguish of our profession" (p. 1).

But does commonplaceness necessarily have to be the anguish of our profession? By no means must this be the case if we recognize and acknowledge not only how ordinary our treatment tools seem to be but also how pervasively these everyday activities that become our treatment tools are intertwined with the health and well-being of all humankind. What other profession can claim that its tools are in the real world among real people here, there, and everywhere? The tools may be similar in some respects all over the world and different in other respects in various societies and cultures, but they are always directed ultimately to existence, subsistence, and coexistence.

With recognition and acknowledgment, however, comes our professional responsibility to build a base of knowledge about activities both as natural human phenomena and as links to health. Our explorations into these realms have so far been sporadic at best, so this book, *The Texture of Life,* is doubly welcome, first because it is one of the few texts devoted unequivocally to inspecting and describing activities and second because it links activities to the process of clinical intervention, a first step in demonstrating the importance of activities as therapeutic tools.

But we still have a long way to go. We urgently need an activities database from an occupational frame of reference. With our present knowledge, we have little systematic information about what people in the real world do every day; how, when, how often, with whom, and where these activities are done; and from whom and how these activities are learned. We need to know how activities as natural human phenomena manifest themselves in different societies, cultures, and other subgroups and in persons belonging to those groups. Until now, most of what we know about human activities has resulted largely from information that we have extrapolated from our own experiences combined with activities histories that we have gleaned from our clients. To have at our disposal more objective, general, and systematic data about those natural human phenomena we call "activities" would certainly lend greater legitimacy to our tools and would additionally serve as a social basis for research.

Similarly, we urgently need a knowledge base related to the links between activities and health. In this area, we are in a somewhat better position. We already have a perfectly structured hypothesis waiting to be tested (Reilly, 1962), an operational (versus semantic) definition of activities that serves not only to include but also to delimit the range of our concerns, and a theoretical construct, activities health, that emanates from an emphasis on what persons can do, not on what they cannot do (Cynkin & Robinson, 1990). The latest contribution vital to our in-depth investigations probes the meaning of activities (Fidler & Velde, 1999). Each study serves as a guide to further exploration and provides a framework for increasingly sophisticated theoretical speculation and interpretation.

At the end of this century, we have come to recognize the central importance of activities to occupational therapy. Perhaps the first years of the new millennium will usher in the "Decade of Activities" in a newer and far more intricate guise as we meet the challenge to uncover the profound beneath the commonplace. This we must do to survive.

Simme Cynkin, MS, OT, FAOTA

References

Cynkin, S., & Robinson, A. M. (1990). *Occupational therapy and activities health: Toward health through activities.* Philadelphia: Lippincott.

Fidler, G. S., & Velde, B. P. (1999). *Activities: Reality and symbol.* Thorofare, NJ: Slack.

Reilly, M. (1962). Occupational therapy can be one of the great ideas of 20th century medicine, 1962. Eleanor Clarke Slagle lecture. *American Journal of Occupational Therapy, 16,* 1–9.

Acknowledgments

For all of their joint and individual efforts in the preparation of this book, the Editors sincerely thank the faculty and staff members of the Department of Occupational Therapy at New York University. We especially thank the authors and contributors to this work, both those who are faculty and graduate students at New York University and those colleagues who work at other universities and sites. Among those who contributed greatly to the book but whose names do not appear elsewhere is Shu-Hwa Chen, who prepared many of the final manuscripts and figures and checked references. The Editors are in her debt.

Marie-Louise Blount profoundly appreciates the love and support of Elena and Wesley Blount, who have made all of her endeavors worthwhile. Jim Hinojosa thanks both of his parents, who instilled in him a love for engagement in purposeful, meaningful activity. Additionally, he thanks Dr. Anne C. Mosey, who provided the insight that would refine his thinking about activity and occupational therapy.

We are indebted to our clients because they reaffirm our beliefs about the value of active engagement and the meaningfulness of occupational therapy. Finally, we are indebted to our students, current and former, who are the reason for writing this book. We continually learn the value of what we do from them.

Contributors

Beverly Bain, EdD, OT, FAOTA, is Adjunct Associate Professor, Department of Occupational Therapy, New York University, New York, New York.

Paulette F. Bell, MA, OT, is Admissions Director, Professional Program, Department of Occupational Therapy, New York University, and in private practice, New York, New York.

Marie-Louise Blount, AM, OT, FAOTA, is Clinical Associate Professor, Department of Occupational Therapy, New York University, New York, New York.

Wesley G. Blount, is Editor, New York, New York.

Karen A. Buckley, MA, OT/L, is Clinical Assistant Professor, Department of Occupational Therapy, New York University, New York, New York.

Ann Burkhardt, MA, OTR/L, BCN, is Director of Occupational Therapy, New York Presbyterian Hospital, and Associate Clinical Professor, Columbia University, New York, New York, and Clinical Associate, Mercy College, Dobbs Ferry, New York.

Lisa Cyzner, MS, OTR, is Doctoral Candidate, Department of Occupational Therapy, New York University, New York, New York, and in pediatric private practice, Long Island, New York.

Mary V. Donohue, PhD, OT, FAOTA, is Clinical Associate Professor, Department of Occupational Therapy, New York University, New York, New York.

Beth K. Elenko, MA, OTR, is Doctoral Candidate, Department of Occupational Therapy, New York University, New York, New York, and private contractor, Early Intervention, Queens, New York.

Ellen Greer, MA, OT, CpsyA, is Doctoral Candidate and Adjunct Faculty, Department of Occupational Therapy, New York University, and in private practice, New York, New York.

Sharon A. Gutman, PhD, OTR, is Assistant Professor, Division of Occupational Therapy, Long Island University, Brooklyn, New York.

Prudence Heisler, MA, OT/L, is Assistant Fieldwork Coordinator, Department of Occupational Therapy, New York University, Special Programs in Occupational Therapy Services (SPOTS), New York, New York.

Jim Hinojosa, PhD, OT, FAOTA, is Professor, Department of Occupational Therapy, New York University, New York, New York.

Paula Kramer, PhD, OTR, FAOTA, is Professor and Chair, Department of Occupational Therapy, Kean University, Union, New Jersey.

Sheama S. Krishnagiri, PhD, OTR, is Assistant Professor, Department of Occupational Therapy, Virginia Commonwealth University, Richmond, Virginia.

Deborah R. Labovitz, PhD, OTR/L, FAOTA, is Professor and Chair, Department of Occupational Therapy, New York University, New York, New York.

Paula McCreedy, MEd, OT/L, is Clinical Assistant Professor, Department of Occupational Therapy, New York University, Special Programs in Occupational Therapy Services (SPOTS), New York, New York.

Jane Miller, MA, OTR/L, is Post Professional Admissions Director, Department of Occupational Therapy, New York University, New York, New York.

Bernadette Mineo, PhD, OTR, is in Private Practice, Long Beach, New York.

David L. Nelson, PhD, OTR/L, FAOTA, is Professor, Department of Occupational Therapy, Medical College of Ohio, Toledo, Ohio.

Laurette J. Olson, MA, OTR, BCP, is Occupational Therapy Consultant, Mamaroneck Union Free School District, Mamaroneck, New York, and Professional Associate, Coordinator of the Adolescence and Occupational Therapy Practice Module, Graduate Program in Occupational Therapy, Mercy College, Dobbs Ferry, New York.

Anita Perr, MA, OT, ATP, is Clinical Assistant Professor, Department of Occupational Therapy, New York University, New York, New York.

Sally E. Poole, MA, OT, CHT, is Clinical Assistant Professor, Department of Occupational Therapy, New York University, New York, New York, and Co-Owner, Hands-On Rehab, Valhalla, New York.

Elizabeth A. Roarty-O'Herron, MS, OTR, is Senior Occupational Therapist, South Oaks Hospital, Amityville, New York, and Teaching Associate, Mercy College, Dobbs Ferry, New York.

Joyce Shapero Sabari, PhD, OTR, BCN, is Associate Professor and Chair, Occupational Therapy Program, State University of New York, Health Science Center at Brooklyn, Brooklyn, New York.

Dalia Sachs, PhD, OT(I)R, is Senior Lecturer, Department of Occupational Therapy, Haifa University, Haifa, Israel.

Julie Jepsen Thomas, PhD, OTR/L, FAOTA, is Associate Professor and Chair, Department of Occupational Therapy, Medical College of Ohio, Toledo, Ohio.

1

Purposeful Activities Within the Context of Occupational Therapy

Jim Hinojosa, PhD, OT, FAOTA
Marie-Louise Blount, AM, OT, FAOTA

Activities—what we do, the foundation of much of our routine, enterprise, and art in the world—have a unique place in the context of occupational therapy. The importance of activities in occupational therapy is a varied landscape, one with multiple meanings.

In this chapter, we address some of the more fundamental of these meanings, and we establish that occupational therapy's application of these meanings is the core of the profession and an integral part of practice. We show that occupational therapy practitioners apply the various ideas analyzed in chapter 2 to describe their reasoning and their practice. The labels used are not always the same, and the ideas behind the labels are not necessarily uniform. We believe that the varying labels and ideas represent an important aspect of our thinking as well as a richness in the methods that we use, and we should therefore examine these ideas and develop our understanding of their potential for practice.

If *purposeful activity* refers to portions of occupations and encompasses various behaviors and performances (American Occupational Therapy Association [AOTA], 1993), then discussing, delimiting, and understanding the behaviors and tasks that are part of it are necessary, as is appreciating the occupations under which it is subsumed (i.e., having a definition does not necessarily simplify one's understanding of a phenomenon or the issues that it raises).

We suggest, therefore, adopting the "pluralistic approach" advocated by Mosey (1985). We advocate continued attention to questions raised by Henderson, Cermak, Coster, Murray, Trombly, and Tickle-Degnen (1991), who examined some of the dilemmas regarding our uses of and preferences for ideas surrounding purposeful activity. These authors additionally suggested that we embrace a multidimensional view of purposeful activity, both as an entity and as a therapeutic modality.

Because purposeful activity is the core of occupational therapy, we must understand the many modes in which we use that term. As Henderson and associates (1991) pointed out, both purposefulness and its varied meanings are "attributes of persons and not of activities" (p. 370). We support their belief that occupational therapy services can and do include approaches and methods other than purposeful activity.

As noted in chapter 2 of this book, numerous approaches exist in occupational therapy for using the term *purposeful activity* and other terms that we often substitute for it. As noted by Henderson and associates (1991), a wide range of types and levels of activities exist that occupational therapy practitioners use in practice. One dimension of these ranges is that from low level (e.g., reaching for an object) to high level (e.g., a simulated work activity). Other dimensions, however, involve ranges of activities from simple to complex that may include a continuum from gross (e.g., an assembly toy in which a client places a smaller plastic ring on top of a larger plastic ring) to fine (e.g., attaching a small nut to a bolt and screwing it in place) and a continuum from very brief (performing a time-limited activity once) to more lengthy (in which a client carries out demanding work or leisure activity in a concentrated fashion for an hour or more). The reader should consider other aspects of activities that range from simple to complex by identifying not only polar ends of a given continuum but also various stages of complexity that exist along the continuum.

Henderson and associates (1991) were justifiably concerned that occupational therapy practitioners realize that the person performing the activity, sometimes aided by the occupational therapy practitioner (often with the collaboration of the client to accomplish or move toward a legitimate therapeutic goal), invests meaning (purposefulness) into an activity. These authors stated that, in acute care settings and in any situation where remediation of disability is the goal of intervention, activities or segments of activities may be the means to attain a purpose or goal. Their view, which we share, is that all activities have the potential to be meaningful and purposeful. Several variables, such as the person performing the activity, the context within which the activity occurs, and when in the course of a program or series of activities the practitioner introduces the activity, affect the activity's meaningfulness and purposefulness.

Other techniques (such as performing an activity in a group or stabilizing a joint while performing an activity), as noted by these same authors (Henderson et al., 1991), contribute to the effectiveness of an activity. Although not purposeful activity per se, these are legitimate methods that the occupational therapy practitioner uses to facilitate or enhance the activity.

The same authors identify another dimension of activity that relates to occupational therapy (i.e., the history of the use of activity in the profession) and that leads to certain historical and traditional applications of activity as well as more contemporary expressions of choices of or applications of activity. Chapter 2 discusses some of these issues. Henderson and associates (1991) were concerned not only with the ways in which occupational therapy practitioners view and use activities but also with the ways in which practitioners investigate an activity's therapeutic aspects. The key point in this discussion is the multiple and varied meanings that occupational therapy practitioners apply to the concept of purposeful activity. For everyone, activities represent the core and the texture of our daily lives. For occupational therapy practitioners, purposeful activities have additional meaning.

Occupational Therapy: The Profession's Mandate

Before examining the tools that a profession uses, we must consider the purpose and focus of a profession. Professions exist to apply knowledge for the benefit of the members of society (Kielhofner, 1992; Mosey, 1981, 1992). Although each profession has a unique purpose, professions often overlap in the services they provide and the tools that they use as part of their interventions to benefit members of a society. A profession's practice is grounded in the society in which it exists. Therefore, a profession's practice may vary depending on the region of the country, the city, or the culture in which the practice is located. These differences in a profession's practices often create tension for the members of the profession who would like to believe that all members practice in the same manner with the same goals.

All members of a distinct profession share specialized training and a unique expertise. They likewise share a common philosophy and a code of ethics. The philosophical beliefs of occupational therapy outline how we view the person, the society, and persons within the context of their environments. Occupational therapy's philosophical orientation heavily influences the tools that we use to intervene with clients as occupational therapy practitioners. Chapter 2 in this text discusses the foundational beliefs of occupational therapy as they relate to one of occupational therapy's most important tools—purposeful activity. No profession, however, is unique in "owning" a philosophical orientation or the tools that its practitioners use.

The Representative Assembly of the AOTA approved an association policy related to the philosophical base of occupational therapy in 1979. In this statement, AOTA (1979) articulated the profession's basic beliefs about human nature and adaptation. Furthermore, the policy stated that occupational therapy practitioners believe in the importance of purposeful activity to facilitate the adaptive process. Adoption of this statement highlighted the importance of purposeful activity, which was synonymous with occupation. This relationship between purposeful activities and occupation has been a major philosophical topic within the profession. The following definitions are intended to delineate the terms as the authors use them in this book.

Occupation

"Occupations are the ordinary and familiar things that people do every day" (Christiansen, Clark, Kielhofner, Rogers, & Nelson, 1995, p. 1015). The meaningful groupings of activities that humans engage in as part of their daily lives are occupations. These occupations give life meaning, and occupational therapy practitioners have broadly categorized them into work, self-care, and play and leisure areas. The person who is engaging in the activity and the circumstances around which the person performs the activity defines the range of activities that is included in any one occupation. For example, eating can be work or pleasure at a state fair, work at a business lunch, and self-care at home.

Many important dimensions of an occupation make it a unique classification for occupational therapy practitioners. First, and most important, occupations have personal, specific meaning to the person (see Box 1). This personal meaning is variable and involves contextual, temporal, psychological, social, symbolic, cultural, ethnic, and spiritual dimensions. Second, occupations involve mental abilities and skills. They may or may not have an observable physical dimension. Third, the occupations that a person engages in define him or her. Fourth, as the person interacts with his or her environment, matures, or responds to life conditions, the person's preferred occupations are likely to change (AOTA, 1997).

Purposeful Activity

"Purposeful activity refers to goal-directed behaviors or tasks . . . that the individual considers meaningful" (AOTA, 1993, p. 1081). Humans engage in purposeful activities as part of their daily life routines. Purposeful activities are tasks or experiences in which the person actively participates. While engaged in a purposeful activity, the person directs his or her attention to the task (AOTA, 1993). Purposeful activities are one of the foundational elements of an occupation. Unique combinations of purposeful activities link together with the person's personal meanings to form that person's occupations. Purposeful activities are goal directed in that they involve active participation and require coordination of a person's physical, emotional, and cognitive systems. *Goal directed* means that the person actively engages in actions to meet a personal purpose or need; it does not mean that the end product must be a physical outcome. In occupational therapy, purposeful activities are an important therapeutic tool. Practitioners use them alone to address a specific need or in patterns or groups to help a person develop meaningful occupations (AOTA, 1997).

Linking Purposeful Activity and Occupation

AOTA's Uniform Terminology (1994) defines occupational therapy's area of expertise or domain of concern as encompassing performance components, performance areas, and performance contexts. These broad areas delineate differences between occupational therapy and other professions. The principal concern of occupational therapy is to maintain, restore, or facilitate a person's ability to function within his or her daily occupations. We have broadly defined daily occupations to include active participation in self-maintenance, work, and leisure and play activities. The ability to engage in these occupations requires that the person be able to complete many purposeful activities.

Occupational therapy practitioners use a wide variety of strategies and tools in their practice that they select to be consistent with well-defined theoretical bases or rationales. No one universally accepted way exists in which occupational therapy practitioners conceptualize practice. Some view practice on the basis of a model, others suggest paradigms, and others use frames of reference. In this book, we do not address the issue of how practitioners conceptualize practice. We accept that many scholars use different organizational structures and view practice differently. What is important is that each of the models, paradigms, or frames of reference provides the guidelines for the selection and use of therapeutic tools. Each occupational therapy practitioner selects from a wide assortment of tools in which he or she is both knowl-

---

Box 1
Personal Hierarchy of Needs

An important concern of educators is what motivates humans and how this interrelates with the development of human potential. Maslow, the founder of humanistic psychology, proposed that a person's gratification of needs is the most important single principle underlying development. He proposed seven levels of needs: physiological, safety, belongingness and love, esteem, self-actualization, knowing and understanding, and aesthetics. The way humans fill these needs is by engaging in meaningful activities. Reflect on the last two days and list how you satisfied your personal needs in the categories identified in Maslow's hierarchy.

- Physiological needs (food, drink, sleep, and survival)

- Safety (avoidance of danger and anxiety, desire for security)

- Love and belongingness (affection, feeling wanted, roots in a family or peer group)

- Esteem (self-respect, feelings of adequacy, competence, mastery)

- Self-actualization (striving for or using talents, capacities, potential)

- Knowing and understanding (curiosity, learning about the world)

- Aesthetic (experience and understand beauty for its own sake)

After completing the list, consider the following.

- What needs did you not meet?

- Which activities contributed to the satisfaction of your needs?

- What does the list suggest about your health status?

Note. From *Educational Psychology: Principles and Applications*, by J. A. Glover, R. H. Bruning, and R. W. Filbeck, 1983, Glenview, IL: Scott Foresman. Copyright 1983 by Scott Foresman. Adapted with permission.

edgeable and competent for practice. Specialization of practice has resulted in some occupational therapy practitioners using different tools than other practitioners do. Whatever tools an occupational therapy practitioner chooses to use, we all share a common goal that the person will be able to engage in activities of daily living (ADL), work, and play and leisure activities.

Tools of the Profession

With advancements in knowledge and technology, the practices and concerns of a profession change over time. Thus, a profession changes its priorities and practices in response to changes in society. This continuous change ensures that a profession remains viable and is responsive to the needs of the society that it serves. Occupational therapy's evolution in response to changes in society, knowledge, and technology has contributed to a viable, dynamic profession that continues to meet its mandate from society. These changes have been difficult for some occupational therapy practitioners. For example, we have replaced the early extensive use of crafts with new modalities such as manual manipulation, computer adaptation, or physical activity. Practitioners may view some changes in the importance and use of a modality as not consistent with the philosophical base of the profession. Some occupational therapy practitioners continue to believe that "true" occupational therapy must involve active engagement in an activity.

Occupational therapy's mandate has always been to enable clients to engage and participate in their own daily life activities. The trends and concerns of medicine influence occupational therapy, which a health care profession (Christiansen, 1991). Although medicine continues to affect the evolution of the profession, other more recent changes in society seem to be having a greater influence. In response to societal change, occupational therapy has moved into education and community-based service delivery models. This change in society's priorities has led to an increase in the number of practitioners working in education-based practices and a change in the site of practice to schools and community settings (Kramer & Hinojosa, 1993). These shifts in the site of practice and service delivery models are evident in other areas of practice. In the 1990s, a shift from clinic settings to more integrated community, classroom, and home settings occurred. These changes were responses to numerous internal influences (e.g., growth in knowledge, advances in technology) and external influences (e.g., social and government policy, payment practices).

This chapter presents views of purposeful activities as they relate to occupational therapy practice today and defines and outlines the relationship between the major constructs of the profession: occupation, purposeful activity, and occupational performance. Furthermore, this chapter provides the framework for the rest of the book.

Occupational Therapy's Intervention Tools

The application of any frame of reference (model, practice guidelines, paradigm) involves the use of various intervention strategies and tools. Tools are items, means, methods, or instruments that professionals use in practice in a theoretically pro-scribed manner to bring about change. A profession's tools change with evolving knowledge, technological advances, and the changing needs of clients. Occupational therapy practitioners use various tools depending on the particular frame of refer-ence. Mosey (1986) identified six major legitimate tools in occupational therapy: nonhuman environment, conscious use of self, activity analysis and adaptation, pur-poseful activities, activity groups, and the teaching–learning process. In addition to these tools, the profession has other tools that are specialized and often are specific to one frame of reference (Hinojosa & Kramer, 1993).

One of the major issues related to tools is that many practitioners consider the tools of the profession to be exceptionally important. Some even consider the tools to be symbolic of the profession as a whole (Hinojosa & Kramer, 1993). This impor-tance may be a result of the tangible aspects of legitimate tools and may be because practitioners use tools daily as they interact with clients (Mosey, 1986). In addition, many practitioners view the tools of their profession as unique. In reality, however, the legitimate tools are not unique, and many professions may share them. What is unique is the way that a specific profession applies the tools. In occupational therapy, this uniqueness lies in how practitioners use the tools together in the application of the specific frame of reference.

Activities

Each day, we engage in numerous activities as part of our lives. We perform some of these activities to meet our self-care needs. We perform some activities because we enjoy them. Other activities result from our responses to others' expectations or to circumstances that require them. Thus, activities are the things that we do. They are the building blocks that we use to construct our lives. Occupational therapy evolved from the realized importance of how we occupy our time as human beings. This con-cern with occupations is central to our beliefs about what we do and believe as occu-pational therapy practitioners. From our perspective as occupational therapy practitioners, activities are the actions that humans take to accomplish a goal or func-tion. Activities consist of groupings of actions or tasks that a person does as part of accomplishing the goal or fulfilling the expected or required function. Activities are purposeful when they are meaningful to the person who is completing the task or action. Tasks are the component parts of some activities. We can combine one or more tasks together to become one activity. When we view a pattern of daily activities together that has meaning for the person, we categorize the activities as occupations. Thus, activities are the fundamental basis for occupations (Kramer & Hinojosa, 1995).

From this perspective, both activities and the consequent occupations are fundamental and are an essential part of life. Our daily activities and occupations define who and what we are. Engagement in purposeful activities gives our lives meaning. In defining our domain of concern, we, as occupational therapy practitioners, typically view activities as part of occupations (e.g., we divide activities into ADL, work activities, or play and leisure activities). By viewing activities in this manner, we think about activities as they relate to the end result for the person who engages in that particular purposeful activity. Thus, the same activities may fit into several occupations depending on the goal of the activity, the developmental status of the person, and the specific circumstances and the context in which he or she performs the activity. The following example illustrates this point. Writing may be "work" for a school-aged child at camp who has to write a letter home to his parents. For a young person, writing a letter to a girlfriend may be a leisure activity. For an adult, writing a shopping list may be an ADL. In these examples, note that the activity is writing. The occupations for which writing is an activity component are work, leisure, and ADL. For the professional author who writes, writing may be an occupation, the essential core of his work. In this scenario, the professional author engages in numerous writing activities that together are an occupation. The following discussion outlines the unique view we share related to purposeful activities and occupations.

ADL

Each day, all humans engage in many daily living occupations. These occupations consist of self-care activities, which are the means that we use to interact and respond to our life demands and needs. Not all self-care activities are interesting or enjoyable. In fact, we consider many basic self-care activities to be boring, routine, and unexciting. These ordinary daily self-care activities, however, are basic to our survival as social human beings. We should not minimize the importance of the ability to engage in these activities. Our ability to take care of ourselves and meet our daily needs is vital to our existence. The ability to feed ourselves, dress ourselves, and take care of our own toileting needs provides valued independence. As mundane as many self-care activities can be, they are critically important to self-esteem and self-worth. A wide range of factors including individual attributes and abilities, culture, context, developmental status, and socioeconomic status determines the multitude of purposeful activities categorized as self-care.

Work or Productive Activities

The occupations of work or productive activities consist of the numerous activities that humans engage in to support themselves and their family members, to fill time in a socially acceptable fashion, to give expression to their interests, to apply their education and training, to maintain important social status, to alleviate stress, to mitigate loneliness, or to avoid doubts about life's purposes, to name a few possibilities.

Work is an obligation for many persons, but, in our society, work is not usually a requirement for children, some students, some persons with disabilities, and most persons who have retired. We devote much of our time to work and productive activities. In addition to time spent working, we devote much of our time to preparing for work and traveling to and from work. Many persons have more than one job. Activities involved in work are extremely varied. Many American workers must adjust to the demands of large, formal organizations and complex technology. Work activities are central to the lives of most adult men and women and become a key focus in what makes many persons' lives meaningful.

Play or Leisure Activities

Play or leisure occupations include a wide range of activities in which one engages for intrinsic pleasure (because they are fun). These occupations can range from solitary activities such as reading a book to physically demanding sports. An important characteristic of play or leisure activities is that the person chooses to engage in them because he or she wants to. As with self-care activities, a wide range of factors including individual attributes and abilities, culture, context, developmental status, and socioeconomic status determines play or leisure purposeful activities.

As occupational therapy practitioners, we are concerned with the wide range of activities in which clients engage. Activities are fundamental and normal for all humans. Purposeful activities define what and who you are. They allow us to express feelings, and they have personal and social meaning. We learn from engaging in purposeful activities and receive satisfaction from them. From a purposeful activity, a person can explore interests, satisfy needs, determine and evaluate capacity and limitations, meet personal and interpersonal needs, and cope with life.

Purposeful Activities as a Tool of Intervention

Occupational therapy practitioners use purposeful activities as a tool of intervention. Therefore, we must have more than a mere appreciation for them. We must have in-depth knowledge of purposeful activities as the foundation of occupation, which is a core concept in our profession. We must understand the value and benefit of purposeful activities as therapeutic media. Part of using purposeful activities as a therapeutic tool is understanding the component elements of purposeful activities. In addition, because of the characteristics of purposeful activities, we must take a broader view of them within the context of the person's life, abilities, and life circumstances.

Why do we use purposeful activities? Occupational therapy practitioners have always used activities as part of their interventions with clients. Although specific activities have changed and will continue to change, the six basic reasons that we choose to use purposeful activities are relatively constant.

1.   Purposeful activity builds on the person's abilities and leads to achievement of personal and functional goals. For an activity to be purposeful, it must have four qualities. First, the person must direct the activity toward a goal that he or she considers important. Second, the participant must be actively engaged in the activity because he or she wants to be. Third, the activity must have personal meaning for the participant (Evans, 1987; Gilfoyle, 1984; Mosey, 1986; Nelson, 1988). The purposefulness of an activity is always grounded in the person who is doing the activity and the situational context in which he or she performs the activity (Henderson et al., 1991). Finally, the person must be capable and have the knowledge, skills, and abilities to engage in the activity.

2.   Purposeful activity offers the person opportunities for effective action. Activity involves doing something to achieve an end goal. Therefore, the person must be an active participant. The completion of the activity results in something, which may be a physical outcome (e.g., finishing a chore) or a more intellectual achievement (e.g., writing a letter). The person must be personally involved in actively performing the activity.

3.   Purposeful activities provide opportunities for the person to achieve mastery of the environment, and successful performance promotes feelings of personal competence. By skillfully selecting the appropriate activity, we can coordinate the person's capabilities, potential, desires, and the particular tasks. The appropriate purposeful activity provides an opportunity for a person to master skills, accomplish a goal, and build self-confidence. Accomplishment of the various tasks leads to the person having successful experiences and ultimately to the accomplishment of purposeful activities. These accomplishments when grouped together develop into achievement of occupations. A person who can master washing his or her face (purposeful activity) and then bathe (purposeful activity) gradually may become capable of independently completing his or her own self-care (occupation). This person's feelings about and mastery of the environment become realized as he or she engages in purposeful activities (washing, bathing) as part of the intervention plan.

4.   When engaged in a purposeful activity, the person directs his or her attention to the goal rather than to the processes required for achievement of the goal. One major value of engagement in a purposeful activity is that the person's attention is not on the specific tasks but rather is on the accomplishment of the activity and the end goal. For example, a child who is playing with a doll is less likely to attend to increased upper-extremity range of motion, cognitive challenges, or psychosocial interaction imposed by the practitioner. The child's goal is to have fun while engaging in an imaginary activity. If an adult concentrates on making a sandwich, he or she may not focus on the pain or limited range of motion associated with arthritis.

5.   Engagement in purposeful activity within the context of interpersonal, cultural, physical, and other environmental conditions requires and elicits coordination

among the person's sensory, perceptual, motor, and cognitive systems and his or her emotions. The nature of being involved in an activity, which has a goal, has anticipated outcomes and involves several tasks, leads to engagement in a purposeful activity, and occurs in complex interactions between the person and his or her environment. Although a practitioner can control the degree of each factor to some extent, the nature of selecting an activity that is meaningful requires multiple levels of processing. The complex interaction of factors that stem from involvement in a specific purposeful activity enhances the therapeutic value of purposeful activities.

6.   Engagement in purposeful activity provides direct and objective feedback concerning performance both to the occupational therapy practitioner and to the person. Finally, occupational therapy practitioners use purposeful activities because, by actively engaging a person in the activity, the practitioner and the person receive feedback about the person's own action. The person receives feedback both while performing the activity and from the result of the actions. Because the purposeful activities are part of real-life occupations, they provide additional insight into the potential of the person to engage in occupations successfully. Feedback from real-life, meaningful activities provides valuable information that we cannot obtain from simulated or fabricated tasks.

These six reasons provide a rationale that occupational therapy practitioners have always used to justify their use of purposeful activities. Although the types of activities have continually changed, occupational therapy practitioners are committed to using meaningful, real-life purposeful activities as a tool for evaluation and intervention.

Occupational Therapy Practitioners Examination and Use of Purposeful Activities

To use purposeful activities as part of our intervention, we examine the use of them from several perspectives. The following discussion outlines some of the general characteristics of purposeful activities that we consider as we use them as evaluation and therapeutic tools.

Goal of the Activity for the Person

Each person has his or her personal goals for engaging in an activity. These goals may be immediate or long term. The goals vary depending on the purpose that the person has for doing the activity and the time he or she has to do it. For the occupational therapy practitioner, the person's goal for engaging in the activity is an important factor to consider when judging performance. We often assume that, when the goal for engaging in the activity comes from the person, he or she has greater investment and values the activity. Likewise, we often assume that, if the person is completing the activity for someone else, he or she may not put forth the same effort or have the same investment in the activity. These assumptions, however, may not be true. When analyzing a person's performance of a task or completion of an activity, a practitioner must carefully consider the person's motivation to perform as only one influencing factor.

Meaning and Value of the Activity for the Person

As occupational therapy practitioners, we use activities in evaluation and intervention that have personal value and meaning for the person. When we select activities to use with a client, we choose activities that are important to that person on the basis of such factors as his or her personal attributes, culture, lifestyle, and life situation. For example, when working with children, we frequently choose play activities that are meaningful and appropriate to them. If the child has a physical limitation, comes from a Hispanic background, and lives in a large metropolitan area, we carefully consider each of these factors when selecting a specific activity.

Required Knowledge, Abilities, and Skills To Engage in the Activity

Every purposeful activity has knowledge, abilities, and skills that are necessary to be able to perform the activity effectively. As practitioners, we use our understanding of activity and task analysis to determine what is necessary to engage in the activity. On the basis of this analysis, we select activities that match the person's abilities.

Objects, Articles, or Paraphernalia That the Activity Requires

Most purposeful activities involve the use of objects, articles, or paraphernalia to accomplish the various tasks. As practitioners, we examine the materials that are essential to the task. At times, we modify, adapt, or change the materials required, but we try to maintain the integrity of the purposeful activity. A key point of an activity analysis is to determine which materials the activity actually requires and to what extent they are necessary.

Actions Required To Engage in the Activity

Although persons perform many activities in specific ways, often we can modify, adapt, or change them if necessary. The actions an activity requires are the structure, rules, organization features, and timing of each task in the activity. In addition, persons may need to perform actions in a specific way or order in a set amount of time. Occupational therapy practitioners examine activities related to the actions necessary to engage in them and complete them. This requires adept activity analysis skills.

Level of Participation That the Activity Requires With the Human Environment

Although all purposeful activities require that the person who is engaged in the activity participate, many activities necessitate the participation of other humans. Depending on the activity, participants can be a specific person (e.g., mother, spouse, family member, friend), an acquaintance (e.g., peers, colleagues, health care providers), or a stranger. Sometimes the activity demands that the persons involved have particular knowledge or skills. The specific activity and its context may influence the degree of participation of all the participants. Practitioners carefully examine the degree and quality of participation necessary for the entire activity and its component tasks.

Level of Participation With the Nonhuman Environment That the Activity Requires

As discussed previously, most purposeful activities involve the use of objects, articles, or paraphernalia. Beyond these, the nonhuman environment includes pets and other animals that may be critical to the activity. Purposeful activities that involve interaction between the nonhuman elements of the environment and the persons included in the activity may vary in terms of the degree of involvement. Again, as with the human environment, practitioners carefully examine the degree and quality of participation necessary for the entire activity and its component tasks.

Context in Which Persons Perform the Activities

Performance of a task or an activity can be context dependent. The context within which the persons performs an activity includes physical, social, cultural, and temporal factors.

Purposeful Activities in Evaluation and Intervention

The person's actual performance in purposeful activities and other evaluation data help in developing a comprehensive intervention plan. The person's actual performance in purposeful activities provides insight into the person's ability to engage in occupations and function in his or her real world.

By definition, prescription of purposeful activity is specific to the person. Thus, the practitioner selects activities on the basis of the needs of the person, the person's abilities and disabilities, and the inherent characteristics of the activity. Once the practitioner selects the activity, he or she grades or adapts the chosen activity to promote successful performance or to elicit a particular response.

Purposeful activities have the potential to facilitate a client's mastery of a new skill, restore a deficient ability, provide the client with a means for compensating for a functional disability, maintain health, and prevent dysfunction. During intervention, we select activities or modify them in response to the dynamic changes of the person and provide opportunities for gradual development of skill and related therapeutic benefits. Aspects of the purposeful activity that we manipulate as part of the intervention include sequence; duration; procedures of the task; the person's position; the position of the tools and materials; the size, shape, weight, or texture of materials; the nature and degree of interpersonal contact; the extent of physical handling by the practitioner during the performance; and the environment in which the person performs the activity. We discuss all of these elements in detail in further chapters.

Summary

Occupational therapy practitioners use purposeful activities to restore function and to compensate for functional deficits (AOTA, 1993). Before using a purposeful activity as part of an intervention plan, we complete an analysis of the activity relative to the situational context of the person (activity analysis). This includes identifying the essential information, abilities, skills, and proficiencies necessary to complete each task. We consider the age, occupational roles, cultural background, gender, interests, and preferences of the person. By scrutinizing the context and circumstances encompassing the performance of the activity, we skillfully select purposeful activities within the conditions of the frame of reference to guide the intervention. By using activity synthesis, we implement purposeful activities that are appropriate for the client. ■

References

American Occupational Therapy Association. (1979). Policy 1.12: Occupation as the common core of occupational therapy. In *Policy Manual of the American Occupational Therapy Association*. Rockville, MD: Author.

American Occupational Therapy Association. (1993). Position Paper: Purposeful activity. *American Journal of Occupational Therapy, 47,* 1081–1082.

American Occupational Therapy Association. (1994). Uniform terminology for occupational therapy—Third edition. *American Journal of Occupational Therapy, 48,* 1047–1054.

American Occupational Therapy Association. (1997). Statement—Fundamental concepts of occupational therapy: Occupation, purposeful activity, and function. *American Journal of Occupational Therapy, 51,* 864–866.

Christiansen, C. (1991). Occupational therapy intervention for life performance. In C. Christiansen & C. Baum (Eds.), *Occupational therapy: Overcoming human performance deficits* (pp. 3–43). Thorofare, NJ: Slack.

Christiansen, C., Clark, F., Kielhofner, G., Rogers, J., & Nelson, D. (1995). Position Paper: Occupation. *American Journal of Occupational Therapy, 49,* 1015–1018.

Evans, K. A. (1987). Definition of occupation as the core concept of occupational therapy. *American Journal of Occupational Therapy, 41,* 627–628.

Gilfoyle, E. M. (1984). Transformation of a profession. 1984 Eleanor Clarke Slagle lecture. *American Journal of Occupational Therapy, 38,* 575–584.

Glover, J. A, Bruning R. H., & Filbeck, R. W. (1983). *Educational psychology: Principles and applications.* Glenview, IL: Scott Foresman.

Henderson, A., Cermak, S., Coster, W., Murray, E., Trombly, C., & Tickle-Degnen, L. (1991). The Issue Is—Occupational science is multidimensional. *American Journal of Occupational Therapy, 45,* 370–372.

Hinojosa, J., & Kramer, P. (1993). Legitimate tools of pediatric occupational therapy. In J. Hinojosa & P. Kramer (Eds.), *Frames of reference for pediatric occupational therapy* (pp. 25–33). Baltimore: Williams & Wilkins.

Kielhofner, G. (1992). *Conceptual foundation of occupational therapy.* Philadelphia: F. A. Davis.

Kramer, P., & Hinojosa, J. (1993). *Frames of reference for pediatric occupational therapy.* Baltimore: Williams & Wilkins.

Kramer, P., & Hinojosa, J. (1995). Epiphany of human occupation. In C. B. Royeen (Ed.), *AOTA self-study series: Human occupation* (Lesson 8). Bethesda, MD: American Occupational Therapy Association.

Mosey, A. C. (1981). *Occupational therapy: Configuration of a profession.* New York: Raven Press.

Mosey, A. C. (1985). A monistic or a pluralistic approach to professional identity? 1985 Eleanor Clarke Slagle lecture. *American Journal of Occupational Therapy, 39,* 504–509.

Mosey, A. C. (1986). *Psychosocial components of occupational therapy.* New York: Raven.

Mosey, A. C. (1992*). Applied scientific inquiry in the health professions: An epistemological orientation.* Rockville, MD: American Occupational Therapy Association.

Nelson, D. L. (1988). Occupation: Form and performance. *American Journal of Occupational Therapy, 42,* 633–641.

2

Perspectives

Beth K. Elenko, MA, OTR
Jim Hinojosa, PhD, OT, FAOTA
Marie-Louise Blount, AM, OT, FAOTA
Wesley Blount

As much as the use of purposeful activity and occupation have always defined occupational therapy, the literature has not fully discussed the philosophical concepts about purposeful activities that theorists use to define the profession. Needless to say, many differing theoretical approaches have grown and transformed as the profession has grown and transformed over the years. Although each theorist has added to the body of knowledge from a differing perspective, these differing approaches have led to multiple realities in the ways in which we view occupational therapy, with each relevant term taking on a different meaning with each new theorist. At the same time, to carve out unique vantage points, frequently a theorist will ignore the definitions of others or subtly redefine the scope of others' work.

With the broadening range of occupational therapy's areas of practice, a continual need exists for expanding the concepts that define the profession. What began as a limited range of arts and crafts activities later involved the rehabilitation of soldiers, then pediatric therapy and the role of play, and, more recently, spirituality and nonactive occupations of various types. Each expansion brought about a reexamination of the very notion of what constitutes purposeful activities and occupation and of the nuances that distinguish terms as seemingly similar as *occupation* and *purposeful activities*.

Developing an overview of the use of theoretical terms in occupational therapy would be difficult under any circumstances, which may explain why few have attempted to bring the various contributions of the important theorists in the profession together and compare them with one another. First, we believe that nothing substitutes for reading the original works of each of these distinguished contributors.

What we present herein is an overview of the major theorists with summaries of their important contributions to the concepts of purposeful activities and occupation. We believe that with understanding these differing approaches comes perspective and awareness of the important work that has laid a theoretical foundation for the profession. Second, no one "right way" exists to examine the issues of purposeful activities and occupation. We are attempting to develop a taxonomy that will provide consistency in referencing and will add to the body of knowledge in occupational therapy. The profession is a dynamic entity that grows and changes constantly. Any attempt at defining terms must reflect this dynamic change.

Activities: Gail Fidler

As an occupational therapist, an association leader, an educator, and a scholar, Gail Fidler has had a powerful influence on the profession's knowledge and understanding of purposeful activities. Fidler's views and opinions about purposeful activities come from her conviction that doing activities is vitally important and therefore meaningful to persons. In occupational therapy, activities have powerful therapeutic merit. Purposeful activities are at the core of occupational therapy practice. From Fidler's perspective, *purposeful activities* and *occupation* are synonymous terms for the same construct (Fidler, 1996).

Fidler recognized that, if society is to value occupational therapy and the use of activities as authentic therapeutic modalities, then occupational therapists need a conceptual rationale for using activities. Furthermore, occupational therapists must develop methods for empirically examining activities and their value. In observing that the occupational therapy literature only involved the appeal, interest factors, and popularity of activities, Fidler (1948) argued that occupational therapists needed a scientific method for analyzing activities. She proposed activity analysis as one approach to learn more about activities. Activity analysis gives therapists a means to examine activities by dividing the activity into component parts. Understanding the component parts of an activity provides the information that a therapist needs to match a specific activity to a client's needs. Thus, therapists can match the activity to the needs of the client and the objectives of treatment (Fidler, 1948). This original activity analysis is the foundation for many activity analyses in practice today.

After proposing a structure for examining activities and emphasizing the importance of matching the activity to the client's needs and the objectives of treatment, Fidler turned her attention to the therapeutic value of active involvement in doing activities in task groups (Fidler, 1969). In 1954, with her husband, Jay Fidler, she published a book titled *Introduction to Psychiatric Occupational Therapy*. This text included an extensive discussion of the use of activities in psychiatric settings and provided a conceptual rationale for using purposeful activities for all occupational therapists. Analyzing the component parts of an activity provides the information that therapists require to correlate the client's needs, interests, and abilities. Furthermore, occupational therapy impels the person to develop skills through an action-oriented learning experience. Fidler and Fidler (1954) introduced occupational therapists to the psychodynamic properties of activities. They related some aspects of the activity to then-contemporary psychodynamic beliefs, including motion, procedures, materials, creativity, symbols, hostile and aggressive components, control, predictability, narcissism, sexual identification, dependence, reality testing, and group relatedness. They stressed the importance of human and nonhuman environments in understanding and performing activities.

In 1978, Fidler and Fidler provided a theoretical rationale for purposeful activities. They selected the word *doing* because it would

> convey the sense of performing, producing, or causing. It is purposeful action in contrast to random activity in that the action is directed toward the intrapersonal (testing a skill), the interpersonal (clarifying a relationship), or the nonhuman (creating an end product). Doing is viewed as enabling the development and integration of the sensory, motor, cognitive, and psychological systems; serving as a socializing agent; and verifying one's efficacy as a competent, contributing member of one's society. (p. 305)

Knowledge about activities provides the basis on which an occupational therapist selects a particular activity that matches the client's therapeutic needs, learning readiness, intact functions, and values. The therapist then plans and implements an action learning experience to allow the client to develop skills (Fidler & Fidler, 1978). Purposeful activities provide opportunities and means for a person to achieve mastery and competence, and the following beliefs support their use.

■ A person's social environment affects the value of any single activity. Each society has its own values and norms that determine how the members of that society view the activity. Each societal group considers some activities to be more important than others. For a person to be competent in his or her social group, he or she must able to do the necessary activities. Consequently, all activities have social relevance.

■ Each person is a unique neurobiological and psychological being. As such, each person must have his or her own level of mastery and competence to be able to engage in and complete an activity. Each person's makeup determines whether the person receives gratification, pleasure, and satisfaction from participation in an activity, which highlights the importance of matching an activity to the person.

■ An activity has real and symbolic personal meaning for the person that is grounded in a social and cultural context.

■ Each activity has its own specific actions and its level of sensory integration, motor, cognitive, psychological, and social components.

■ Activities can motivate, promote development, teach, and remediate dysfunctions. We can harness the therapeutic power of an activity when a client is ready to learn or to be stimulated and when we match the activity with his or her socio-cultural values, norms, and personal characteristics. This match may be at the real or symbolic level.

■   Activities that result in an end product have the added value of verifying performance, mastery, and competence.

■   During an activity, a person receives feedback from interacting with human and nonhuman environments. This feedback provides information about the person's skills, abilities, and competence (Fidler, 1981).

Recently, Fidler (1996) introduced the Life Style Performance Model to provide a comprehensive picture of a person's activities, abilities, needs, interests, capacities, and self-expectations with his or her human and nonhuman worlds. This model highlights the interrelatedness of person, environment, activity profile, and quality of life. The model describes four activity domains: activities concerned with self-care and self-maintenance, personally referenced pleasure and intrinsic gratification, societal contribution, and interpersonal engagement. The model describes the importance of a balance among daily life activities. We can achieve this balance by understanding that a person's lifestyle is a configuration of activity and his or her patterns of doing. When a person has a healthy activity pattern, he or she is a contributing member of society. The role of an occupational therapy practitioner is to work with a client toward a healthy activity pattern. The quality of one's life is extremely important, and the occupational therapy practitioner must have a holistic view of practice (i.e., receive direction from the client). In this model, purposeful activity

> means a personally referenced action that is concerned with testing a skill, ability, or level of competence or an activity that is focused on clarifying a relationship and discerning the nature of one's relatedness to another person (or persons) or to one's nonhuman world . . . activity is understood to reference any act or series of interconnected acts requiring the active engagement of a person's mind and body in the pursuit of a discernible outcome. (Fidler, 1996, p. 141)

This model advances the use of meaningful, purposeful activities as a powerful therapeutic medium.

Activities Health: Simme Cynkin

Simme Cynkin (1979) has provided perspective on the fundamental nature of activity as a therapeutic response to dysfunction. In this perspective, the value of activities as fundamental to humans is the basis for occupational therapy. Activities are part of our human existence, and Cynkin believes that the very presence of activities in our daily lives promotes our physical and mental well-being. Cynkin has four assumptions about activities.

1.   Activities of many kinds are the essence of human existence on the basis of the interactions of the person and the environment. Activities center on survival, subsistence, and coexistence.

2.   Activities are a culmination of acceptable norms of behaviors that a sociocultural system of values and beliefs defines.

3.   Acceptable and unacceptable variations exist in individual activities.

4.   A person's engagement in meaningful activities leads to a satisfying way of life and personal fulfillment (Cynkin, 1979; Cynkin & Robinson, 1990).

Cynkin and Robinson's (1990) assumptions result from a historical perspective: activity has always defined human existence, and activities are basic to human survival. By drawing on the works of Piaget and Reilly, Cynkin and Robinson centralized human nature and a person's humanity around the performance of various activities, both personal and interpersonal. To this foundation, the authors added the notion of differing sociocultural norms and differing values that various societies have concerning particular activities.

By building on the notion that persons can change, Cynkin and Robinson (1990) further argued that persons can change behavior related to activity and that behavioral changes can improve functioning in the person. Furthermore, the person can learn to improve function, and the learning process can take place in various ways, both direct and indirect.

The importance of these assumptions, and the framework that Cynkin and Robinson developed from them, is that they contribute to a foundation for the teaching of ideas behind occupational therapy. "Early occupational therapy was founded on the belief that being engaged in activities promotes mental and physical well-being and that, conversely, absence of activity leads . . . at worst to deterioration or loss of mental and physical functioning" (Cynkin & Robinson, 1990, p. 4). Although theorists like Fidler developed ways of analyzing activity, Cynkin provided an important additional link by placing activity in a context of overall human behavior to provide a greater understanding of its therapeutic importance. Cynkin offered the strongest method possible to give the occupational therapy student not only the tools to assist in restoring function but also the philosophical structure that underlies the importance of activity in everyday life.

Occupational Behavior: Mary Reilly

Mary Reilly (1966) is a seminal and critical writer and thinker in occupational therapy. Although she has not devoted all of her attention to issues of activity and occupation, her ideas, eventually termed *occupational behavior*, focused attention on the issues of activity and occupation by making concerns about these issues an underlying theme.

Among Reilly's concerns were the impetus to study and investigate the profession to establish clearly its contributions to science. She therefore suggested that a major area for occupational therapy research should be the nature and meaning of activity (Reilly, 1960). The presumption that humans require activity to attain and maintain health is fundamental to the profession's beliefs: "We are becoming more aware of the fact that the interests of man [*sic*] emerge in the gratification of his senses" (Reilly, 1960, p. 208). Indeed, she stressed that investigation of the need to engage in activity should move beyond the traditional reliance of occupational therapy on arts and crafts and into analysis of such activities as the appropriate level for the investigation (Reilly, 1960). She emphasized the physical, sensory, and psychic rewards inherent in activity and spoke against the idea that among various approaches to the use of activity (e.g., subdividing dance from recreation from crafts) is a "best" approach to the application of therapeutic activity.

In her Eleanor Clarke Slagle Lecture, Reilly (1962) further affirmed the centrality of work to human existence. Her thesis in this presentation was that human productivity provides the most life satisfaction and that occupational therapy applies this principle to the maintenance and restoration of health. Occupational therapy intervention ("treatment" in her words) requires that the therapist investigate and address problems persons have in coping with play, work, and school (Reilly, 1962). She rejected the term *activity* to describe how occupational therapists engage clients in this presentation because she had become wary of the increasing use of terms such as *activity therapy* in treatment settings that moved occupational therapy away from seeking to enhance individual human productivity.

As Reilly's approach to the study of occupational therapy became known as *occupational behavior* (Reilly, 1966), she referred back to the core ideas of early occupational therapy thinkers by promoting the idea that a satisfying life requires a balanced approach to work, rest, and play. Occupational therapy, appropriately applied, would establish a setting to address all of these aspects of life. In describing a model program that addressed all of these aspects, she included exercise programs, required work activities, learning recreational skills, some group activities, social skills, and other activities.

Reilly's interest in occupation and related activities later developed into a special concentration on the occupation of play as it applies to both children and adults (Reilly, 1974). She investigated, along with her students, the development of occupational behaviors during play and the relationship of play to humans' exploration of their environments, their development of competence, and their fulfillment of the drive to achieve.

Her striving to understand the nature and functions of human occupation and to apply this knowledge to occupational therapy intervention led to the development of the Model of Human Occupation and eventually to the school of thought termed *occupational science*.

Model of Human Occupation: Gary Kielhofner

As students of Reilly, Gary Kielhofner and Janice Burke have taken theories on occupational behavior and expanded both the theory's external framework and its organizing principles. Kielhofner continued to refine this theoretical approach, the Model of Human Occupation (Kielhofner, 1995; Kielhofner & Burke, 1980), and he uses the model to observe and explain most aspects of theory related to occupational therapy. Indeed, one of the central tenets of the model is that we can use human occupation for therapeutic benefit, and the model advocates a balanced lifestyle that includes both work and leisure (thus expanding on Reilly's notion of play).

In Kielhofner's view, "occupation is a multifaceted phenomenon that involves the simultaneous operation of biological, psychological, social, and ecological factors" (Kielhofner, 1985, p. xvii). Like most of his definitions, his notion of occupation relies on multiple levels of explanation to allow for as many aspects within a framework as necessary to explain the multitude of possibilities inherent in human behavior.

Kielhofner (1995) began his model by developing historical perspectives on human behavior within the context of systems theory. From this, he posited that human beings are an example of an open system, that is, that human activity involves taking in information (or input), synthesizing the information, and then creating output. The important quality of an open system, he argued, is the opportunity for feedback, which involves responses to the output that allow the person to make changes and, with the same input, create a different output (Kielhofner, 1995).

Within the person, Kielhofner and Burke (1980) noted several components and determinants that affect human behavior, including volition, habituation, and performance. *Volition* refers to the impulses that cause the person to value certain types of occupation, including personal causation (the knowledge of self), values (ideas of what is good, right, important), and interests (the disposition to find particular occupations pleasurable). *Habituation* refers to the normative definitions that the person places on occupation and encompasses roles (publicly recognized positions or society's input) and habits (the private regulation of behavior). *Performance* deals with the person's skills in performing occupations, containing communication, following a process, and using perceptual-motor skills (Kielhofner, 1995; Kielhofner & Burke, 1980).

After determining the internal structures that comprise individual behavior, Kielhofner then dealt with the external aspects of human occupation, including determining whether the person is functional or dysfunctional and thus needs therapeutic intervention. Just as function in his view has three levels of exploration, competence, and achievement, Kielhofner viewed dysfunction as having three corresponding levels of inefficiency, incompetence, and helplessness. He emphasized that we should view both function and dysfunction as processes, not static states. For occupational dysfunction to exist, Kielhofner explained that the person in his or her social group would not meet expectations for productive and playful participation.

Furthermore, the person "does not fulfill the urge to explore and master" (Kielhofner, 1985, p. 64) his or her environment.

By using this model, Kielhofner developed ideas about the optimal use of therapy in treating dysfunction and worked to fit the model into larger contexts, such as the *Conceptual Foundations of Occupational Therapy* (Kielhofner, 1992). Kielhofner does not engage in the debate regarding terms like *activity* or *occupation* as much as he ignores the debate altogether. Occupation is the central concept that he uses in developing theories regarding occupational therapy, but more fundamentally, the person's role in the complex process of human occupation defines what persons and, following his model, therapists will do to improve human function. Kielhofner's detailed model, with its emphasis on human behavior, aids greatly in establishing a psychological framework for the human need for occupation in daily life.

Occupational Form and Occupational Performance: David Nelson

David Nelson (1994) has become particularly interested in the term *occupation* and its meaning for occupational therapists. His principal contribution to this perspective has been semantic and includes developing a nomenclature to delimit the use of the term *occupation* by occupational therapists. The nomenclature Nelson developed provides names or symbols to describe what he viewed as essential terms for understanding the therapeutic discipline of occupational therapy.

Nelson (1994) divided the term *occupation* into what he views as its essential aspects, form and performance. *Form* concerns the objects and circumstances that make the occupation possible. Forms can be a game, a building in which an occupation takes place, a piece of equipment, a piece of music, or another person. Forms are essential to the way in which the specific occupation takes place.

Performance, on the other hand, is what the person does to carry out the occupation. Nelson stipulated that performance, in this sense, must be voluntary. "The 'doing' is the occupational performance, and the 'something' to be done is the occupational form" (Nelson, 1994, p. 11). Performance then is playing the game, constructing the building, lifting the weight for exercise, playing the music, or teaching something to the other person. Again, myriad performances are possible depending on the relevant occupations.

Nelson (1994) viewed occupation as the relationship between an occupational form and an occupational performance. Many possible variations exist in a given occupation, which include diverse occupational forms and differences in performances, which themselves may be as variable as the persons who are performing the occupation. If the occupation is eating a meal, the occupational forms, at a simple level, may be breakfast, lunch, or dinner. The occupational performances may be as divergent as that of a baby eating as much oatmeal as he or she "feeds" to the high chair tray and the room versus a diet-conscious woman 20 years of age who picks carefully at the low-fat foods on her plate. Many variables come into play, including duration, certainty of outcome, and intricacy.

Nelson (1994) further subdivided the term *occupational form* into a physical dimension and a sociocultural dimension. The physical dimensions are factors that we can measure and describe. They include the things involved in and the physical characteristics of the occupation, which additionally involve the temporal aspects of the occupation. In this sense, the form of a piece of music, for example, may include in its physical dimensions the musical composition itself, the piano, the concert hall, and the length of time the piece takes to play.

The sociocultural dimension includes all of the social and cultural practices, expectations, and settings involved. For the occupation described above, let us use the example of a contemporary, atonal classical music piece played on an electronic keyboard in a museum in Bucharest, Romania. All of these aspects help define the piece's sociocultural dimension.

Another delineation that Nelson applied to occupations is his distinction between overt and covert occupations. *Overt occupations* describe a performance that actually takes place and is observable if observers are present. *Covert occupations* are imagined occupations, and these play an important part in Nelson's ideational structure. The musical form described above, in the sense that no one observed it taking place, may be covert. Nelson included habitual occupational performances in his nomenclature, which are accustomed performances that require little conscious attention. The human being carrying out (or thinking about) the occupation is the link between the form and the performance. As such, the various abilities of the human being, as the occupational therapist views them (Nelson, 1994), influence the technique and fashion in which the person carries out the occupation.

Nelson likewise discussed the meanings inherent in and applied to occupations in his work. Nelson divided this aspect of the structure into perceptual and symbolic meanings. The perceptual aspects pertain to all of the physical dimensions embodied in the occupational form (e.g., sound, texture, time), whereas the symbolic aspects relate to the sociocultural dimensions that may include linguistic, cognitive, and emotional issues. Nelson includes immediate and past experiences in his construct of meaning. Another term that occupational therapists apply to tasks, doing, or occupation is purpose. According to Nelson (1994), *purpose* is the desire for a certain "outcome" embodied in an occupational performance. Purpose is the reason for the actions a performer takes and, according to Nelson, provides the "energy" to act. As is true with meanings, any given occupation may have more than one purpose. Not only may a given person have more than one purpose for performing an occupation, but also many persons may each have different purposes for performing the same occupation. Nelson (1994) subdivided purpose into several frameworks. One subdivision is that of the intrinsic or extrinsic purpose. "Intrinsic purpose involves doing something for its own sake, as in wanting to explore the situation or wanting to master the situation" (Nelson, 1994, p. 24). Reading a novel for enjoyment is an example of an intrinsic motivation. Extrinsic motivation, on the other hand, is a purpose or motivation found outside of the occupation itself. Reading a textbook for the purpose of passing an examination is an example of an extrinsic motivation. Another subdivision of the term *purpose* for Nelson and for other occupational therapists is that of conscious and unconscious purposes. Unconscious purposes, of course, are those of which we are not aware. The best example, according to Nelson, are purposes involved with habitual occupations that we perform routinely with little thought unless the situation in which we do them changes in some relevant way.

By viewing occupations as a series of steps, Nelson (1994) applied the term *impact* to describe the effect that completion of one step has on the performance of the next step. For example, purchasing fabric and using a pattern to cut out a jacket are steps that have an effect on the actual construction of the jacket. Nelson introduced the term *adaptation* to describe changes in the person performing an occupation caused by carrying out that very occupational performance. Referring back to the example of making the jacket, by completing the construction of the jacket, the person who accomplished this may experience much satisfaction at his or her sewing prowess and has a garment to wear.

Understanding therapeutic occupations, according to Nelson (1994), requires the same set of ideas about occupational performance described above. The occupational therapy practitioner and the occupational therapy student must have a structure and process in which to perceive occupation to move onto therapeutic application. Nelson termed that process *occupational synthesis*, which is the designing of an occupational experience that will have therapeutic impact. The recipient of service is a collaborator in the therapeutic process. A person recuperating from a serious leg fracture may work with the occupational therapy practitioner to incorporate progressively longer periods of standing, walking, and bending at the hip while playing his favorite game, billiards.

Nelson deliberately avoided the term *activity*. In his view and in the view of others, the term *activity* is not specific enough because it is sometimes applied to other than human enterprises and because it is not always purposeful. He pointed out that terms like *molecular activity* and *solar activity* (Nelson, 1994, p. 42) clearly do not refer to human enterprises and that *activity* can refer to any kind of liveliness (see also Darnell & Heater, 1994). This approach clearly does not comport with the terminology in this book, but it does represent a school of thought within the profession and, as such, should be a familiar point of view.

Another important contribution of Nelson and his students has been an intense effort to study and measure the concepts that he has developed and advocated, including a series of published works beginning in 1987 (Bloch, Smith, & Nelson, 1989; DeKuiper, Nelson, & White, 1993; Hsieh, Nelson, Smith, & Peterson, 1996; Lang, Nelson, & Bush, 1992; Miller & Nelson, 1987; Nelson et al., 1996; Sietsema, Nelson, Mulder, Mervau-Scheidel, & White, 1993; and Yoder, Nelson, & Smith, 1989).

Occupation: Charles Christiansen and Carolyn Baum

Charles Christiansen and Carolyn Baum bring together differing theories of activity and occupation to lay a theoretical framework for teaching practice. In *Occupational Therapy: Overcoming Human Performance Deficits* (Christiansen & Baum, 1991), they proposed an occupational performance hierarchy that centered on "*the activity*, which consists of specific goal-oriented behaviors . . . directed toward the perform-ance of a task" (p. 28). The emphasis on activities regarding the performance of tasks creates the theoretical basis for occupational therapy as a way to treat dysfunction or disability. The work of previous authors serves in this context as a way to take ideas about activity and apply them to the practice of occupational therapy. By contrast, in *Occupational Therapy: Enabling Function and Well-Being* (Christiansen & Baum, 1997), the second edition of their work, the authors focus much more on the devel-opment of a definition of occupation and move away from both the term *activity* and the notion of *disability*. The revisions to the text allowed for the incorporation of newer ideas from different theorists but underscored the difficulty of taking the dif-fering approaches and blending them into a coherent whole. Like Kielhofner, Christiansen and Baum developed a model in the second edition that they referred to at the start of each chapter and that attempted to encompass all possible facets of human performance in an arrow-shaped form that points to "well-being," and each chapter within the text presents a part of this triangular model. By using the ideas developed by Law and her Canadian colleagues (see the section "Client-Centered Occupational Therapy: Mary Law" in this chapter), they emphasize the client-cen-tered approach with a resulting deemphasis in specific practice solutions to problems and a greater focus on the client's needs and perceptions. This deemphasis of specific treatments for dysfunction incorporates the occupational science model's focus on wellness and healthy occupational performance.

Although the multiplicity of changes makes what specific stance Christiansen and Baum prefer to take editorially regarding terms like *occupation* and *activity* unclear, the two volumes exemplify the contemporary dilemmas facing practicing therapists in bridging and balancing the differing theoretical expectations in the pro-fession. Placing occupation into a sociocultural context that emphasizes the role of the person in society is an important concept, but without practical methods of addressing dysfunction, students may not completely understand the role of the occupational therapy practitioner in promoting wellness.

Client-Centered Occupational Therapy: Mary Law

In conjunction with various collaborators, Mary Law has focused on the relationship between the practitioner and the "person receiving services" or client to develop an approach called *client-centered occupational therapy* (Law, 1998). This approach to occupational therapy brings together several areas of observation and research from occupational therapy and other disciplines. As an early basis for the client-centered approach, Law and Mills (1998) cited psychologist Carl Rogers, who emphasized the need for therapists to work with clients in developing solutions to problems rather than "directing" the course of therapy. Law and Mills consider the views of persons with disabilities and their feelings regarding treatment.

The client-centered approach resulted in a series of guidelines for practice produced by the Canadian Association of Occupational Therapists (1991). Law and associates (1994) produced the Canadian Occupational Performance Measure (COPM), an assessment designed to measure "a client's self-perception of occupational performance" (p. 191). Although the authors subsequently referred to the pilot testing as covering a "broad spectrum" of clients and environments, the subjects were mostly persons more than 60 years of age in inpatient geriatric facilities. Thus, the client-centered approach may better facilitate the subjects' ability to evaluate their own conditions and treatment needs versus a population less able to indicate self-awareness or occupational needs, such as children with developmental disabilities. In fact, contributors to *Client-Centered Occupational Therapy* discussed the various ways of interpreting the term *client*. The client is not only the person receiving therapy but also is "someone who wishes to make a change through the process of therapy" (Pollock & McColl, 1998, p. 91) (i.e., possibly the caregiver or parent). A frequent example in the works of these authors and Law is that of the patient with Alzheimer's disease who may be unable to communicate needs; the *client* is the spouse (and the term *spouse* is the one most often used in this example) giving care. As in the client-centered approach, the caregiver's role is the one that changes.

In Law's approach, the client defines activity and occupation, and the client's needs are foremost in the development of interventions created through the partnership between the client and the therapist. This may seem somewhat reflexive because an evaluation model would always require that the client's needs are part of the determination of appropriate therapy. What is important to Law and her colleagues, however, is that the evaluation comes from the client, and the client always evaluates the value of the therapy best. The therapist serves as a facilitator who aids the client in identifying areas of concern and assists in developing a plan to address these areas (and, in theory, those areas alone). One of the central concepts of client-centered practice is that occupational therapy service delivery is flexible and individualized, and the very flexibility and mutability of using occupation and activity make determining a specific approach to using occupation as a means of therapy in the client-centered practice difficult. Law and Mills (1998) acknowledged the lack of specific methodologies in client-centered therapy.

The focus of client-centered occupational therapy is on changing the overall approach to therapy from a medical model. In the medical model, clients perceive therapists to be all-knowing, and therapists evaluate treatment on the basis of generalized goals such as "independence at all costs" (Law, 1998, p. 71; see also Baum & Law, 1997). In the client-centered approach, the focus is on the client's finding meaning in everyday occupations and the development of active collaboration between the occupational therapist and the client to resolve occupational performance problems (Baum & Law, 1997). Specific assessments and treatment plans are not involved because the client-centered approach makes those determinations part of the larger client–therapist process of developing a relationship. Lacking such specifics, however, makes a comparative evaluation of the value of the client-centered approach difficult.

Occupational Science: University of Southern California, Department of Occupational Science and Occupational Therapy

Occupational science is the study of occupation and its role in human experience. Clark and associates (1991) defined occupation as "chunks of culturally and personally meaningful activity in which humans engage that can be named in the lexicon of culture" (p. 301). The study of occupation is grounded in a Model of Human Subsystems That Influence Occupation. Similar to Kielhofner's Model of Human Occupation, this model is an open system model that includes feedback to allow the person to make changes in occupational behavior. Occupational science as a discipline encompasses the studies of human and nonhuman occupation and occupational behavior, with noted zoologist Jane Goodall serving as a University of Southern California occupational science faculty member.

Because of the focus on generalized concepts regarding occupation and not on specific uses of purposeful activities in therapeutic settings, occupational science publications deal with the theoretical issues that we compare in this chapter. Anne Cronin Mosey (1992) has suggested that we should "partition" occupational science from occupational therapy because such a separation would serve to clarify the role of the discipline from that of the profession. Although the two areas of study may not benefit from a total separation, the notion of occupational science is far broader than the use of occupation for therapeutic benefit, and the very expansiveness of its scope suggests a substantial philosophical difference in method and application from occupational therapy as we understand it.

Occupational science provides a philosophical as well as theoretical basis for our understanding of purposeful activity. Purposeful activities are embedded within this definition of occupation. A person's participation in meaningful and socially valued activities is core to the moral philosophy of occupational therapy (Zemke & Clark, 1996). This belief results from the fact that, as occupational therapists, we focus on the everyday things that persons must do. Some researchers have immersed themselves in the study of these occupations of daily living that we engage in during our lifetime. Henderson (1996) stated that confusion exists between occupation and purposeful activity. She described occupation similarly to Clark and associates (1991) as chunks or units of culturally and personally meaningful activity within the stream of human behavior. Each level of occupation further subdivides into smaller ones. Theorists have not agreed on the vocabulary used, and the terms are interchangeable. Henderson believes that practitioners equate these terms in the field of occupational therapy, and therefore we must seek to understand further the interrelationships to distinguish the levels of occupations in which we engage.

We define purposeful activities in relation to particular activities, and we accept the notion that adaptations can occur in our activities. Human beings have a self-reinforcing power to challenge themselves in an array of adaptive strategies to improve quality of life. This is most relevant after disability, when occupations in which clients engaged previously require adaptation for participation (Frank, 1996).

An important milestone for human beings in occupational science is play. Play is a purposeful vehicle for change, one that truly encompasses the traditional definition of purposeful activity. The literature on play and purposeful activity correlate and are the root of much of what we discuss in the therapeutic process. Play, as a purposeful activity, encompasses much of what occupational science involves. Through childhood play exploration, the act of doing results from the activities that a child carries out daily. Play is an important occupation beginning at childhood and continuing throughout the life span. Play has its importance in the ability to interact with our environment, and thus children use it to cope when changes occur (Burke, 1996).

Occupational science research often attempts to take theories of occupation and broaden their context to create enhanced possibilities for study and application. Occupational science examines concepts such as adaptation, work, and play (on the basis of Reilly's themes) for their value as parts of human culture, not in areas of specific application. Often, occupational therapy is a reference point for developing larger thematic statements. At the graduate level, an occupational therapy student may find a text like *Occupational Science: The Evolving Discipline* (Zemke & Clark, 1996) a useful set of readings for contemplating the larger cultural implications of activity and occupation. Because the text contains few practical strategies, practitioners may not find these writings directly applicable to practice.

Legitimate Tools: Anne Cronin Mosey

Anne Cronin Mosey (1968) proposed that occupational therapists develop and use frames of reference to guide their evaluation and interventions. Frames of reference provide therapists with an organized theoretical knowledge base for practice. Occupational therapists use various means to implement their interventions that Mosey labeled the profession's *legitimate tools*. Legitimate tools are the means that a professional uses to accomplish a goal and include activities, actions, instruments, modalities, methods, and processes (Mosey, 1981). This perspective of a profession having legitimate tools acknowledges that, although many professions use the same therapeutic modalities, no one profession "owns" them. Although professions share tools, each profession uses them in unique ways that society authorizes. This dynamic view of a profession's legitimate tools means that a profession's tools change as the profession evolves.

Before her classification of legitimate tools, Mosey identified the unique therapeutic value of activities to assist persons with mental illness to become part of their communities and to engage in their daily lives (Mosey, 1973). In this text, *Activities Therapy*, Mosey described the power of doing an activity as a means for a person to learn new skills and behaviors. She underscored the potential of learning through doing; purposeful "activities are used to provide familiar life situations in which participants are assisted in identifying faulty patterns of behavior and the ideas, feelings, and values that support these faulty patterns" (Mosey, 1973, p. 2). Activities provide therapists with a means to understand the person and a method to assist the person in participating in the tasks at hand. Important aspects of using activities therapeutically are that they involve the here and now, they are action oriented, and they involve learning through doing. Mosey (1973) emphasized the notions of satisfaction and enjoyment of the activity and the therapeutic benefit to the client.

In 1986, Mosey proposed that occupational therapists have six primary legitimate tools: nonhuman environment, conscious use of self, the teaching–learning process, purposeful activities, activity groups, and activity analysis and synthesis. In her extensive discussion of purposeful activities as a legitimate tool, Mosey (1986) described the characteristics important for occupational therapy evaluation and intervention. Therapists develop expertise and skills in using these therapeutic tools as part of their basic professional education and ongoing postprofessional education (Mosey, 1986, 1996).

Mosey (1986) defined purposeful activities as a "doing process that require the use of thought and energy and are directed toward an intended or desired end result" (p. 227). The characteristics of purposeful activities she proposed include the following.

- Persons who are engaged in purposeful activities are aware of the reason for doing the activities.

- Persons participate in purposeful activities at their own free will and are not coerced.

- Purposeful activities have a planned end result that is not necessarily a material product.

- Purposeful activities have the potential to be symbolic.

- Purposeful activities are universal in that they exist as part of the human experience of interacting with our environments. Humans participate in purposeful activities throughout their daily lives.

- Purposeful activities are ordinary in nature.

- Purposeful activities are essential to the development of humans in all aspects of their development.

■ Purposeful activities are

made up of elements that can be identified, holistic, able to be manipulated, promoting differential responses, able to be graded, facilitating communication, having a focusing organizing effect, emphasizing doing, frequently involving the nonhuman environment, varying on a continuum from conscious to not conscious/unconscious, varying on a continuum from simulated to natural. (Mosey, 1986, p. 241)

Mosey included purposeful activities as one of occupational therapy's major legitimate tools until 1996, when she proposed a different categorization of the profession's legitimate tools by placing purposeful activities within subcategories of a revised taxonomy. This new taxonomy consists of an interpersonal process, activity process, and physical modalities. Interpersonal process includes conscious use of self and activity groups. Activity process includes elements of performance areas and stimulus–response activities. Physical modalities include atmospheric elements, technological products, and physical agents (Mosey, 1996). Thus, her revised taxonomy did not include purposeful activity itself as a separate legitimate tool but included activity as a subcomponent of other tools. This categorization may reflect the trend in occupational therapy of not using specific purposeful activities and instead focusing on the foundation for participation in occupations.

Summary

The nature of purposeful activities and occupation as a concept for study and theory presents inherent difficulties and always has in that, unlike with other treatment modes, the cause and effect in treatment is less easy to quantify and measure. Theories of activity and occupation must encompass the broadest possible range of human possibilities and experience, but at the same time, practitioners must be able to apply them in incredibly small and specific ways and always remain as practical and applicable in real situations as possible. We respect and acknowledge these theorists for taking on such a daunting task and developing such a variety of thoughtful, considered approaches to the questions at the heart of occupational therapy. Again, nothing can substitute for reading the works of these authors in their original words.

Some of these concepts continue like a running thread through the works of theorists whose conclusions can vary widely. Fidler, Kielhofner, and Law all speak of the involvement of the person receiving treatment as, in various ways, fundamental to the success of therapeutic intervention. Such continuous emphasis, drawn out over time, can stand as an important concept that each occupational therapy practitioner should bear in mind.

At the same time, important, unique ideas set these theorists apart from one another. For the practicing therapist, one strategy for processing and incorporating the work of various theorists is to study more than one but to find the one that best matches the therapist's area of practice. Reilly's focus on pediatrics, Law's focus on gerontological issues, and Kielhofner's focus on mental health all offer ways to incorporate theoretical concepts into specific areas of practice. The works of Fidler (in defining ways to think about activity), Nelson (in deriving a nomenclature), and Cynkin (in developing a notion of how to teach activity theory) stand as important guideposts regarding how theorists in occupational therapy approach writing and thinking about these issues.

The terms we present herein and the ways in which they are defined deal with important theoretical issues, but the questions they raise are provocative and open to debate. One of the most central questions concerns who is doing the defining of these concepts: Who determines what is a meaningful outcome? What constitutes a purposeful activity? And whose purpose should it serve?

Most importantly, occupational therapy continues to grow and evolve by bringing out new ideas in a rapidly changing field. The profession has room for many perspectives and a need to reexamine constantly established thought in the face of newly developed concepts and theories. In dealing with the complexities of human occupation and purposeful activities, occupational therapy takes on tremendous challenges and offers substantial rewards. The search for understanding the role of occupation and purposeful activities in human existence remains ongoing. ■

References

Baum, C., & Law, M. (1997). Occupational therapy practice: Focusing on occupational performance. *American Journal of Occupational Therapy, 51,* 277–288.

Bloch, M. W., Smith, D. A., & Nelson, D. L. (1989). Heart rate, activity and affect in added-purpose versus single-purpose jumping activities. *American Journal of Occupational Therapy, 43,* 25–30.

Burke, J. (1996). Variations in childhood: Play in the presence of chronic disability. In R. Zemke & F. Clark (Eds.), *Occupational science: The evolving discipline* (pp. 413–418). Philadelphia: F. A. Davis.

Canadian Occupational Therapy Association. (1991). *Client-centered guidelines for the practice of occupational therapy.* Toronto, Author.

Christiansen, C., & Baum, C. (Eds.). (1991). *Occupational therapy: Overcoming human performance deficits.* Thorofare, NJ: Slack.

Christiansen, C., & Baum, C. (Eds.). (1997). *Occupational therapy: Enabling function and well-being* (2nd ed.). Thorofare, NJ: Slack.

Clark, F., Parham, D., Carlson, M., Frank, G., Jackson, J., Pierce, D., Wolfe, R., & Zemke, R. (1991). Occupational science: Academic innovation in the service of occupational therapy's future. *American Journal of Occupational Therapy, 45,* 300–310.

Cynkin, S. (1979). *Occupational therapy: Toward health through activities.* Boston: Little, Brown.

Cynkin, S., & Robinson, A. (1990). *Occupational therapy and activities health: Toward health through activities.* Boston: Little, Brown.

Darnell, J. L., & Heater, S. L. (1994). The Issue Is—Occupational therapist or activity therapist: Which do you choose to be? *American Journal of Occupational Therapy, 48,* 467–468.

DeKuiper, W. P., Nelson, D. L., & White, B. E. (1993). Materials-based occupation versus imagery-based occupation versus rote exercise: A replication and extension. *Occupational Therapy Journal of Research, 13,* 183–197.

Fidler, G. S. (1948). Psychological evaluation of occupational therapy activities. *American Journal of Occupational Therapy, 2,* 284–287.

Fidler, G. S. (1969). The task-oriented group as a context for treatment. *American Journal of Occupational Therapy, 23,* 43–48.

Fidler, G. S. (1981). From crafts to competence. *American Journal of Occupational Therapy, 35,* 567–573.

Fidler, G. S. (1996). Life-style performance: From profile to conceptual model. *American Journal of Occupational Therapy, 50,* 139–147.

Fidler, G. S., & Fidler, J. W. (1954). *Introduction to psychiatric occupational therapy.* New York: Macmillan.

Fidler, G. S., & Fidler, J. W. (1978). Doing and becoming: Purposeful action and self-actualization. *American Journal of Occupational Therapy, 32,* 305–310.

Frank, G. (1996). The concept of adaptation as a foundation for occupational science research. In R. Zemke & F. Clark (Eds.), *Occupational science: The evolving discipline* (pp. 47–55). Philadelphia: F. A. Davis.

Henderson, A. (1996). The scope of occupational science. In R. Zemke & F. Clark (Eds.), *Occupational science: The evolving discipline* (pp. 419–424). Philadelphia: F. A. Davis.

Hsieh, C. L., Nelson, D. L., Smith, D. A., & Peterson, C. Q. (1996). A comparison of performance in added-purpose occupations and rote exercise for dynamic standing balance in persons with hemiplegia. *American Journal of Occupational Therapy, 50,* 10–16.

Kielhofner, G. (Ed.). (1985). *A Model of Human Occupation: Theory and application.* Baltimore: Williams & Wilkins.

Kielhofner, G. (1992). *Conceptual foundations of occupational therapy.* Philadelphia: F. A. Davis.

Kielhofner, G. (Ed.). (1995). *A Model of Human Occupation: Theory and application* (2nd ed.). Baltimore: Williams & Wilkins.

Kielhofner, G., & Burke, J. (1980). A Model of Human Occupation, Part 1: Conceptual framework and content. *American Journal of Occupational Therapy, 34,* 572–581.

Lang, E. M., Nelson, D. L., & Bush, M. A. (1992). Comparison of performance in materials-based occupation, imagery-based occupation, and rote exercise in nursing home residents. *American Journal of Occupational Therapy, 46,* 607–611.

Law, M. (Ed.). (1998). *Client-centered occupational therapy.* Thorofare, NJ: Slack.

Law, M., Baptiste, S., Carswell, A., McColl, M. A., Polatajko, H., & Pollock, N. (1994). *Canadian Occupational Performance Measure* (2nd ed.). Toronto: Canadian Association of Occupational Therapists.

Law, M., & Mills, J. (1998). Client-centered occupational therapy. In M. Law (Ed.), *Client-centered occupational therapy* (pp. 1–18). Thorofare, NJ: Slack.

Miller, L., & Nelson, D. L. (1987). Dual-purpose activity versus single-purpose activity in terms of duration on task, exertion level, and affect. *Occupational Therapy in Mental Health, 7,* 55–67.

Mosey, A. C. (1968). Recapitulation of ontogenesis: A theory for practice of occupational therapy. *American Journal of Occupational Therapy, 22,* 426–432.

Mosey, A. C. (1973). *Activities therapy.* New York: Raven Press.

Mosey, A. C. (1981). *Occupational therapy: Configuration of a profession.* New York: Raven Press.

Mosey, A. C. (1986). *Psychosocial components of occupational therapy.* New York: Raven Press.

Mosey, A. C. (1992). The Issue Is—Partition of occupational science and occupational therapy. *American Journal of Occupational Therapy, 46,* 851–853.

Mosey, A. C. (1996). *Applied scientific inquiry in the health professions: An epistemological orientation* (2nd ed.). Bethesda, MD: American Occupational Therapy Association.

Nelson, D. L. (1994). Form and function. In C. B. Royeen (Ed.), *AOTA self-study series: The practice of the future: Putting occupation back into therapy* (Lesson 2). Bethesda, MD: American Occupational Therapy Association.

Nelson, D. L., Konosky, K., Fleharty, K., Webb, R., Newer, K., Hazboun, V. P., Fontaine, C., & Licht, B. (1996). The effects of an occupationally embedded exercise on bilaterally assisted supination in persons with hemiplegia. *American Journal of Occupational Therapy, 50,* 639–646.

Pollock, N., & McColl, M. (1998). Assessment in client-entered occupational therapy. In M. Law (Ed.), *Client-centered occupational therapy* (pp. 89–106). Thorofare, NJ: Slack.

Reilly, M. (1960). Research potentiality of occupational therapy. *American Journal of Occupational Therapy, 14,* 206–209.

Reilly, M. (1962). Occupational therapy can be one of the great ideas of 20th century medicine, 1962 Eleanor Clarke Slagle lecture. *American Journal of Occupational Therapy, 16,* 1–9.

Reilly, M. (1966). A psychiatric occupational therapy program as a teaching model. *American Journal of Occupational Therapy, 22,* 61–67.

Reilly, M. (Ed.). (1974). *Play as exploratory learning.* Beverly Hills, CA: Sage.

Sietsema, J. M., Nelson, D. L., Mulder, R. M., Mervau-Scheidel, D., & White, B. E. (1993). The use of a game to promote arm reach in persons with traumatic brain injury. *American Journal of Occupational Therapy, 47,* 19–24.

Yoder, R. M., Nelson, D. L., & Smith, D. A. (1989). Added-purpose versus rote exercise in female nursing home residents. *American Journal of Occupational Therapy, 43,* 581–586.

Zemke, R., & Clark, F. (Eds.). (1996). *Occupational science: The evolving discipline.* Philadelphia: F. A. Davis.

3

Occupations and Their Dimensions

Sheama S. Krishnagiri, PhD, OTR

Occupations are patterns of culturally and personally meaningful activity in which humans engage (Clark et al., 1991). These occupations include the ordinary things that we do every day (e.g., shopping, eating, gardening, making love). Yerxa (1998) further clarified this definition by stating that occupation is self-initiated, self-directed, adaptive, and organized. In other words, persons are not born with a preset agenda of daily occupations. They learn, become habituated, and make conscious decisions regarding what they will or will not do. The person's organizing and orchestration of daily occupations enables adaptation to occur in biological, social, and physical realms and thereby facilitates survival.

The above definition has as its basic feature the subjective and experiential nature of occupation. Any occupation may have a culturally recognizable nature of sociocultural and physical characteristics. Nelson (1988) termed this *occupational form*. Until a person engages in the occupation, experiences it, and perceives its personal meaning, however, it is not an occupation. According to Bruner (1990), the subjective experiences of the person and applying meaning to one's actions within the environment occur through a culturally shaped narrative about who we are and how we fit into the social world. Our concept of self reflects both individual idiosyncrasies and the requirements of social living.

For example, consider the occupation of playing tennis. This occupation generally involves a racket, at least one tennis ball, an opponent, a tennis court, appropriate dress and shoes, appropriate weather (if the court is outdoors), and the knowledge and intent to play within the rules. Persons may undertake this occupation for pleasure or for competition. In a parallel occupation in another cultural situation, Dennis, an inner-city youth 11 years of age who loves the game, hits old tennis balls back and forth with a neighborhood friend. His court consists of a deserted parking lot with a cracked uneven surface and boundaries marked by chalk. The net consists of a string tied to a fence at one end and a garbage can at the other end. On days when his friend is willing to play, Dennis enjoys playing a set or two; otherwise, he practices by hitting the ball against the wall of the parking lot over and over again every afternoon after school. He makes a game out of hitting the same spot on the wall from different angles. The exhilaration he feels when he scores a difficult point against his opponent makes him feel like he is "just like Pete Sampras on TV." Dennis, who has been saving money to buy himself a new racket and balls, has been interested in the game ever since he saw it on television when he was 9 years of age. He first began playing with a flat piece of wood and then graduated to the racket that he now uses, which he found in the trash. Someday, when his mother will allow him, he will travel across town and play on the public tennis court, perhaps with a new racket. When asked what he would like to be when he grows up, he replies, "I don't know . . . maybe a tennis player."

For Dennis, the reality of playing tennis involves the particular elements described above, even if they are different from the occupational form generally necessary for playing tennis. What makes tennis an occupation for him is the meaning he derives from engaging in it. This meaningfulness arises out of his desire to play, his choice of making tennis his primary afterschool activity, his adaptation of the environment to mimic the prescribed form for tennis, and his excitement and enjoyment when playing. The adaptation of the occupational form to his needs and desires shapes his narrative of himself, thereby defining the meaning of his actions. By engaging in the occupation of playing tennis, Dennis's growth physically, socially, and mentally will shape who he is and who he is becoming. All of the other occupations in which Dennis engages affect who he is and who he is becoming (e.g., being a student, doing his share of the chores as a family member, watching television). All of us continue to evolve as a result of our individual experiences in various occupations in which we engage throughout our day. In fact, "the experience of individual occupations and their blend shape, in part, a person's perception of the quality of life" (Yerxa, 1998, p. 367).

As the example of Dennis indicates, understanding the occupations of a human being involves understanding various dimensions of the occupation and of the person's engagement in it. Little empirical research exists regarding occupations or their dimensions. To better understand the nature of this complex phenomenon, perspectives from the persons doing the occupation and the interpretation of external observers are both necessary. Occupation has various dimensions, including the cognitive, physical, spiritual, emotional, and contextual (AOTA, 1995). This chapter presents the author's views about the various dimensions to consider when studying and comprehending human occupation with the caveat that this classification is not a treatise on the subject but only a tool to convey the complexity of the phenomenon. The author discusses the biological, temporal–spatial, sociocultural, psychological, and spiritual dimensions. These dimensions are not mutually exclusive. Given the complexity and the interconnectedness of the various systems within the human being, the material in one dimension may fit into another dimension as well. The point is not the term under which an aspect of occupation is discussed but that the aspect is included when trying to comprehend human occupation.

Biological Dimension

The biological dimension includes all aspects of human occupation concerned with the needs, drives, abilities, and limitations of the person at the physiological level and at the organism level. Scholars from various disciplines have hypothesized that action and activity serve a vital function in the evolution and survival of species. In the human, several characteristics and capacities are necessary for adaptation to the environment and for developing occupational behaviors. The most important of these are upright walking, hand dexterity, stereoscopic vision, communication, and socialization (Campbell, 1988). An assumption related to the biological development of human occupations is that the emergence of any characteristic is grounded in its functional use. In other words, our ability to walk, jump, dance, climb, or manipulate objects with our fine motor skills is at once the reason for the development of the particular structure and shape of our limbs and conversely the result of the structure and shape of the limbs. These physical capabilities, along with the development of the cerebral cortex and its higher-level functions in the human including thinking, imagining, learning, and judging (Kolb & Whishaw, 1990), facilitate the human being's performance of complex occupational behaviors. These behaviors in turn allow the adaptation and survival of the species in various environments. On the basis of the idea that humans have an innate biological drive to engage in occupation, Wilcock (1998) proposed four functions for occupation in species survival and individual health. The first function is to provide for immediate bodily needs of sustenance, self-care, shelter, and safety. The second function is to develop skills (i.e., social structures and technology aimed at superiority over predators and the environment). The third function is to maintain health by a balanced exercise of personal capacities. The last function of occupation in survival and individual health is to enable individual and social development so that each person and the species will flourish.

Some occupations are directly and observably related to survival, such as eating and self-care occupations or jobs to then gain access to shelter, whereas others such as dancing and singing are not. Persons best perform occupations, however, when their underlying biological capacities are intact. Each person has different capacities that result in varying abilities to engage in and perform occupations. The biological considerations in the performance of an occupation are many and are all equally important.

To begin, we must examine structural integrity. Are all physiological structures present, and do they relate to the performance of the occupation? Is the neurophysiology supporting these structures functional? A lack of or some change in the structures may impede proper functioning and thereby affect the performance of the occupation.

The next consideration is whether the functional capacity of the structure has developed. In other words, are the physical parts integrated with the neurophysiology? How far has the function developed? Has the skill matured to the level necessary for performing the tasks of the occupation? In this case, the developmental age of the person in various areas becomes an important indicator of his or her physical and cognitive capacities. In an extreme example, the complete lack of coordination secondary to head trauma may make completing tasks in any familiar occupation impossible.

In addition to the structure and function at this basic level, research has shown that genetics and gender have an effect on the capacities of persons to perform tasks (Gagne, 1991; Jones, 1992; Scarr, 1980). For example, persons who are born with an extra chromosome, number 21 (Down syndrome), may develop variant structures and neurophysiology that may affect their performance of activities. Some researchers have reported that gender differences affect behavior and therefore possibly affect engagement in occupation (Kolb & Whishaw, 1990).

Another important biological consideration is the development of some form of communication. Bruner (1972) hypothesized that language is an outgrowth of mastering the skills of action and perceptual discrimination. As our anatomy and physiology changed and we developed into more complex beings who use social structures, our speech and language increased in complexity. This led to more complex occupational behaviors: language-requiring occupations (Wilcock, 1998). For a person to participate actively in society, he or she must be able to communicate and use symbols (Chomsky, 1986). A person is able to engage successfully in occupations when the person's skills match the level of occupational performance required.

Another aspect of the biological dimension is the ability to learn and adapt. Learning and adaptation can occur through engagement in occupation. Learning and adaptation affect physiological structures and are influenced by the environment. Biological factors such as genetics, disease, and trauma may influence learning and adaptation. Alternatively, conditions in the environment may impede or nurture the physiological capacity to learn and adapt. Awareness of the physiological capacity to learn and adapt is crucial in understanding a person's performance of an occupation.

Sleep, the basic rest activity, influences a person's occupational performance. Sleep is when the body is able to repair and recuperate from the day's activities. Sleep research has shown that, without the appropriate amount of sleep, symptoms such as irritability, blurred vision, and decreased coordination may occur that consequently affect occupational performance (Creighton, 1995; Pierce, 1991). Sleep, or the lack of it, may affect homeostasis in the body. Homeostasis is the balance of the internal environment in the body. As we know from physiology, homeostasis is basic to the proper functioning of the nervous system (Kolb & Whishaw, 1990). Genetic factors, disease, and stress can interfere with homeostasis. Malfunctioning of the nervous system resulting from such variables will decrease the effective performance of occupations.

Another aspect of the biological dimension to consider when discussing human occupation is the level of arousal and consciousness. *Level of arousal* refers to the state of being awake and ready to accept sensory input. To choose and consequently to engage in the occupation, one must be conscious and awake. Level of arousal is linked to changes in the chemical balances within the internal environment of the body as well as cognitive and emotional states. For example, changes in hormonal levels resulting from pregnancy, disease, or other imbalances affect moods and behavior (Hilman, Bowers, & Valenstein, 1993).

Each of the factors above influences a person's engagement in an occupation (i.e., choosing to and having the ability to perform the occupation). Some publications relating occupation directly to one or more of the biological aspects include Farnworth's (1995) exploration of skill as an issue in unemployment and employment, Zemke and Horger's (1995) examination of the hand as a tool for adaptation, Pierce's (1997) notions about object play in infants, and Goodall's (1996) work regarding the occupations of chimpanzee infants and mothers.

Exercise 1

Choose a leisure time occupation. Identify the physical structures and functions or skills necessary to perform the occupation. Are your skills appropriate for the occupation? What effect does heredity or gender have on your performance, if any? What might be the consequence for your performance if you are lethargic or lack proper sleep? Does the occupation require any communication or language skills?

Temporal–Spatial Dimension

The temporal–spatial dimension includes the time and space aspects of human occupation. For the sake of clarity, this chapter first discusses the temporal aspects and then moves on to the spatial aspects of occupation. The temporal aspects of the dimension involve three major types: the temporal nature of the occupation, the temporal nature of the person engaging in it, and the temporal nature of the environment around the person.

Temporal Nature of the Occupation

The temporal nature of the occupation relates to the length of the occupation: when it begins, when it ends, the pace or tempo of activities within the occupation, and the routines and schedules within the occupation. For example, when playing tennis, the beginning is when the two parties agree to begin the game. The game ends when the parties reach the agreed goal (e.g., after two out of three sets or after an hour of rallying). In a professional match, specified times mark the beginning of the match, the time between the end of one point and the beginning of the next point, and so forth. Generally, the rules of the game dictate how play proceeds and set its pace.

Temporal Nature of the Person Engaging in the Occupation

The second type of temporality relates to factors that affect the temporal nature of the person. The temporal nature of the person refers to the person's sense of past, present, and future. In other words, when one performs an activity and creates a memory, one interprets the experience and shapes the future. Ongoing interpretations of the experience enable one to reshape the future continually. This gives the person a sense of where he or she is going and the sense that the experience of living allows the realization of future possibilities (Clark, 1997). A person's occupations are imbued with meaning in relation to one's sense of the past and present.

This aspect of temporality includes various biological rhythms such as the circadian rhythms, day–night cycle, or the hormonal cycle. Evidence exists that biological rhythms affect performance of activities. For example, when working in an assembly line on the night shift, increased fatigue and poor performance are common (Gordon, Cleary, Parker, & Czeisler, 1986; LeFevre, Hedricks, Church, & McClintock, 1992).

Another aspect of the temporal nature of the person involves the capability of the person. In other words, the person's physical structure and skill enable him or her to control the pace of an activity. In the example of the tennis match, at the discretion of the person, the players may increase or decrease the pace of the game depending on their skill and stamina. Capability is likewise evident in a person's cognitive skills. For example, can a person organize a daily round of activities? Can Tina, a college student 20 years of age, manage her time between attending classes, studying, working at a pizza parlor, having fun with her boyfriend and friends, and doing necessary self-care and household chores? To manage, Tina must decide which occupations are most important to her. Then she must organize her daily routines to accomplish her goals. Her individual patterns for using time affect her choices of activities and occupations and how she engages in them. In summary, the temporal nature of the person encompasses biological rhythms; a sense of past, present, and future; abilities; and the subjective experience of time.

The subjective experience of time is yet another aspect of the temporal nature of the person. Simply put, if persons are having fun or find an occupation rewarding, then they may perceive time as moving swiftly; however, if they find an activity as too challenging or boring, then they may perceive time as moving rather slowly.

Temporal Nature of the Environment Around the Person

The last type of temporality is the temporal aspect of the environment. This includes the physical environment, seasonal cycles such as summer and fall, or institutional cycles such as the fiscal year. Certain occupations are involved in these changes such as planting vegetables in the spring, skiing in the winter, or working on taxes. Social calendars and clocks may dictate the performance of an occupation. Simple examples include being a student and paying attention to the teacher when the bell sounds at 8:30 a.m., working Monday through Friday but not on the weekend, young adults dancing all night long with friends on a Saturday night, or dining at 8 p.m. for older adults because they all agreed on the time.

Context of Space

Space involves the immediate and global physical area well as the tools and objects contained in that space. The *immediate physical space* refers to the proximal environment of the person. This may range from the immediate work space in which the person performs an occupation to a slightly larger area such as the office, the home, or the beach. A larger conceptual space may be the city, the mountains, or the east coast. Each person perceives space and its boundaries according to his or her own world view and the occupation in which he or she is engaged. For example, a painter's immediate space may include the area in which he or she sits with an easel and paints. If the painter is painting a landscape from a photograph, the space boundaries are limited. On the other hand, if the painter is painting and viewing the landscape itself, the boundaries of space are vast.

Generally, the immediate space is important when examining an occupation. Considerations important to understanding the fit between the physical space and the occupation include size, configuration, and locale. Basketball usually requires a basketball court and a hoop. Classroom teaching usually requires a room large enough to seat everyone comfortably, a lectern, and a chalkboard. Although such environments may be optimal for these occupations, they are not necessarily essential. Another element of space is the objects and tools necessary to engage in the occupation. Playing basketball usually requires a basketball. Classroom teaching requires desk chairs, chalk, and writing implements. Again, these objects may be optimal for these occupations, but they are not essential. Additionally, the appropriateness of the shape and size of the immediate space and the objects and tools within it may be important to support full engagement in the occupation. The unique combination of these various aspects of time and space may affect the adequacy and meaningfulness of the performance of the occupation. The following are several studies within the occupational therapy literature directly relating occupation to one or more temporal or spatial aspects: Primeau's (1998) examination of the orchestration of work and play occupations within families, Ludwig's (1998) study of routines in older women, White's (1996b) exploration of temporal adaptation in the intensive care unit, Segal's (1995) study of routines and schedules in families that have a child with a disability, Pierce's (1997) examination of objects in an infant's space and the consequent effect on infant and toddler play, Mailloux's (1996) work on the occupational therapy center as an enriched environment, and Dear's (1996) work involving the time, space, and geography of homeless persons.

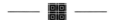

Exercise 2

Pick your favorite occupation and determine the length and pace of the activity as well as the beginning and end. Do socially and culturally accepted rules or norms define a pace for the activity, a space for the activity? Does time seem to move at a different speed when you are doing this activity? At what time of year do you usually do it? Are you able to perform this occupation as you want to, or are you having difficulty fitting it into your schedule? Are you aware of any of your biological rhythms that may be affecting your engagement in this occupation? Are the size and area in which you perform the occupation appropriate? Are the objects and tools appropriate?

Sociocultural Dimension

The biological and the temporal–spatial dimensions of occupation are strongly identified with the person as an individual. The human, however, is a social animal and is a member of a complex, interlinked social structure in which each link affects the person to some degree. The sociocultural dimension of occupation considers relationships with others within the immediate social environment and those that result from commonly valued behaviors and characteristics of the culture or subculture to which the person belongs.

This chapter discusses objects in the environment in the temporal–spatial dimension from the viewpoint of whether they were appropriate and useful for performing the occupation. In this section, the consideration concerns how persons relate to objects. For example, if one wants a particular boat, this desire may influence his or her actions and choices of occupations. The person may spend time in a paid job to earn the money to buy the boat, spend leisure time reading about boats, or take lessons in boat maintenance. After he or she purchases the boat, depending on the cathexis that develops, the bond that the person feels for the boat may influence the person's choice of occupations. The person's emotions not only influence this choice but also the levels of engagement in the occupation and the performance of it.

Human beings and animals are animate objects in the sociocultural environment. They are different from physical objects in that they have biological drives, wants, and abilities and are capable of responding to the person and each other. This reciprocity and communication may elicit a negotiation between persons regarding the performance of an occupation. Occupations may be solitary or shared. For example, playing tennis requires two players; hence, it is a shared occupation and requires negotiation of many details. On the other hand, teaching is a solitary occupation for the person but requires another person performing a complementary occupation, that of student. This relationship requires negotiation of some details. Other occupations are performed alone but within the temporal–spatial or a cognitive realm of another person, and these may require some negotiation. For example, performing self-care activities in a bathroom that roommates share requires negotiation of time, although the person performs the occupation completely alone. The cognitive realm includes one's thoughts while performing an occupation such as considering what someone else may think about one's performance or action.

These relationships can be of several types, and each influences the negotiations in a different way. These include familial relationships both nuclear (e.g., parent–child relationships or siblings) and more extended relationships such as grandparents–grandchildren, uncles and aunts, nephews and nieces, and cousins. Outside family relationships include friendships of the same gender and opposite gender, romantic relationships, coworker relationships, employer–employee relationships, neighbors, and acquaintances. Each of these relationships has different levels of influence on a person's engagement in an occupation. For example, in shopping for her summer wardrobe, Julie, a teenager in high school, said that her close friends influence her choice of when, where, and for what to shop. Her mother's opinion and influence are limited to setting limits on the money Julie spends. Other relatives, neighbors, or acquaintances have little or no influence on this choice. In relation to her performance as a student, the multiple influences include the teacher as well as her parents and grandparents.

In addition to these individual relationships, society as a whole promulgates rules and regulations about acceptable behavior. Groups within the society, on the basis of various factors including race, gender, and geography, have evolved particular values, traditions, and rituals related to behavior. Societal expectations are unwritten but influence to a large extent what the occupational form of a particular occupation is and how persons generally performed it within that culture. The prevailing form of the occupation then highly influences the person living in that culture. His or her unique physical and mental makeup, combined with the circumstances surrounding any given moment, will determine how much the person follows the prescribed format. Getting together with family to cook and share a turkey every Thanksgiving holiday, aspiring to higher education in Asian cultures, men mowing the lawn and taking out the garbage, and attending a formal dance called a prom in the United States during the senior year of high school are all examples of values, trends, and traditions that influence the choice and performance of occupations. Alongside these culturally sanctioned symbols, values, and traditions are standards of conduct, of right and wrong action. These are the ethics and morals of society. They represent norms for behavior expected of a person. In other words, when making the choice to engage in an occupation or how to perform it, one's membership in society and socialization to follow the morals and ethics of that society limit him or her. These morals and ethics not only come from what society has set as a standard but also from organized religion and the person's beliefs. In fact, all of these standards are interrelated.

The formalization of the rules and regulations of society into written laws and institutions is another level of organization that affects individual occupation. These institutions include the political system, the legal system, the economic system, the educational system, and other overarching systems. We are all familiar with these systems and can determine how they guide our choice of occupations as well as our performance. A simple example is fishing in the lake instead of fishing in the river. The choice resulted from laws against fishing in the river on the basis of environmental considerations.

Sociocultural influences operate at various levels and interact reciprocally. These factors influence one's engagement in occupations. To understand occupations fully, one must examine the sociocultural dimension and related factors. Some recent works that directly examine the relationship between these factors and occupation are Pendleton's (1996) examination of the occupation of needlework, Moore's (1996) article on feasting as an occupation and the emergence of ritual from it, Krishnagiri's (1994) exploration of mate selection, and Dunlea's (1996) study of mothers and blind infants and their coadaptation.

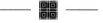

Exercise 3

By using the same occupation as in the previous exercise, identify the various levels of sociocultural influences on your choice and performance of your occupation. Include which persons, animals, or objects in your life influence you and how. Think about the neighborhood you live in, your race and gender, and the culture you live in and examine how they may have influenced your performance. Have you made moral and ethical choices in doing this occupation? Additionally, examine the larger society and determine whether any of the systems, institutions, and symbols under which you live affect your choices and performance.

Psychological Dimension

The *psychological dimension* refers to all the emotional and cognitive aspects of human occupation. Emotions are the affective subjective component of psychological function. Sarafino's (1990) interpretation of Freud's work described emotions as the investment of psychic energy in an external object, whereas neo-Freudians view emotions as a function of human interaction in the context of culture. Behaviorists define emotions in terms of observable manifestations. Finally, cognitive theorists view emotions as the consequence of a mental appraisal of the current situation (Sdorow,

1990). Emotions range from more positive constructs such as happiness, ecstasy, and joy to more negative constructs such as sadness, anger, bitterness, and jealousy.

Appreciation of emotions requires consciousness of physiological responses of the body such as tears and increased heartbeats. Additionally, language and moral judgments affect the feelings that we interpret as emotions (Harre, Clarke, & DeCarlo, 1985; Sarafino, 1990). These physiological and behavioral elements affect and are affected by action. Hence, the state of one's emotions can affect the choice and performance of an occupation. For example, if Enrico is anxious before an examination, his blood pressure may increase as well as his heart rate. This physiological state may cause him to be nervous and perform poorly on the exam. The performance on the exam, which is a part of his student role, may affect his motivation to continue to stay in school or may make him work harder and concentrate on becoming a better student.

Cognition is the acquisition, organization, and use of knowledge and encompasses perception, memory, attention, pattern recognition, problem solving, reflection, learning, and anticipation (Neisser, 1976). Each of these mental processes plays a major role in the interactions of a person with his or her environment. *Perception* is a basic process out of which all the others emerge. The perceiver takes in information and then processes, transforms, recodes, and assimilates it and generally provides structure and meaning to what may otherwise be chaos, which can loosely be termed *schema*. The results of organizing and assimilating the information with previous experiences and current circumstances are actions and thoughts. These systematic organizations and plans for action are termed *cognitive maps* (Schmidt, 1988).

Perceptions and the resultant schema are subject to the effects of time and development. As humans age, they perceive more, and perceptions change and become more complex. For example, with growth, maturity, and practice resulting in expert knowledge, a person who plays expert chess will, when shown a board with a game in progress for a few seconds, be easily able to recollect where all the pieces stood on the board. This ability stems from perceiving the information in more complex patterns on the basis of relationships and not from simple memory. Higher-level cognitive functions enable the person to juggle various occupations and still attend to each of them appropriately. In addition to what one can perceive in the immediate environment, culture provides additional information. Thus, perceptions and experience affect behavior. On the basis of behavioral patterns, humans develop expectations and anticipate others' behaviors. These anticipations prepare them for action and its consequences and motivate them positively or negatively. Sometimes humans develop sets of behaviors that result from temporal and spatial factors. For example, playing horseshoes may well motivate someone to engage in a horseshoes competition when the opportunity arises.

As some persons mature, the ability for future orientation and more goal-directed action may develop and increase in capacity. This requires other higher-level cognitive functions like motivation and imagination and the use of the basic mental processes of perception, memory, learning, problem solving, and so forth. These higher-level functions require several cognitive maps for action. The higher-level functions, which work on the basis of removing schemas from the context in which they are embedded and connecting them to other possible contexts, provide the impetus for various behaviors and actions within any given occupation. For example, the ability to imagine using a different ingredient than that used in a traditional recipe and anticipating the outcome results in a dissimilar approach to performing the occupation.

At the core of these concepts related to mental processes is the belief that the choice of action is never free of the information from which it results (Neisser, 1976). Therefore, one's engagement in occupation depends on the functioning of these cognitive processes. Given that each person's perceptual history is unique, which leads to individualized schemas and cognitive maps, the way he or she engages in the occupation may be unique and uniquely meaningful to him or her.

In summary, emotions and cognitive processes, both the basic and higher-level ones, have a strong influence on the choice of engagement and the method of engagement in occupation. Research in the psychological dimension as it relates to occupation is beginning to emerge. Some examples include Jackson's (1995) work on sexual orientation, White's (1996a) work on emotions and narrative in the occupations of Miles Davis, and Pierce's (1991) work on organizational capacities and temporal orientation.

Exercise 4

Think about your various engagements in an occupation of your choosing and identify changes in your performance of it secondary to the emotions you may have been experiencing at the time. Think of times when you are angry, sad, joyful, or jealous. Can you anticipate how your engagement in the occupation would change when you are feeling these emotions? Now consider learning a new occupation: What cognitive processes are you aware of while learning to engage in this occupation? If you had poor memory, how would this affect your favorite occupation? How would the ability to anticipate or the lack of such an ability affect the performance of your occupation?

Spiritual Dimension

Spirit is the essence or true nature of the person, something that is expressed through all actions (Egan & Delaat, 1994). According to Polkinghorne (1988), spirituality is the manifestation of this self and guides one through life.

> We achieve our personal identities and self-concept through the use of the narrative configuration, and make our existence into a whole by understanding it as an expression of a single unfolding and developing story. We are in the middle of our stories and cannot be sure how they will end; we are constantly having to revise the plot as new events are added to our lives. Self, then, is not a static thing or a substance, but a configuring of personal events into an historical unity which includes not only what one has been but also anticipations of what one will be. (p. 150)

The spiritual self consists of the personal experiences of meaning in everyday life (Urbanowski & Vargo, 1994). A person may view this spirituality in several ways. Some view spirituality as part of a religious orientation, whereas some interpret it as just a feeling or sense of meaning. Others do not believe in spirituality at all.

Finding purpose and meaning in what one does is linked to narrative knowledge, storymaking, and storytelling. *Narrative knowledge* refers to what one thinks one did in which settings in what ways for what reasons (Polkinghorne, 1988). Storytelling and storymaking are expressions of that knowledge and the need to make sense of it within the culture in which one lives (Bruner, 1990; Clark, 1993; Mattingly, 1991). Understanding the stories of the person's experience then is the key to understanding purpose and meaning in individual occupations. For example, others may view a person who is engaged in paid employment as a carpenter as merely working. In the view of the person, however, the story may interpret the occupation as more than just making a living and may include providing for the family, making a home, or creating a beautiful piece of art. Imbuing the occupation with these particular purposes and meanings may even relate to the spiritual nature of the person.

Narrative knowledge, the harbinger of meaning and purpose, is a constantly changing phenomenon. Several factors can modify knowledge and consequently its expression, including the history of experiences, reflections, anticipations, perceptions, and motivations. These are all mental processes that may help to derive meaning and purpose for the person in an occupation. Narratives are grounded in the culture in which the person lives. For example, if the person lives in a religious home but a highly sectarian culture, the types of reflections, perceptions, and motivations that are typical for that culture and a specific religion may influence his or her narrative knowledge of a particular activity. The expressions of his or her experience and the meaning he or she finds in the activity therefore will involve these same connotations. Individual histories, physiology, and other idiosyncrasies will likewise greatly influence the narrative knowing and storytelling.

In summary, the spiritual dimension reflects individualized expressions of meaning in experience. Several works in recent years have explored occupations and aspects of the spiritual dimension, including Frank's (1994) work on the personal meaning of self-care occupations, Jackson's (1996) work on living a meaningful existence in old age, and a host of articles in the special issues of the *American Journal of Occupational Therapy* and the *Canadian Journal of Occupational Therapy* on spirituality in 1997.

—— ▦ ——

Exercise 5

Consider one of the occupations you have used in preceding exercises. What meaning do you derive from this occupation? How does the way you perform it differ from the way others perform it? What makes it your occupation? What enjoyment do you receive from this occupation?

_____

Summary

Occupations are complex dynamic phenomena occurring in the stream of time that we cannot explain simply by describing their objective characteristics. Because humans engage in occupations, the factors that they introduce as performers of the occupations are necessary for a true understanding of occupation. This chapter describes preliminarily the various aspects of occupation to consider along five major dimensions: biological, temporal–spatial, sociocultural, psychological, and spiritual. Intense scrutiny of any of these concepts shows that many more variables exist that require explanation and consideration. At this time, the most central and important of these concepts appears to be the subjective meaningful experience of the person, which infuses the performance of the occupation with the spirit of that person. The performance of any individual activity would not in and of itself possess all of the aspects described in this chapter regarding occupation. The activity when viewed as part of a larger grouping of related activities that have meaning in the culture, however, would possess these characteristics. ■

References

American Occupational Therapy Association. (1995). Position paper: Occupation. *American Journal of Occupational Therapy, 49,* 1015–1018.

Bruner, J. (1972). Nature and uses of immaturity. *American Psychologist, 27,* 687–708.

Bruner, J. (1990). *Acts of meaning.* Cambridge, MA: Harvard University Press.

Campbell, B. G. (1988). *Humankind emerging* (5th ed.). New York: Harper Collins.

Chomsky, N. (1986). *The origins of language: Its nature origin and use.* New York: Praeger.

Clark, F. (1993). Occupation embedded in a real life: Interweaving occupational science and occupational therapy. 1993 Eleanor Clarke Slagle lecture. *American Journal of Occupational Therapy, 47,* 1067–1078.

Clark, F. (1997). Reflections on the human as an occupational being: Biological need, tempo, and temporality. *Journal of Occupational Science, 4,* 86–92.

Clark, F. A., Parham, D., Carlson, M. E., Frank, G., Jackson, J., Pierce, D., Wolfe, R. J., & Zemke, R. (1991). Occupational science: Academic innovation in the service of occupational therapy's future. *American Journal of Occupational Therapy, 45,* 300–310.

Creighton C. (1995). Effects of afternoon rest on the performance of geriatric patients in a rehabilitation hospital: A pilot study. *American Journal of Occupational Therapy, 49,* 775–779.

Dear, M. (1996). Time, space, and the geography of everyday life of people who are homeless. In R. Zemke & F. Clark (Eds.), *Occupational science: The evolving discipline* (pp. 107–114). Philadelphia: F. A. Davis.

Dunlea, A. (1996). An opportunity for co-adaptation: The experience of mothers and their infants who are blind. In R. Zemke & F. Clark (Eds.), *Occupational science: The evolving discipline* (pp. 227–241). Philadelphia: F. A. Davis.

Egan, M., & Delaat, M. D. (1994). Considering spirituality in occupational therapy practice. *Canadian Journal of Occupational Therapy, 61,* 95–101.

Farnworth, L. (1995). An exploration of skill as an issue of unemployment and employment. *Journal of Occupational Science: Australia, 2,* 22–29.

Frank, G. (1994). The personal meaning of self-care occupations. In C. Christiansen (Ed.), *Ways of living: Self-care strategies for special needs* (pp. 27–49). Rockville, MD: American Occupational Therapy Association.

Gagne, F. (1991). Toward a differential model of giftedness and talents. In N. Colabango & G. Davis (Eds.), *Handbook of gifted education* (pp. 65–80). Boston: Allyn & Bacon.

Goodall, J. (1996). Occupations of chimpanzee infant and mothers. In R. Zemke & F. Clark (Eds.), *Occupational science: The evolving discipline* (pp. 31–42). Philadelphia: F. A. Davis.

Gordon, N. P., Cleary, P. D., Parker, C. E., & Czeisler, C. A. (1986). The prevalence and health impact of shift work. *American Journal of Public Health, 76,* 1225.

Harre, R., Clarke, D., & DeCarlo, N. (1985). *Motives and mechanisms: An introduction to the psychology of action.* New York: Methuen.

Heilman, K. M., Bowers, D., & Valenstein, E. (1993). Emotional disorders associated with neurological diseases. In K. M. Heilman & A. E. Valenstein (Eds.), *Clinical Neuropsychology* (3rd ed.). New York: Oxford University Press.

Jackson, J. (1995). Sexual orientation: Its relevance to occupational science and the practice of occupational therapy. *American Journal of Occupational Therapy, 49,* 669–679.

Jackson, J. (1996). Living a meaningful existence in old age. In R. Zemke & F. Clark (Eds.), *Occupational science: The evolving discipline* (pp. 339–362). Philadelphia: F. A. Davis.

Jones, S. (1992). Genetic diversity in humans. In S. Jones, R. Martin, & D. Pillbean (Eds.), *The Cambridge encyclopaedia of human evolution* (pp. 264–267). New York: Cambridge University Press.

Kolb, B., & Whishaw, I. Q. (1990). *Fundamentals of human neurophysiology* (3rd ed.). San Francisco: Freeman.

Krishnagiri, S. (1994). *Mate selection as an occupation.* Unpublished doctoral dissertation, University of Southern California, Los Angeles.

LeFevre, J., Hedricks, C., Church, R. B., & McClintock, M. K. (1992). Psychological and social behavior of couples over a menstrual cycle: "On the spot" sampling from everyday life. In A. Dan & L. Lewis (Eds.), *Menstrual health in women's lives* (pp. 75–82). Chicago: University of Illinois Press.

Ludwig, F. M. (1998). The unpackaging of routine in older women. *American Journal of Occupational Therapy, 52,* 168–175.

Mailloux, Z. (1996). The occupational therapy center as an enriched environment. In R. Zemke & F. Clark (Eds.), *Occupational science: The evolving discipline* (pp. 171–176). Philadelphia: F. A. Davis.

Mattingly, C. (1991). The narrative nature of clinical reasoning. *American Journal of Occupation Therapy, 45,* 998–1005.

Moore, A. (1996). Feasting as occupation: The emergence of ritual from everyday activities. *Journal of Occupational Science: Australia, 3,* 5–15.

Neisser, U. (1976). *Cognition and reality.* New York: Freeman.

Nelson, D. L. (1988). Occupation: Form and performance. *American Journal of Occupational Therapy, 42,* 633–641.

Pendleton, H. M. (1996). The occupation of needlework. In R. Zemke & F. Clark (Eds.), *Occupational science: The evolving discipline* (pp. 287–295). Philadelphia: F. A. Davis.

Pierce, D. E. (1991). Cognition: Temporal orientation and organizational capacity. In C. B. Royeen (Ed.), *Neuroscience foundations of human performance* (Lesson 9, pp. 1–44). Rockville, MD: American Occupational Therapy Association.

Pierce, D. E. (1997). The power of object play with infants and toddlers at risk for developmental delays. In L. D. Parham & L. Fazio (Eds.), *Play in occupational therapy for children* (pp. 86–111). St. Louis: Mosby.

Polkinghorne, D. E. (1988). *Narrative knowing and the human sciences.* Albany, NY: State University of New York Press.

Primeau, L. (1998). Orchestration of work and play within families. *American Journal of Occupational Therapy, 52,* 188–195.

Sarafino, E. P. (1990). *Health psychology: Biopsychosocial interactions.* New York: Wiley.

Scarr, S. (1980). *Race, social class and individual differences.* Hillsdale, NJ: Erlbaum.

Schmidt, R. A. (1988). *Motor control and learning: A behavioral emphasis.* Champaign, IL: Human Kinetics.

Sdorow, L. (1990). *Psychology.* Dubuque, IA: William C. Brown.

Segal, R. (1995). *Family adaptation to a child with attention deficit hyperactivity disorder.* Unpublished doctoral dissertation, University of Southern California, Los Angeles.

Urbanowski, R., & Vargo, J. (1994). Spirituality, daily practice, and the occupational performance model. *Canadian Journal of Occupational Therapy, 61,* 277–284.

White, J. (1996a). Miles Davis: Occupations in the extreme. In R. Zemke & F. Clark (Eds.), *Occupational science: The evolving discipline* (pp. 259–273). Philadelphia: F. A. Davis.

White, J. (1996b). Temporal adaptation in the intensive care unit. In R. Zemke & F. Clark (Eds.), *Occupational science: The evolving discipline* (pp. 363–371). Philadelphia: F. A. Davis.

Wilcock, A. (1998). *An occupational perspective on health.* Thorofare, NJ: Slack.

Yerxa, E. (1998). Occupation: The keystone of a curriculum for a self-defined profession. *American Journal of Occupational Therapy, 52,* 365–372.

Zemke, R., & Horger, M. (1995). The hand: A tool for adaptation. In C. B. Royeen (Ed.), *Hands-on: Practical intervention for the hand.* Bethesda, MD: American Occupational Therapy Association.

4

Activity Analysis

Karen A. Buckley, MA, OT/L
Sally E. Poole, MA, OT, CHT

The concept that man must use his mind and body to maintain health and well-being was documented as early as 2600 B.C. The ancient Chinese, Persians, and Greeks understood that a mutually dependent relationship exists between physical and mental health and well-being. Egyptians and Greeks viewed diversion and recreation as treatment for the sick. Later, the Romans recommended activity for persons who were mentally ill (Hopkins & Smith, 1978).

Many centuries later, in Europe and the United States, activity and occupation became treatment modalities for persons with mental and physical illness. In 1798, Benjamin Rush, the first American psychiatrist, advocated the use of domestic occupations for their therapeutic value. Weaving, spinning, and sewing were occupations that Rush considered to be therapeutic because of their interest to the patients of the era and because of their social and cultural relevance (Dunton & Licht, 1957). In the United States during the 18th and 19th centuries, occupations were used to care for persons with mental illness. In 1892, Edward N. Bush, superintendent of a psychiatric hospital in Maryland, wrote the following.

> The benefits of occupation are manifold. Primarily, even the most simple and routine tasks keep the mind occupied, awaken new trains of thought and interests, and divert the patient from the delusions or hallucinations which harass and annoy him. (as cited in Dunton & Licht, 1957, p. 9)

In addition to the use of occupations in psychiatric treatment during the 18th and 19th centuries, early documentation indicates that occupations helped to build muscles and improve joint range. In 1780 in France, Clement-Joseph Tissot (Dunton & Licht, 1957) described the beneficial use of arts and crafts and recreational activities to mediate the physical effects of chronic illness. In his work, he cites shuttlecock, tennis, football, and dancing as activities that promote range of motion for all joints of the upper and lower extremities. In this early literature concerning the use of occupations or activities, few details exist about the precise methodology for selecting activities to address specific problems. Activities appear to have been selected for their cultural, social, recreational, and diversional characteristics.

In the early 1900s, occupational therapists embraced the Arts and Crafts Movement, which was a backlash against the social ills that some believed were the result of the Industrial Revolution (Reed, 1986). The Arts and Crafts Movement promoted a simpler life in which persons performed activities at a slower pace than in factory production, in which the process was as important as the end product, that valued the creative spirit, and that valued manual learning versus intellectual learning alone (Reed, 1986). Before World War II, few reports in the literature indicate that therapists selected activities on any basis other than intuition (Creighton, 1992; Reed, 1986).

At the end of World War I, two factors strongly influenced occupational therapists' use of activities and related occupations. First, the end of the Arts and Crafts Movement in the United States and in Europe meant that many activities were not valued in the same way. Second, therapists found themselves treating patients who were exhibiting both physical and psychological trauma resulting from the war. Therapists began selecting activities on the basis of the patient's particular deficits and needs. Therapists began to carefully analyze each patient's deficits and used a problem-solving approach to determine which specific activity would be appropriate. Therapists used activities because of their characteristics, but no formal analysis was part of the therapist's treatment routine. Therapists and physicians, however, began to look beyond the profession of occupational therapy to gain knowledge about activity analysis.

During this early development of the profession of occupational therapy, at least two men outside of the profession, Frank Gilbreth and Jules Amar (Creighton, 1992), influenced activity selection and subsequent intervention. Gilbreth, an engineer by training, studied jobs to identify the most productive and least fatiguing methods of job performance. Gilbreth's work, which industry accepted, examined the worker, the environment, and motion. While visiting hospitals in Europe to study physicians and how they work, Gilbreth became acquainted with the research of Jules Amar, a French physiologist. The French government commissioned Amar to study how to prepare wounded soldiers effectively for reentry into the workforce. As a physiologist, Amar measured the physiological requirements of a job. Amar's work influenced Gilbreth by showing Gilbreth the possibilities of applying motion studies to the reeducation of returning wounded veterans. Gilbreth presented his work at the 1917 annual meeting of the National Society for the Promotion of Occupational Therapy (NSPOT), which led to the eventual inclusion of the concept of activity analysis into the field of occupational therapy. In 1919, occupational therapy textbooks began to incorporate activity analysis (Creighton, 1992).

The years between World War I and World War II saw the establishment of the American Occupational Therapy Association (AOTA), formerly NSPOT, and the further development of the profession in general. AOTA encouraged therapists to establish departments and published guidelines to help them do so. In addition, AOTA published guidelines to assist therapists in the appropriate selection of activities. Crafts were the treatment activities of choice, although "crafts" did include work-related and recreational activities (Creighton, 1992). In 1922 and 1928, AOTA published guidelines promoting the analysis of crafts for psychiatric occupational therapy and for physical restoration.

World War II took women out of the home and into the workforce and took occupational therapists from traditional roles to new real-life circumstances. As a result of improvements in medical and surgical care, veterans were surviving severe physical injuries and living with permanent disabilities. Occupational therapists began to specialize in the practice area of physical disabilities. Again, occupational therapists referred to the work of Gilbreth, now carried on by his wife Lillian, who proposed that engineers and rehabilitation professionals work together to assist soldiers with disabilities (Creighton, 1992). At the same time, the U.S. Army developed its own manual of therapeutic activities (War Department, 1994), which described activities to improve joint range of motion and strengthening of all extremities. The military, in fact, "divided" the body so that occupational therapists worked with the upper body and physical therapists worked with the lower body (Hinojosa, 1996). The occupational therapy profession still follows many policies and procedures set by the military.

Immediately after World War II in 1947, Sidney Licht published an article advocating the use of a more precise method for analyzing activity for occupational therapists working with physical disabilities. He believed that craft analysis examined the "psychomotor values, economic factors, tempo, or other inherent characteristics" (Licht, 1947, p. 75). When therapists analyze the tools or activities for the motions involved, he termed this *kinetic analysis*. Many of his ideas continue to influence practice in the area of physical disabilities. Contemporary occupational therapists who are concerned about muscle contraction, range of joint motion, precision and accuracy of intervention, ergonomics of body mechanics, and control variants continue to use the criteria for examining motion that Licht originally proposed for kinetic analysis.

Occupational therapists in physical medicine apparently became interested in activity analysis before therapists working in mental health. Fidler (1948) proposed that occupational therapists working in psychiatric occupational therapy must use scientific analysis of activities.

> While the functioning of a personality is certainly not as quantifiable as a muscle, the use of activity for the psychiatric patient should be more scientifically allied with the principles of dynamic psychiatry and treatment objectives than it is at the present. (p. 284)

Fidler proposed an outline for activity analysis to help occupational therapists meet the goals or aims of treatment so that occupational therapy in psychiatry could, in fact, move from diversion to the level of therapy.

Activity Analysis: Definition and Purpose

Activity analysis is the process of closely examining an activity to distinguish its component parts (Mosey, 1986). A careful examination allows a skilled occupational therapy practitioner to select the most therapeutic and appropriate activity from the activities available. A careful examination ensures that the activities that an occupational therapy practitioner selects are relevant and correspond to the client's needs. Originally in occupational therapy, activity analysis was rudimentary and focused almost exclusively on the product and not on the process of analysis. Gradually, the process of analysis has become more important than the end product. Today, activity analysis is an important tool that occupational therapists use to analyze activities and to examine the process and outcome of intervention. Activity analysis is an important tool that occupational therapy practitioners use as part of deductive reasoning in whatever frame of reference or approach they use with clients.

Activity analysis enables occupational therapy practitioners to determine an activity's therapeutic properties so that they can make an appropriate match between the interests and abilities of the client and the activity that will meet his or her health needs (Mosey, 1986). Activity analysis is a process of determining the component parts of an activity so that a practitioner can use an activity in a way that will meet the intervention goals. Llorens' (1993) definition of activity analysis exemplified the broadened scope of current thinking. Llorens (1993) defined activity analysis as

> a process by which the properties inherent in a given activity, task or occupation, may be gauged for their ability to elicit individual intrinsic and extrinsic motivation and to fulfill patient needs in occupational performance and performance components. Occupational therapists use activity analysis in activity selection for guiding and evaluating activity use by the patient. (p. 199)

Without this process, occupational therapy practitioners cannot use activities therapeutically.

In practice, however, occupational therapy practitioners sometimes concern themselves with analyzing the activity into too many minute, insignificant pieces and thus lose the "wholeness" of the activity. Whenever completing an activity analysis, occupational therapy practitioners must keep in mind the total activity and the occupations underlying the activity. Today, AOTA's (1994) Uniform Terminology provides a framework for activity analysis that allows analysis of the small components without losing the whole. The Uniform Terminology fits the small pieces into one of three general categories: performance areas, performance components, and performance contexts.

In the interest of looking at the whole, some scholars have suggested that occupational therapy practitioners give one category preference over another. Cynkin and Robinson (1990) proposed that occupational therapy practitioners begin an activity analysis with the performance context. Trombly and Scott (1977) proposed that practitioners analyze performance areas first. Hinojosa and Kramer (1998) argued that an analysis should begin in the area (performance component, performance area, performance context) that is most appropriate to the client and his or her needs. For example, a therapist who works in a hand therapy practice would begin with an analysis of the activity grounded in the performance components. In this example, the practitioner selects activities on the basis of how the activities address performance component deficits.

Occupational Therapy Perspectives on Activity Analysis

Extensive literature exists in our profession regarding activity analysis. In occupational therapy professional education, students spend much time on activity analysis by learning how to conduct an analysis by dividing an activity into its component parts. Traditionally, occupational therapy students learn to analyze an activity by focusing on the performance components that comprise the individual tasks. This process often leads students not to consider the whole activity and the context in which a person usually performs it. This microanalysis may result in not attending to the important occupation associated with the activity. As discussed above, many forms related to activity analysis result from Uniform Terminology and follow the outline of performance components or performance areas. Students learning how to do activity analysis must be able to identify not only that the component is functional but also to what extent it is functional and the way it is functioning in the context of the activity. The following section outlines this process by focusing on an analysis that examines activities within the context in which the person performs them.

Activity Analysis in Occupational Therapy

Occupational therapy practitioners have an organized conceptual approach to activity analysis that views the activity as a whole and then breaks it down into component parts. The following section outlines one method of completing an activity analysis. Each section has drawn from various sources within the occupational therapy literature. Many of the ideas herein have become common knowledge within occupational therapy. Hence, determining who originated the idea or concept is impossible (Allen, 1987; Ayres, 1983; Kremer, Nelson, & Duncombe, 1984; Llorens, 1973, 1986; Neistadt, McAuley, Zecha, & Shannon, 1993; Nelson, 1996; Pedretti & Wade, 1996; Willoughby, King, & Polatajko, 1996).

The following is a suggested framework for occupational therapy students and practitioners to follow when analyzing performance components. Like many other forms of activity analysis, this example follows the Uniform Terminology (AOTA, 1994). The activity analysis begins with a description of the activity and each of its fundamental tasks (i.e., the steps necessary to complete the activity). The occupational therapy practitioner and student describe the activity and the way in which a person generally performs it under usual circumstances. When the analysis is part of intervention, the occupational therapy practitioner should keep in mind the whole person. The practitioner appraises the activity relative to the context of the client who will perform it and the activity's associated performance areas.

The Activity

Activity:

Relationship to tasks:

Tasks (steps required to perform the activity):

1.

2.

3.

Materials, tools and equipment (availability, cost, source):

Safety precautions and contraindications:

Time needed to complete: hours: minutes: seconds:

■   Is this an activity that the person must complete in one session?

■   Is this an activity that the person can perform over time?

■   Can the activity naturally be divided so that the person can perform it over time?

■   Do the steps in the activity require that the person perform it over a period of time?

The Person

A person performs the activity. Thus, in the activity analysis, the occupational therapy practitioner must consider the person, including his or her interests and goals. Roles:

■   Present:

■   Past:

■   Future:

Relevance and meaningfulness (historical or current personal and social relevance):

■ Current:

■ Past:

■ Future:

■ Values and interests:

■ Culture:

Rating Performance Components

On the basis of the performance components of Uniform Terminology (AOTA, 1994), the occupational therapy practitioner evaluates the level of influence that each component has on a person's ability to do the activity. In other words, what effects do the performance components have on the activity? Eventually, the occupational therapy practitioner must understand how a deficit in a performance component affects or challenges the person to complete the activity. Another reason for analyzing an activity is to elicit the potential for providing stimulation or opportunities to use the specific performance component element. The numerical scale for rating the influence of each component is a five-point scale.

0   This component has no effect or influence on the ability to do the activity.

1   The component has only a minimal effect or influence on the ability to do the activity. The activity would not substantially stimulate or address the performance component element.

2   The component has a moderate effect or influence on the ability to complete the activity. If a client has a deficit, compensation may be necessary for the client to perform the activity. The activity would present a challenge to the performance component element.

3   The component has a major effect or influence on the ability to complete the activity. The activity would be extremely difficult to complete if the client has a deficit in this performance component. The activity would present a major stimulation or opportunity to address the performance component element.

4   This component has a major effect or influence on the completion of the activity. A performance component deficit in this area would seriously affect the person's ability to do the activity. Such a person would most likely not be able to complete the activity. The activity would present a major stimulation or opportunity to address this performance component element.

The observation section describes special circumstances or concerns. This section provides a space to include any other comments a practitioner or student has regarding the influence of the performance component on completion of the activity.

In the following section, we define each of performance components and provide several questions to assist in the activity analysis relative to the specific performance component. These questions help occupational therapy practitioners understand the role the performance component has in completing the activity. The questions are not definitive but are a "jump start" when considering each performance component. After considering each question, the occupational therapy practitioner rates the influence and writes observational notes.

Performance Component	Observations:			
Level of Influence				
0	1	2	3	4

Sensorimotor Components

The sensorimotor components include the ability to receive input, process information, and produce an output from the senses. The sensorimotor component involves sensory awareness and sensory processing relative to tactile, proprioceptive, vestibular, visual, auditory, gustatory, and olfactory senses. Although occupational therapy practitioners segregate sensory modalities during evaluation, no purposeful activity is purely tactile, auditory, or vestibular. Thus, an occupational therapy practitioner must develop a synopsis of the sensory characteristics of the entire activity that considers all the sensory requirements and sensory demands. This final synopsis is more meaningful and relevant than focusing on any individual sensory system. After completing an examination of all the sensory characteristics of the activity, the occupational therapy practitioner's ultimate goal is to interpret how all the sensory systems relate to each other by answering the following questions: Is one sensory system more important than another? Can the person compensate for a deficit in one sensory system by heightening the use of another? Can we teach clients to compensate if they have a deficit in a sensory system? Finally, if the client performs the activity with compensatory techniques, will that compromise the activity and its meaning to the client?

Sensory

Sensory Awareness

Sensory awareness of an activity is the degree to which the activity requires that a person be able to accept and discriminate input from various sensory sources. The nature of the materials included in the activity, the environment in which the person performs the activity, and the consequences of the actions required during the completion of the activity influence sensory awareness.

■   What sensory systems must be intact to complete the activity?

■   Does the activity require that the person register sensory information?

■ How quickly must the person register information to engage in the activity safely and efficiently?

Sensory Awareness					Observations:
Level of Influence					
0	1	2	3	4	

Sensory Processing

A person's central nervous system processes sensory information and integrates it so that the person can make an adaptive response. Sensory processing is the internal mechanism that the person uses to process and respond to sensory input. Sensory processing may influence the client's ability to reach a calm state of alertness and thus influence the person's ability to engage in and complete the activity. Each activity presents unique sensory processing requirements. Thus, the ability to organize and integrate multiple sensory processes during performance of an activity is critical (adequate response).

■ Does the activity require the person to make changes on the basis of sensory input?

■ Is continuity of performance dependent on the ability to proceed on the basis of sensory input?

■ Does the ability to cease performance result from sensory processing (e.g., physical discomfort or a problem with the activity)?

■ What degree of sensory modulation does the activity require?

■ Is response to sensory input important to activity performance?

■ Will an aversive response influence the performance (e.g., defensiveness)?

■ Will a diminished response influence the activity?

Sensory Processing					Observations:
Level of Influence					
0	1	2	3	4	

Tactile stimulation. Tactile stimulation involves interpreting light touch, pressure, temperature, pain, and vibration through skin contact and receptors.

■ Does the activity require the client to hold objects gently?

■ Is the amount of force and pressure important (e.g., styrofoam cup, plastic cup)?

- Are the materials at room temperature, or do they require heat or cooling?

- Does the activity require the client to appreciate vibration (i.e., tools that are electric and require control in relation to the vibratory responses)?

- Does the activity require tactile discrimination?

- Are body parts always within the visual field? When should the person rely on tactile input?

- Are the tactile properties of the activity noxious (e.g., defensiveness, overload, localization)?

- Is the ability to localize tactile input part of the task?

Tactile Stimulation					Observations:
Level of Influence					
0	1	2	3	4	

Proprioceptive stimulation. Proprioceptive stimulation involves interpreting stimuli originating in muscles, joints, and other internal tissues that give information about the position of one body part in relation to another.

- Does the activity stretch or compress joints and tissues (e.g., elongation, shortening, compression)?

- Is weight bearing part of the activity (lower extremities or upper extremities)?

- What is the degree of pushing, pulling, and lifting that occurs during the activity (e.g., gross or fine)?

- Is the ability to assume and maintain posture important in performing the activity?

- Do movements and positioning of the extremities occur outside of the visual field (e.g., reaching in or out)?

Proprioceptive Stimulation					Observations:
Level of Influence					
0	1	2	3	4	

Vestibular input. Vestibular input involves interpreting stimuli from the inner ear receptors regarding head position. Vestibular input contributes to appropriate righting and equilibrium reactions, automatic postural responses, and maintaining posture and movement during activity performance.

■ Does the activity require quick movements of the head or body (relational or canals)?

■ Does the activity require postural change in relation to gravity (acceleration and deceleration) (e.g., sit to stand, vertical or horizontal changes)?

■ Does the activity require cocontraction?

■ Does the activity require coordinated eye movements?

■ Does the activity require postural background movements (e.g., adequate extension, ability to dissociate head, neck, and arm movements)?

Vestibular Input					Observations:
Level of Influence					
0	1	2	3	4	

Visual reception. Visual reception involves interpreting stimuli through the eyes, including peripheral vision, acuity, and awareness of color and pattern.

■ Does the activity require the person to fixate on a stationary object (visual fixation)?

■ Does the activity require slow, smooth movements of the eyes to maintain fixation on a moving object (visual tracking)?

■ Must the person rapidly change fixation from one object in the visual field to another (scanning) (e.g., locating a misplaced utensil while cooking, locating a dropped object while participating in a sport)?

■ What degree of discrimination of fine detail is necessary to perform the activity?

■ What degree of accommodation is necessary?

■ Does the activity require changes in focus (e.g., near to far)?

Visual Reception					Observations:
Level of Influence					
0	1	2	3	4	

Auditory stimulation. Auditory stimulation involves interpreting and localizing sounds and discriminating background sounds.

■ Does the activity require the person to listen to sounds and interpret their meaning?

Musical notes

Verbal instructions

Verbal communication

Warning sounds (alarm buzzers)

Functional sounds that assist the person in monitoring the environment (e.g., water running, food frying, opening sounds, closing sounds, traffic)

■ Does the activity produce loud or harsh sounds during performance (e.g., hammering, power tools)? Could these sounds be stressful to a person?

■ Does the activity environment require the person to discriminate or suppress background sounds?

■ Does the activity require attention to soft sounds or low tones (degree of auditory detail or auditory processing) (e.g., instructions, commands, communication)?

■ Does the person use or rely on sound while moving (e.g., search for a source of sound and move toward it)?

Auditory Stimulation					Observations:
Level of Influence					
0	1	2	3	4	

Gustatory stimulation. Gustatory stimulation involves interpreting tastes.

■ During the activity, does the person need to interpret taste to enhance or contribute to performance (e.g., eating skills, oral motor responses)?

■ Does the taste or texture elicit an aversive response (e.g., an alerting and calming influence)?

Gustatory Stimulation					Observations:
Level of Influence					
0	1	2	3	4	

Olfactory stimulation. Olfactory stimulation involves interpreting odors.

■ Does the activity contain odors that the person may interpret as noxious?

■ Does the activity involve odors that may be alerting (e.g., burning) or calming?

■ How may the scents affect someone who is hypersensitive to odors?

Olfactory Stimulation					Observations:
Level of Influence					
0	1	2	3	4	

Perceptual Processing Components

Perceptual processing components involve organizing sensory input into meaningful patterns and consists of 12 components: stereognosis, kinesthesia, pain response, body scheme, right–left discrimination, form constancy, position in space, visual closure, figure–ground perception, depth perception, spatial relationships, and topographical orientation.

Stereognosis. Stereognosis involves identifying objects through proprioception, cognition, and the sense of touch.

■   Does the activity require the hands or feet to identify or manipulate objects without relying on the sense of vision (e.g., reaching into a bag to find specific objects related to a task, reaching into a pocket to find a coin, reaching into a drawer)?

■   Do aspects of the activity require visual vigilance that may necessitate that the person find, manipulate, or reach for objects outside of the visual field (e.g., sewing on a machine, use of machinery)?

Stereognosis					Observations:
Level of Influence					
0	1	2	3	4	

Kinesthesia. Kinesthesia involves identifying the excursion and direction of movement.

■   Does the activity require movements to be coordinated over multiple joints (e.g., shoulder, elbow, wrist, fingers)?

■   Does the activity require the use of one side of the body (unilateral) or both sides of the body (bilateral)?

■   Does the activity require postural adjustments on the basis of patterns of movements of the limbs (e.g., symmetrical, asymmetrical, reciprocal)?

■   Does the activity require visual vigilance such that the person must rely on this ability to execute various movements without the aid of vision (e.g., swinging a bat at a baseball, playing tennis, playing basketball)?

■   Does the activity require the person to change directions of movements (quick, slow, precise) (e.g., fingers during typing)?

Kinesthesia					Observations:
Level of Influence					
0	1	2	3	4	

Pain response. Pain response involves interpreting noxious stimuli.

■   Does the activity pose any danger that the person may prevent from his or her ability to interpret noxious stimuli?

■   What senses are important in the activity (e.g., tactile, olfactory)?

■   Does participation in the activity result in any excessive stress on any part of the body?

■   Do any of the tasks result in a product that the person may consider offensive or painful (e.g., smoke)?

Pain Response					Observations:
Level of Influence					
0	1	2	3	4	

Body scheme. Body scheme involves acquiring an internal awareness of the body and the relationship of body parts to each other. This component is closely related to kinesthesia and proprioception because it requires integration of sensation from muscles and joints.

■   Does the activity require that the person have an appreciation for his or her body and be able to sense how body parts work together (e.g., playing basketball)?

■   Does the activity require the person to have an internal awareness of body actions that must happen in a specific sequence (e.g., ballroom dancing)?

Body Scheme					Observations:
Level of Influence					
0	1	2	3	4	

Right–left discrimination. Right–left discrimination involves differentiating one side of the body from the other.

■ What degree of bilateral coordination is necessary to perform the activity?

■ Must the person be able to use or apply right–left concepts?

■ Does the activity require that the person be able to follow verbal or written directions that require actions to the left, right, or both sides of the body?

■ Does the activity involve tools that require bilateral coordination and use of one hand as an activator and the other as an assist?

■ Does the activity require the person to differentiate between right and left on another person (e.g., in demonstrated instruction for aikido, karate, or dancing)?

Right–Left Discrimination					Observations:
Level of Influence					
0	1	2	3	4	

Form constancy. Form constancy involves recognizing forms and objects as the same in various environments, positions, and sizes.

■ Does the activity occur in two or three dimensions?

■ Does the activity require the person to respond to changing representations of objects?

■ Does the activity require the person to move in relation to tools?

■ Do the materials change form (e.g., laundry [folded clothes], cooking)?

■ Docs the activity require the person to locate tools in different orientations?

■ During the performance of the activity, does the person change position relative to the activity?

■ Are varying sizes of tools necessary to perform the activity?

Form Constancy					Observations:
Level of Influence					
0	1	2	3	4	

Position in space. Position in space involves determining the spatial relationship of figures and objects to self and other forms and objects.

■ Does the activity require the person to determine front, back, top, bottom, beside, behind, under, or over?

■   Does the activity require the person to understand the relationship between action and his or her body?

Position in Space					Observations:
Level of Influence					
0	1	2	3	4	

Visual closure. Visual closure involves identifying forms or objects from incomplete presentations.

■   Does the activity require that the person complete tasks in which the object or image is hidden from view?

■   Does the activity require that the person complete activities in which the image is incomplete?

Visual Closure					Observations:
Level of Influence					
0	1	2	3	4	

Figure–ground perception. Figure–ground perception involves differentiating between foreground and background forms and objects.

■   Does the activity require that the person be able to select an object or image from a competing condition (e.g., word search games, find hidden objects)?

■   Does the activity require that the person be able to discriminate two- or three-dimensional figures to complete tasks?

■   Does the activity require that the person be able to discriminate objects from a cluster of objects (e.g., food in a refrigerator, clothes in a closet, an object in a junk drawer)?

■   Must the person be able to distinguish a figure or word from a page with multiple images?

Figure–Ground Perception					Observations:
Level of Influence					
0	1	2	3	4	

Depth perception. Depth perception involves determining the relative distance between objects, figures, or landmarks and the observer and changes in planes and surfaces.

- Does the activity require the person to step down or up?

- Must the person make precise movements with the arms and legs to complete the activity?

- Must the person reach distances to acquire objects or complete activity?

- Must the person place body parts (e.g., foot, arms) in relation to changing elements of the environment?

- Do aspects of the activity occur in different planes?

Depth Perception					Observations:
Level of Influence					
0	1	2	3	4	

Spatial relationships. Spatial relationships involve determining the position of objects relative to each other.

- Does the activity require the use of spatial concepts (e.g., manipulation, take apart, put together)?

- Does the activity require the use of constructional materials?

- Does the activity require that the person estimate sizes?

- Does the activity require that the person judge distances?

- Does the activity require that the person move through surroundings?

- Does the activity require orientation of shapes, sizes, or designs (e.g., organization of tools and materials for safety and efficiency)?

- Does the activity require attention to detail in positioning?

Spatial Relationships					Observations:
Level of Influence					
0	1	2	3	4	

Topographical orientation. Topographical orientation involves determining the location of objects and settings and the route to the location.

- Does the activity require the person to use maps or other guides?

- Must the person be familiar with the surroundings to complete the activity?

- Does the activity require the person to use verbal maps or directions?

■   Does the activity rely on the person's ability to identify visual landmarks or routes?

■   Does the activity require the person to use mental representations of surroundings (e.g., cognitive mapping)?

Typographical Orientation					Observations:
Level of Influence					
0	1	2	3	4	

Neuromusculoskeletal Components

Neuromusculoskeletal components involve the subcomponents of reflex, range of motion, muscle tone, strength, endurance, postural control, postural alignment, and soft-tissue integrity.

Reflex

Reflex involves eliciting an involuntary muscle response to sensory input.

■   Does the activity elicit or inhibit reflexes?

■   Does reflex integration affect performance of the activity?

■   Does the activity naturally incorporate patterns of movement that require "traditional reflex patterns?"

■   Does the activity have the potential for the person to use "primitive reflex" patterns?

■   Does the activity use repetitive movement?

Reflex					Observations:
Level of Influence					
0	1	2	3	4	

Range of Motion

Most activities that involve a physical action require some degree of active range of motion (or moving body parts through an arc).

■   During the activity, which joints are static, and which joints are active?

■ During the activity, what degree of movement is necessary (e.g., beginning range, middle range, end range)? This factor is very detailed in worker rehabilitation or in a biomechanical approach.

■ What movements does the activity require of the head, neck, trunk, and limbs?

■ Does the activity or any task require the person to control movements at multiple joints (e.g., swinging a bat involves the shoulder, elbow, wrist, and hand)?

■ What type of muscular contractions are necessary during active movement?

Isometric to hold a joint position and maintain tension?

Isotonic with shortened muscles to cause a change in joint position (e.g., muscle shortening and muscle tension [concentric], muscle lengthening and muscle tension [eccentric])?

Is simultaneous contraction of agonist and antagonist necessary to hold a joint or limb in position (cocontraction)?

Range of Motion					Observations:
Level of Influence					
0	1	2	3	4	

Muscle Tone

Muscle tone involves the degree of tension or resistance in a muscle at rest and in response to a stretch.

■ What degree of postural tone in the trunk is necessary to perform the activity?

■ Does the activity require frequent positional changes of the trunk?

■ Are movements with the assistance of or against gravity?

■ How does the type of muscular contractions used during movement affect the tone in the extremities?

■ Does the person need to hold his or her limbs against the forces of gravity (e.g., stability, cocontraction)?

■ Does the person need to use his or her arms for postural support (e.g., weight bearing cocontraction for stability)?

■ What degree of concentric and eccentric contraction is necessary (reversal of movements)?

Muscle Tone					Observations:
Level of Influence					
0	1	2	3	4	

Strength

Strength involves the degree of muscle power when movement is resisted, as with objects or gravity.

■   What degree of muscle power is necessary to perform the task or activity?

■   How does gravity influence the performance of the activity?

■   What resistance do the objects, tools, and so forth provide?

A passive activity with no physical exertion?

An active activity with muscle contraction or motion with no external assistance or resistance?

An active assistive activity with muscle contraction and motion with external assistance?

A resistive activity that uses gravity, weight, or tension to increase muscle tension?

Strength					Observations:
Level of Influence					
0	1	2	3	4	

Endurance

Endurance is sustained cardiac, pulmonary, and musculoskeletal exertion over time.

■   What is the duration of the activity (time)?

■   What degree of exertion is necessary to perform the activity under normal conditions?

■   How repetitive is the activity?

■   Are positional changes necessary?

■   Are portions of the activity resistive?

■   What is the fatigue level on completion?

Endurance					Observations:
Level of Influence					
0	1	2	3	4	

Postural Control

Postural control involves using righting and equilibrium reactions to maintain balance during functional movements.

■   Must the person maintain alignment of the trunk and limbs?

■   Does the position of the head change frequently?

■   Must the person stabilize himself or herself against the forces of gravity when engaged in the activity (e.g., lean forward, lean back, lean to the side)?

■   While engaging in the activity, do changes in the base of support occur (e.g., two feet to one foot, sit to stand)?

■   Does the activity require that the person be familiar with the demands of the activity so that he or she can anticipate the postural requirements?

■   Does the activity have the potential for a sudden displacement of the center of gravity?

Postural Control					Observations:
Level of Influence					
0	1	2	3	4	

Postural Alignment

Postural alignment involves maintaining biomechanical integrity among body parts.

■   What degree of axial alignment does the activity require?

■   Does the pelvic position change during performance of the activity (e.g., taking off shoes)?

■   Does the activity require frequent changes in alignment (e.g., seated and reading, playing racquetball)?

■   Does the activity require any rapid postural adjustments?

■   What postures are necessary to perform the activity optimally?

Postural Alignment					Observations:
Level of Influence					
0	1	2	3	4	

Soft-Tissue Integrity

Soft-tissue integrity involves maintaining the anatomical and physiological condition of the soft tissues and skin. The client who is unable to move may be at risk for skin breakdown, contractures, or soft-tissue shortening.

■   Does the activity place the person in a static posture in which tissue can become shortened or overly stretched?

Soft-Tissue Integrity					Observations:
Level of Influence					
0	1	2	3	4	

Motor Components

Motor components include gross motor coordination, crossing the midline, laterality, bilateral integration, motor control, praxis, fine motor coordination and dexterity, visual-motor integration, and oral motor control.

Gross Motor Coordination

Gross motor coordination involves using large muscle groups for controlled, goal-directed movements.

■   Does the activity require positional changes?

■   Are the movements necessary for the activity effortless?

■   Which large muscle groups does the person use to perform the activity and to what degree?

■   Must the quality of the movement be precise (e.g., running, swimming, jumping, self-care)?

Gross Motor Coordination					Observations:
Level of Influence					
0	1	2	3	4	

Crossing the Midline

Crossing the midline involves moving the limbs and eyes across the midline sagittal plane of the body.

■ Does the activity require the person to scan the environment to find tools and utensils? If so, how frequently is this necessary?

■ Does the activity require that the person cross the midline of the body with the arms or legs (e.g., dressing)?

■ Does the position of the activity and the person occur naturally when using both sides of the body effectively?

Crossing the Midline					Observations:
Level of Influence					
0	1	2	3	4	

Laterality

Laterality is the use of a preferred or dominant hand or foot.

■ Does the activity or task require a high degree of skill in which the person must use a preferred hand or foot (e.g., cooking, sewing, writing)?

■ Does hand or foot preference influence how smoothly or effortlessly the person performs the activity?

Laterality					Observations:
Level of Influence					
0	1	2	3	4	

Bilateral Integration

Bilateral integration involves coordinating both sides of the body and is a prerequisite for gross and fine motor coordination.

■ How frequently must both sides of the body work together during the activity?

■ Must one side of the body stabilize while the other side assists?

■ Does the activity require fine manipulation while the other side assists?

■ During the activity, must each side of the body simultaneously perform a different function (asymmetrical performance)?

■   Does the activity require that the person use both sides of the body in the same manner (symmetrical performance) (e.g., pushing, pulling)?

■   Does the activity require reciprocal patterns (e.g., bike riding, swimming, running, martial arts)?

Bilateral Integration					Observations:
Level of Influence					
0	1	2	3	4	

Motor Control

Motor control is the use of functional and versatile movement patterns.

■   How frequently does the person use the same movements?

■   Does the activity require repetition? If so, what kind (e.g., putting a puzzle together, catching a ball)?

■   Must the person control numerous joints during the activity (degrees of freedom)?

■   What are the postural control demands of the activity?

■   Does the activity require the person to inhibit movements to be most efficient (e.g., children using scissors)?

■   How familiar must the person be with the activity?

■   Does the activity require constant or variable changes at a fast pace (e.g., dealing cards, jacks)?

■   Does the activity require manipulation of tools or utensils (e.g., the person must control the tool as well as the limb)?

■   Is the pace of the activity externally or internally controlled?

■   Does the activity allow the person to have a preferred pattern?

Motor Control					Observations:
Level of Influence					
0	1	2	3	4	

Praxis

Praxis involves conceiving and planning a new motor act in response to an environmental demand.

- Does the activity require the person to assume a novel position (postural praxis) (e.g., yoga, martial arts, dance routines for the novice)?

- Does the activity require the person to plan movements that are not habitual?

- Does the activity involve the use of new tools or utensils?

- Does engagement require the person to have a plan?

- Does the activity require accurate sensory information? If so, what degree of sensory information is necessary?

- How much experience must the person have with the activity or task?

- Is the activity new and unusual for the person?

- Can the person relate the task to an activity within his or her repertoire?

Praxis					Observations:
Level of Influence					
0	1	2	3	4	

Fine Motor Coordination and Dexterity

Fine motor coordination and dexterity involves using small muscle groups for controlled movements, particularly in object manipulation.

- What degree of isolated finger use is necessary?

- How many grasp patterns must the person use during different functions (e.g., hook, cylindrical, spherical, three-jaw chuck, lateral pinch, tip-to-tip pinch, tripod)?

- Does the activity require in-hand manipulation skills?

- Are the tools or utensils compatible for a left-handed person (e.g., sewing, musical instruments, kitchen devices)?

Fine Motor Coordination and Dexterity					Observations:
Level of Influence					
0	1	2	3	4	

Visual-Motor Integration

Visual-motor integration involves coordinating the interaction of information from the eyes and body movement.

- What degree of eye–hand or eye–foot coordination is necessary (e.g., tracing, copying, pencil tasks, balance beam)?

Visual-Motor Integration					Observations:
Level of Influence					
0	1	2	3	4	

Oral Motor Control

Oral motor control involves control of oral and pharyngeal musculature for controlled movement.

- Does the activity require opening and closing of the mouth?

- Does the activity require the person to maintain a closed mouth?

Oral Motor Control					Observations:
Level of Influence					
0	1	2	3	4	

Cognitive Components

The cognitive components consist of 14 subcomponents that cover a range of skills related to level of arousal, orientation, recognition, attention span, initiation of activity, termination of activity, memory, sequencing, categorization, concept formation, spatial operations, problem solving, learning, and generalization.

Level of Arousal

Level of arousal involves demonstrating alertness and responsiveness to environmental stimuli.

- At what time of day will the person perform the activity?

- Will the time of day influence the arousal level of the person?

- What arousal level is necessary to provide an adequate length of time to complete the activity?

- Do fatigue and pain factors influence arousal level?

Level of Arousal					Observations:
Level of Influence					
0	1	2	3	4	

Orientation

Orientation involves the ability to identify person, place, time, and situation.

■   Orientation to person:

Does the activity relate to lifestyle?

Is the task or activity associated with a role that is meaningful to the person?

Could the person's routines influence the activity (e.g., clean the bathroom on Tuesday or clean the bathroom when it needs cleaning)?

■   Orientation to place:

Does the activity require the person to know where he is she is?

Is the activity associated with a place other than the present situation?

■   Orientation to time: Does the person need to know the exact time and date to engage in the activity or task?

■   Orientation to situation:

What is the relationship between the activity and the person's environment and roles?

Does the person need to know where he or she is to engage in the activity?

Orientation					Observations:
Level of Influence					
0	1	2	3	4	

Recognition

Recognition is the ability to identify familiar faces, objects, and other previously presented material.

■   Does the person need to recognize persons and objects to engage in the activity? Consider the number of persons and objects.

■   Are the objects and persons associated with daily routines?

Recognition					Observations:
Level of Influence					
0	1	2	3	4	

Attention Span

Attention span involves focusing on a task over time.

■   How long must the person attend to the task?

■   Are "down" times (i.e., slow periods) involved?

■   Is vigilance necessary (i.e., high demands, sustained demands)? For how long?

■   Where will the person perform the activity (environment)?

■   Must the person disregard other irrelevant stimuli (e.g., visual, auditory, pets, persons within the activity environment)?

■   Does the physical and social environment influence the ability to attend (e.g., home, workshop, clinic)?

■   Does the activity require the person to shift attention (e.g., frying eggs, making toast, and pouring coffee when cooking)?

Attention Span					Observations:
Level of Influence					
0	1	2	3	4	

Initiation of Activity

Initiation of activity involves starting a mental or physical activity.

■   Does the activity require a "self-start?"

■   Does the person need to plan the start (e.g., use an alarm clock)?

■   How motivating is the activity (e.g., meaningfulness, relevance)?

■   How do the psychological components affect this component?

Initiation of Activity					Observations:
Level of Influence					
0	1	2	3	4	

Termination of Activity

Termination of activity involves stopping an activity at an appropriate time.

- How engaging is the activity?

- Can the person disengage at an appropriate time?

- Is the activity rote and repetitive?

- Is the activity self-limited?

- What is the person's control over engaging and disengaging in the activity?

Termination of Activity					Observations:
Level of Influence					
0	1	2	3	4	

Memory

Memory involves recoding information after a brief or long period of time.

- What are the memory requirements of the activity (e.g., immediate [a minute], short term [longer than a minute but less than an hour], long term [more than an hour])?

- If the activity requires long term-memory, which elements of long-term memory does it require?

  Information related to personal experience (episodic)?

  Factual knowledge of the world (semantic)?

  Knowledge of the world or how to do something (procedural)?

- Is the long-term memory modality specific (e.g., visual, auditory, verbal)?

Memory					Observations:
Level of Influence					
0	1	2	3	4	

Sequencing

Sequencing involves placing information, concepts, and actions in order.

- Does the activity require the person to arrange items in a serial order?

- Does the activity require the person to perform steps in a serial order (e.g., step by step)?

- Does the activity require an understanding of before and after?
- Does the activity require the person to reverse a sequence (e.g., don clothing and then remove clothing, put a toy together and then take it apart)?
- Does the activity allow the person to have personal choice in the manner of sequencing (e.g., morning care, dressing, showering)?

Sequencing					Observations:
Level of Influence					
0	1	2	3	4	

Categorization

Categorization involves identifying similarities and differences among pieces of environmental information.

- Does the activity require the person to group objects according to characteristics (e.g., visual features, tactile features, similarities, differences)?
- Does the activity require mental grouping (e.g., playing cards, different name brands to purchase, price differences, nutritional contents)?
- Does the activity require construction in which the person must understand how parts relate to a whole or break down the whole into its parts?

Categorization					Observations:
Level of Influence					
0	1	2	3	4	

Concept Formation

Concept formation involves organizing various pieces of information to form thoughts and ideas. This component relates to the ability to categorize.

- Does the activity require synthesis of ideas (e.g., formulate a hypothesis in terms of how or why)?
- Does the activity require abstract thought processes?
- Does the activity require symbolic thinking?
- Does the activity require the person to self-question or self-evaluate performance?

Concept Formation					Observations:
Level of Influence					
0	1	2	3	4	

Spatial Operations

Spatial operations involve mentally manipulating the position of objects in various relationships.

■ Does the activity require the person to visualize different perspectives mentally (e.g., two-dimensional diagrams, three-dimensional objects)?

■ Does the activity involve mental visualization of performance (e.g., how close the person is to preferred performances)?

■ Does the activity require that the person visualize how the object or activity should look on completion (e.g., clothing on a hanger or self, how a table will be set for a dinner party, how a cake will look after baking)?

Spatial Operations					Observations:
Level of Influence					
0	1	2	3	4	

Problem Solving

Problem solving involves recognizing a problem, defining a problem, identifying alternative plans, selecting a plan, organizing steps in a plan, implementing a plan, and evaluating the outcome.

■ Is the activity new to the person in which he or she will have to recognize possible solutions to problems?

■ Does the activity incorporate trial-and-error strategies or planned action?

■ What is the level of difficulty during performance?

■ Does the activity require that the person make decisions throughout the performance of tasks?

■ Does the activity allow the person to use alternative strategies during the performance of the activity?

■ Does the activity require the person to evaluate outcome performance?

Problem Solving					Observations:
Level of Influence					
0	1	2	3	4	

Learning

Learning involves acquiring new concepts and behaviors.

- Does the activity provide a structured learning experience?

- Does the activity provide feedback concerning performance?

- Is the activity an unstructured experience requiring spontaneous exploration?

- What type of learning does the activity involve (e.g., motor, verbal, feelings, attitude)?

- Is the activity compatible with the person's leaning style?

Learning					Observations:
Level of Influence					
0	1	2	3	4	

Generalization

Generalization involves applying previously learned concepts and behaviors to various new situations.

- Can the person perform the activity in different contexts (e.g., bathing at the bedside, sponge bathing at the sink, tub bathing)?

- Does the activity provide opportunities to apply learned skills to a new situation?

Generalization					Observations:
Level of Influence					
0	1	2	3	4	

Psychological Skills and Components

Psychological skills involve psychological, social, and self-management skills. Psychological components are values, interests, and self-concept (perceived self-efficacy).

Psychological

Values. Values involve ideas or beliefs that are important to self or others. Which of the following features potentially influence the person's participation or engagement in the activity?

- Does the person place an inferred personal value on the activity?

- What is the personal meaning associated with the activity?

- What is the person's perceived purpose for the activity?

- How does the activity relate to the person's goal?

- To what extent does the activity have social relevance, and is it socially accepted (e.g., family, peers, financial benefit)?

- What inherent praise or rewards are involved with the activity?

- Does the activity meet a desired need?

- Does the activity promote independence or self-reliance?

- Does participation in the activity result in personal enjoyment?

- Does the activity present a personal challenge?

- Will participation in the activity result in a desired personal change?

- Will participation in the activity assist in attaining a personal long-term goal?

Values					Observations:
Level of Influence					
0	1	2	3	4	

Interests. Interests involve identifying mental or physical activities that create pleasure and maintain attention.

- How does the activity stimulate the person?

- Is the activity repetitive?

- Does the activity offer an appropriate degree of challenge (e.g., cognitive, motor)?

- Does the activity include variety?

- What are the possible advantages of participating in the activity?

- What positive feelings does the person associate with this activity (e.g., physical challenge, fellowship with others, intellectual challenge, demonstration of capacity or creativity)?

Interests					Observations:
Level of Influence					
0	1	2	3	4	

Self-concept. Perceived self-efficacy, self-esteem, and self-concept are used interchangeably and are interrelated. *Self-esteem* usually refers to how one evaluates oneself as a person. *Self-concept* is how one describes oneself and includes one's beliefs, ideas, and attitudes about the self. In an activity analysis, the occupational therapy practitioner analyzes the activity relative to the client's perceived self-efficacy.

■   Does the activity enhance the person's ability to deal with life events?

■   Does the activity enhance the person's ability to cope with the change that illness or injury present?

■   Does the activity enhance the person's evaluation of his or her ability to change his or her life?

■   Does the activity enhance the person's satisfaction with a life role?

Self-Concepts					Observations:
Level of Influence					
0	1	2	3	4	

Social Skills

Social skills include the four components of role performance, social conduct, interpersonal skills, and self-expression.

Role performance. Role performance involves identifying, maintaining, and enhancing functions one assumes or acquires in society (e.g., worker, student, parent, friend, religious participant).

■   Does the activity require that the person be familiar with a specific social role (e.g., family, activities of daily living, work and school, play and recreation or leisure)?

■   Does the activity relate to a past, present, or future role?

■   Does the activity incorporate skills that the person may associate with a desired role?

■   Does the person associate the activity with an obligation of a primary role?

Role Performance					Observations:
Level of Influence					
0	1	2	3	4	

Social conduct. Social conduct involves interacting by using manners, personal space, eye contact, gestures, active listening, and self-expression appropriate to one's environment.

- In what type of situation does the activity occur (e.g., one on one, unstructured, parallel, structured activity group, structured verbal group [classroom, club, discharge planning meeting])?

- Does the activity require cooperative behavior?

- What are the accepted personal boundaries of the activity (e.g., a sport, a card game)?

- Does the activity require appropriate interaction with an authority figure?

- Does the activity require the person to initiate and sustain logical conversation?

- Does the activity require the person to assert himself or herself appropriately (e.g., ask questions, make comments)?

- Does the activity offer the person the opportunity to receive negative responses from others?

Social Conduct					Observations:
Level of Influence					
0	1	2	3	4	

Interpersonal skills. Interpersonal skills involve using verbal and nonverbal communication to interact in various settings.

- Does the activity require independence, cooperation, or competition?

- What degree of verbal interaction is necessary?

- During performance of the activity, must the person ask for assistance?

- Does the activity require active verbal participation?

- Does the activity require expression of emotions?

- Does the activity require casual conversation?

- Does the activity require specific nonverbal behavior and appropriate sitting posture (open, relaxed, formal subtle signs of active listening, changes in facial expression)?

- Could engagement in the activity result in criticism?

- Does the activity require the person to assume an unfamiliar interaction style?

Interpersonal Skills					Observations:
Level of Influence					
0	1	2	3	4	

Self-expression. Self-expression involves using various styles and skills to express thoughts, feelings, and needs.

- What types of self-expression (verbal, written, artistic, creative) occur during the activity?

- Does the activity provide the opportunity for imaginative play?

- Does the activity permit different styles of "doing" (e.g., fast or slow tempo, temporal sequence, organization)?

Self-Expression					Observations:
Level of Influence					
0	1	2	3	4	

Self-Management

Self-management consists of coping skills, time management, and self-control.

Coping skills. Coping skills involve identifying and managing stress and related factors.

- Is this a new activity for the person, or is it part of a personal repertoire?

- Does the activity environment influence perceived stress?

- Does the activity provide an appropriate level of challenge without promoting undue stress?

- Could some aspects of the activity contribute to failure or perceived failure?

- Does the activity require "perfection," or does the activity have a range of acceptable performance?

- Are some aspects of the activity externally controlled, or is the activity entirely internally controlled?

Coping Skills					Observations:
Level of Influence					
0	1	2	3	4	

Time management. Time management involves planning or participating in balanced self-care, work, leisure, and rest activities to promote satisfaction and health. This component is global and pertains to the person's lifestyle. Time management is the person's ability to mange "parcels of time" as they relate to the performance of tasks or activities. In this case, time management is a prerequisite to attain an acceptable balance of performance.

- Does the activity require the person to plan and arrange time to complete the activity?

- Does the person perform the activity in one session or several sessions?

- Does the activity include set time restraints for portions of the activity (e.g., bake at 350° for 30 min)?

- Is the activity part of a personal routine that has imposed time restrictions (e.g., morning care: shower 10 min, dress 10 min, grooming 10 min)?

- Does the activity offer the opportunity to make choices about the use of time (e.g., a craft project in which the detailing could require additional time because of increased interest or skill level)?

- Does engagement in this activity require the person to make choices about the use of time?

- What degree of organization and timing is necessary?

- Does the activity require an internal sense of time?

Time Management					Observations:
Level of Influence					
0	1	2	3	4	

Self-control. Self-control involves modifying one's own behavior in response to environmental needs, demands, constraints, personal aspirations, and feedback from others.

- Does the activity or activity environment provide for unexpected "glitches" (e.g., spills, dropping utensils or equipment, nonfunctioning appliances)?

- Does the outcome of this activity lead to attainment of personal aspirations (goals)?

- Will someone criticize the activity performance? Who (an authority figure, peer, friend, family member)?

- Does the activity challenge physical, social, or cognitive abilities?

Self-Control					Observations:
Level of Influence					
0	1	2	3	4	

Exercise 1

Consider the activity of frying an egg for breakfast or folding clothes. Think about the way that you normally do the activity. Follow the process outlined in this section.

The purpose of this assignment is to appreciate that everything that practitioners do is potentially a therapeutic activity. Through the analysis, practitioners learn the component pieces outside of the context of the real world of activities. In practice, occupational therapy practitioners perform activity analysis that considers the client's real activities, the context in which the client performs them, and the meaning that the activities have for the client.

Activity Analysis Within the Context of a Frame of Reference

Activity analysis is a tool that occupational therapy practitioners use to determine the therapeutic potential of an activity and to analyze the activity for therapeutic purposes. As such, activity analyses provide the means for understanding the client and his or her ability to perform specific purposeful activities. Up to this point, we have described activity analysis as a process to examine or analyze specific activities. Occupational therapy practitioners use activity analyses, however, within a frame of reference, a guideline for practice, or a conceptual framework. When an activity analysis occurs within a therapy framework, the framework provides the guidelines under which the occupational therapy practitioner conducts the activity analysis. For example, a client with left hemiparesis will most likely have intact language skills. After screening the client, the therapist determines that the client's standing balance, postural control, and sitting balance are fair and that the client has problems with upper motor control. On the basis of this information, the therapist determines that the neurodevelopmental treatment approach is most appropriate. Given that the client wants to dress himself, the therapist must evaluate his performance of upper-body dressing, which is best done by having the client attempt to dress. The therapist now conducts an activity analysis of the way that the client performs the activity with special attention to the client's neuromotor functioning.

Before observing the client attempting various activities, the therapist conducts an activity analysis of the typical performance of the various purposeful activities involved in upper-body dressing, which involves knowing the component demands of upper-body dressing. The requirements for donning a shirt with buttons are different from those of donning a pullover shirt. In the case of the client with hemiparesis in which neurodevelopmental treatment is guiding intervention, the therapist attends to the motor and sensory demands of upper-body dressing. The therapist uses the frame of reference to guide the focus needed as the client attempts to complete the activity.

Summary

The ability to analyze an activity competently is a critical tool in the repertoire of an occupational therapy practitioner. Without the ability to analyze activities, the practitioner must use trial and error to plan and carry out interventions with clients. This chapter describes the development of activity analysis over the years, and no doubt further development will occur as the profession evolves. The ability to analyze the activity in the context of the person and his or her life, however, will enable the client and practitioner to reach their mutual goals for the client. The chapter includes a comprehensive outline to approach activity analysis for the occupational therapy student and practitioner. Although the activity analysis may seem tedious and difficult for beginning students, these students will gradually integrate the process as a key aspect of clinical reasoning as they use activities as therapeutic interventions. Although we seem to use activity analysis differently in practice from the way it is taught, in reality, occupational therapy practitioners gradually integrate this process into their daily practices. ■

References

Allen, C. A. (1987). Activity: Occupational therapy's treatment method, 1987 Eleanor Clark Slagle lecture. *American Journal of Occupational Therapy, 41,* 563–575.

American Occupational Therapy Association. (1994). Uniform terminology for occupational therapy—Third edition. *American Journal of Occupational Therapy, 48,* 1047–1054.

Ayres, A. J. (1983). *Sensory integration and the child.* Los Angeles: Western Psychological Services.

Creighton, C. (1992). The origin and evolution of activity analysis. *American Journal of Occupational Therapy, 46,* 45–48.

Cynkin, S., & Robinson, A. M. (1990). *Occupational therapy and activities health: Toward health through activity.* Boston: Little, Brown.

Dunton, W. R., & Licht, S. (1957). *Occupational therapy principles and practice.* Springfield, IL: Charles C. Thomas.

Fidler, G. S. (1948). Psychological evaluation of occupational therapy activities. *American Journal of Occupational Therapy, 2,* 284–287.

Hinojosa, J. (1996). Practice makes perfect. *OT Practice, 1,* 34–38.

Hinojosa, J., & Kramer, P. (1998). Evaluation: Where do we begin? In J. Hinojosa & P. Kramer (Eds.), *Evaluation: Obtaining and interpreting data* (pp. 1–15). Bethesda, MD: American Occupational Therapy Association.

Hopkins, H. L., & Smith, H. D. (1978). *Willard and Spackman's occupational therapy* (5th ed.). Philadelphia: Lippincott.

Kremer, A. R., Nelson, D., & Duncombe, L. W. (1984). Effects of selected activities on affective meaning in psychiatric patients. *American Journal of Occupational Therapy, 38,* 522–528.

Licht, S. (1947). Kinetic analysis of crafts and occupations. *Occupational Therapy and Rehabilitation, 26,* 75–78.

Llorens, L. (1973). Activity analysis for cognitive perceptual motor dysfunction. *American Journal of Occupational Therapy, 27,* 453–456.

Llorens, L. (1986). Activity analysis: Agreement among factors in a sensory processing model. *American Journal of Occupational Therapy, 40,* 103–110.

Llorens, L. (1993). Activity analysis: Agreement between participants and observers on perceived factors in occupation components. *Occupational Therapy Journal of Research, 13,* 198–211.

Mosey, A. C. (1986). *Psychosocial components of occupational therapy.* New York: Raven Press.

Neistadt, M., McAuley, D., Zecha, D., & Shannon, R. (1993). An analysis of a board game as a treatment activity. *American Journal of Occupational Therapy, 47,* 154–160.

Nelson, D. (1996). Therapeutic occupation: A definition. *American Journal of Occupational Therapy, 50,* 775–782.

Pedretti, L. W., & Wade, I. (1996). Therapeutic modalities. In L. W. Pedretti (Ed.), *Occupational therapy practice skills for physical dysfunction* (pp. 293–317). St. Louis: Mosby.

Reed, K. L. (1986). Tools of practice: Heritage or baggage. *American Journal of Occupational Therapy, 40,* 597–605.

Trombly, C. A., & Scott, A. D. (1977). *Occupational therapy for physical dysfunction.* Baltimore: Williams & Wilkins.

War Department. (1944). *Occupational therapy.* Washington, DC: U.S. Government Printing Office.

Willoughby, C., King, G., & Polatajko, H. (1996). A therapist's guide to children's self-esteem. *American Journal of Occupational Therapy, 50,* 124–132.

5

Activity Synthesis

Paula Kramer, PhD, OTR, FAOTA
Jim Hinojosa, PhD, OT, FAOTA

The magician's sleight of hand is smooth and sinuous and creates an illusion. The audience watches in awe, trying to reconcile the reality that they know exists with what they see before them. Creating the illusion seems so simple yet is quite complex. In many ways, creating an illusion is much like the activity synthesis that the occupational therapy practitioner creates. Make no mistake, the occupational therapy practitioner does not perform magic, but the practitioner develops and creates activities for the client, activities that are common in everyday life. So much effort goes into the thought process and development of these activities, and that process is as complex as a magician's illusions.

Activity synthesis occurs in everyday life, yet most persons do not conceptualize the development of activities as synthesis. Occupational therapy practitioners, however, view activities and their synthesis in a more complex and theoretical way by building on what humans do on a daily basis. Despite the fact that activity synthesis is central to the art and practice of occupational therapy, few publications specifically discuss this aspect of intervention.

Occupational Therapy Perspectives on Activity Synthesis

Extensive literature in our profession discusses activity analysis. In occupational therapy professional education, practitioners spend much time on activity analysis with little time spent on activity synthesis, which gives the impression to occupational therapy students and practitioners that activity analysis is more important to the intervention process than synthesis. The assumption is that, once the occupational therapy practitioner understands the step or stage of the task that is problematic for the client, intervention can take place, and then the client can complete the task. This assumption may or may not be accurate. Sometimes the practitioner must reconstruct or synthesize the task in a different way to allow the client to be successful. Analyzing the activity is not enough; understanding how one can synthesize an activity is equally important. Both analysis and synthesis are important tools for occupational therapy practitioners.

In Mosey's (1981) discussion of legitimate tools for occupational therapy, she identified activity analysis and synthesis as important tools for therapists. Although she discussed them as separate processes, she stated that together they are the occupational therapy practitioner's means to understand and use purposeful activities. Mosey further maintained that synthesis occurs relative to the specific frame of reference that the occupational therapist selects. Her writings illustrate the complexity of the analysis and synthesis processes. When viewing them as two processes, practitioners use activity analysis and synthesis together for the benefit of the client. In her more recent writings, Mosey described activity analysis and synthesis as a "series of intellectual processes facilitating selection of appropriate tools for problem identification and resolution with clients" (1992, p. 269). She considered this intellectual process to be part of the clinical reasoning and decision-making aspects of practice rather than one of the legitimate tools of the profession (Mosey, 1992). Mosey came to view analysis and synthesis as two intimately connected processes with no clear distinction between where one ends and the other begins (Mosey, 1996).

Nelson's (1997) discussion of occupational analysis as "what occupational therapists do" (p. 15) described the importance of synthesis. Occupational synthesis is grounded in the occupational forms that determine the meaningfulness and purposefulness of an occupation to the person. Nelson believed that the occupational therapy practitioner's expertise is the knowledge of occupational form so that a practitioner can match an occupation to the client's needs and his or her therapeutic goals.

Activity Synthesis in Everyday Life

> All thought, in its early stages, begins as action. The actions which you have been wading through have been ideas, . . . but they had to be established as a foundation before we could begin to think in earnest. (White, 1977, p. 11)

Activity synthesis begins with action or what the client wants or needs to do. The client and the therapist must determine the importance of these actions, think them through, and use this combined thought and action process as the foundation for activity synthesis. Activity synthesis is not unique to occupational therapy; it occurs in everyday life in a much more simplistic form. The way that occupational therapy practitioners understand, analyze, and use activity synthesis, however, is unique. Let us first to explore how synthesis occurs commonly in everyday life.

Synthesizing activities is something that humans take for granted. When one presents a task to a child and encounters resistance from the child, one frequently changes or modifies the task to engage the child and lessen the resistance. For example, many young children do not like clothes put over their heads because this covers their eyes. When the parent turns this activity into a game by saying "Where did Johnny go?" when putting the shirt over Johnny's head, the child will often laugh rather than being frightened. The parent adapted or synthesized the activity for engagement and success.

Humans often modify, adapt, or synthesize activities without thinking. If one is tired when doing a task standing up, he or she will try to find a way to do the same task sitting down. Sometimes modification is as simple as pulling up a chair, and other times it requires moving to another area with a table or counter at a different height so that the person can perform the task sitting down.

Although humans naturally modify activities so that they can complete them successfully, they do not adapt the activity in any organized way. No theoretical rationale exists for the adaptation of the activity; instead, humans rely on what appears to be "common sense" by searching for a simple change in the activity that will bring about success rather than examining the activity as a whole. Occupational therapists, however, use activity synthesis in an organized, theoretical manner.

Activity Synthesis in Occupational Therapy

Occupational therapy practitioners have an organized conceptual approach to activity synthesis. Practitioners view the activity as a whole, then they conduct an activity analysis to break down the task into component parts. The final step in the process is to synthesize or recreate the activity with change, modification, or adaptation to allow the client to achieve success in the task. Synthesis involves more than just the activity; it involves the personal meaning of the activity, the personal interaction, and the context of the activity. Synthesis involves layering all parts of an activity to create a whole. For occupational therapy practitioners, synthesis is complex and requires adapting and grading activities, modifying activities, and creating new activities. Synthesis can be part of an evaluative tool or part of the intervention process. Practitioners can use activity synthesis to evaluate performance within a context, teach a new skill, refine a skill, or maintain the person's functional status or performance ability. The creative process of synthesis requires having a thorough understanding of the activity, visualizing the goal, and knowing the end product one wants to achieve.

Occupational therapy practitioners view synthesis in the context of the person as an occupational being by asking the following questions: Who is the person involved in the intervention process? What occupations are important to this person? How do specific purposeful activities relate to these occupations? Does the accomplishment of a purposeful activity allow this person to engage in or build on meaningful occupations at his or her current stage of life?

The Synthesis Process

Activity analysis is the basis of traditional activity synthesis in which we break down the activity to explore and understand its component parts. Synthesis requires that we reconstruct the activity by incorporating the client's therapeutic goals, areas of strength and limitations, and the therapeutic relationship. We reconfigure the activity such that the client can approach it with minimal fear of failure and with greater potential for success. This section discusses the process of adapting and grading activities, modifying activities, and creating new activities. These processes overlap and may not be mutually exclusive. Although we address each process individually as though it is distinct, practitioners may use one or more processes in combination in practice. As with learning any process, practitioners must appreciate and understand each component (process) in relation to the other components. Through understanding components, one gains a distinct knowledge of the entire synthesis process.

Adapting and Grading

Adaptation involves a change to the environment or the activity and not a change to the person. Adaptation of activities, therefore, involves changing the environment in which the activity occurs or changing the activity itself rather than working to bring about change in the person doing the activity. When a client has difficulty with a task or activity, we adapt that activity for the client. This process begins with an activity analysis that considers the activity, the context in which the person will perform the activity, and the capabilities of the client. After analyzing the activity or completing the activity analysis, we adapt or change the activity to meet the client's abilities so that he or she can perform that activity in a specific context. This adaptation can be as simple as giving the client a spoon with an adapted handle, having the client change his or her position when engaging in the task, or having the client sit down during the activity for energy conservation. Adaptation can involve a more complicated process in which the practitioner changes the activity.

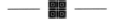

Exercise 1

Think about an activity that you adapted to make your life easier. Reflect on the adaptation. How did you determine the appropriate adaptations? Because you knew your capabilities and had a goal in mind, how did your capabilities and goals influence the way you approached the adaptation?

Exercise 2

Observe children playing in a playground or a schoolyard. Select one activity in which they are engaged. How would you adapt the activity so that a child in a wheelchair could participate?

Grading an activity is a common way of adapting an activity. Grading may involve simplifying the activity, making the activity more complex, modifying the sequence or physical nature of the activity, or modifying the amount of time necessary to perform the task. Simplifying the activity (or grading the activity down) entails making the activity easier in some way for the person. For a child who is learning how to undress himself, grading the activity may involve the child pulling off his socks after the practitioner rolls the sock down off his heel or the child removing his pants after the practitioner has opened the fasteners. In this case, the therapist may do a part of the task for the child and have the child do the remainder of the task. Once the child has accomplished this segment of the task, the practitioner can make the task slightly more difficult and grade the activity "up" rather than "down." Grading a task down allows the client to be successful and gain confidence so that he or she is willing to try more difficult types of tasks, to develop skills, or to build on a previously acquired level of skill development.

Exercise 3

Select an activity that you are competent at doing but that one of your classmates cannot do (e.g., playing chess, playing the piano, or baking). Develop and carry out one teaching session with your classmate. How did you grade the activity so that the other person would have a positive learning experience? How would you grade the activity for a different person?

Whether adapting or grading, the physical nature of an activity frequently changes by modifying the materials in a task. For example, if a child has difficulty building with wooden blocks because they are difficult to grasp and lift, then the child could use cardboard or foam blocks that are lighter and easier to grasp. This adaptation allows the child to play with blocks even though she does not have adequate grasp for lifting. The adaptation is grading the activity down so that the child can use her strength and skills to participate in block building.

Modifying activities. Modifying activities involves altering the sequence or time requirements of the tasks that make up the activity or occupation. Activity modification does not involve changing the activity itself. The purpose and goal of the activity are the same when modifying an activity, but the order or time requirements of the tasks may change. Modifying the sequence of tasks involves changing the order in which the person performs the tasks so that the person can engage more successfully. Practitioners frequently modify the sequence for energy conservation, such as the client changing the order in which he or she performs activities of daily living tasks to avoid walking up and down stairs or back and forth across a room. The client accomplishes the ultimate goal of self-dressing in a more efficient way.

Exercise 4

Think about the way that you accomplish the self-care occupation of getting ready for work in the morning. List the tasks that you do to accomplish each activity (e.g., personal hygiene, selecting clothes, dressing). Select one activity. Consider how you would change the sequence of the tasks if you had to get ready in a shorter period of time.

Time factors. Most activities involve a time factor. The person must complete the activity either within a specified amount of time or at a specific time of day or year for the activity to be functional. In the therapeutic environment, the practitioner can modify the timing of a task or change the time requirements of a task or the activity. The client may use more time to complete the task without repercussion, or the client may dress in the middle of day rather than in the morning. Once a client has mastered an activity within an extended time frame, the practitioner can modify the time requirements of the tasks to decrease the amount of time necessary to do the task. For example, when first working with a child who is learning to don a pullover shirt, allow the child to take as much time as he or she needs. Slowly add a time requirement. After the child has mastered donning the pullover shirt in a reasonable amount of time, ask the child to don a button-down shirt in the same amount of time, even though this type of shirt is more difficult to don. Layer the task of donning and fastening the shirt to make each task more complex than the previous one while using a time requirement as an important component. Many activities are not functional if the person cannot complete them within a specified time frame. By using the above example, a child spending a half hour donning a shirt would not be functional.

Exercise 5

Select an activity at which you excel. Determine how much time you need to perform the activity from beginning to end. Divide the time in half, and perform the activity. How does the time constraint affect your performance? Now double the time that necessary to perform the activity. How does this affect your performance?

Creating New Activities

The most complex type of activity synthesis is creating new activities. This synthesis occurs after the therapist evaluates a client and determines the areas that require intervention; then, in response, the therapist creates an activity specifically for the client. This synthesis requires skill, creativity, and an in-depth understanding of the client.

The activity results from an understanding of the client, his or her interests, and his or her problem areas and goals and has a "just-right" fit for the client. This type of synthesis does not result from activity analysis but rather is person centered (i.e., the activity results from an understanding of the person and his or her needs and goals). In this type of synthesis, the nonhuman environment plays an important role. If the therapist gains an in-depth understanding of who the client is and what is important to him or her in both the human and nonhuman environments, then the therapist can devise activities that will engage the client. If a pet is important to the person and the therapist can involve the care of that pet in an aspect of the intervention, then the client will be more likely to engage in that intervention.

Case Scenario 1

Janet, a woman with multiple sclerosis, uses a wheelchair and resides in a nursing home. Before she came to the nursing home, she raised several dogs that were important to her. The nursing home has a pet therapy dog, and the occupational therapist found that Janet was much more likely to come to group sessions when the therapy dog was present. The occupational therapy practitioner's understanding of Janet's interest in pets allows the practitioner to design activities that will match Janet's interests.

Exercise 6

Determine a goal that you have for a skill that you would like to develop. After selecting the skill, look around your home and develop an original activity that you could engage in that would develop the skill.

Exercise 7

You have accepted a position in a new occupational therapy practice with limited space and materials. All you have in the treatment environment are two chairs and one small table. You have masking tape, a box of colored 1-in. blocks, and two boxes each with 12 pencils (unsharpened) in the supply closet. You have three children scheduled for the day: Steven, a boy 19 months of age with developmental delay functioning at a 9-month developmental level; Shana, a girl 3 years of age with cerebral palsy spastic diplegia; and Kaya, a girl 9 years of age with visual-perceptual processing difficulties. Develop goals for a treatment session for each child and develop an activity by using only the materials, supplies, and environment in your work space.

Connecting Synthesis With Occupation

All of these examples of synthesis require skill on the part of the occupational therapy practitioner. First, practitioners must understand the activity, its importance to the person, and its relationship to the occupations of that person. Why is this activity important to the client? What role will it play in his or her life? How will the activity help him or her engage in meaningful occupations? Accomplishing this goal successfully entails engaging the client and developing a rapport and an understanding of who the client is as a person. Then, by using the creative process, practitioners devise or synthesize activities that meet the needs of the client. If the client has no interest in the activity or does not view it as meaningful to his or her life, then he or she will perform the activity without a personal investment. Furthermore, the client may not be self-motivated to participate in the activity, and this minimizes the therapeutic value of the activity. To be successful, the synthesis of activities must consider the person. Additionally, synthesis will only be effective if the practitioner considers the performance context. The person must be able to do the activity in the real world, not just in the contrived environment of the occupational therapy practice setting.

Importance of Activity Synthesis to Occupational Therapy

When someone has performed a particular task for many years, changing or modifying the way he or she performs that task may be difficult, even if he or she is struggling to complete the activity in the traditional manner. For example, if one is accustomed to preparing a meal while standing at the kitchen counter but has limited standing tolerance, then the person can move meal preparation to the kitchen table so that he or she can complete the task while sitting down. When someone has always done tasks that are important to him or her and can no longer do those tasks in the same manner, making modifications to those tasks is often difficult. For example, when cleaning one's home becomes too strenuous or difficult for one reason or another, some obvious options include receiving assistance from others, cleaning one room each day until all the rooms are clean, or doing minimal cleaning. Some of these options may be more acceptable to some clients than other options. For some clients, receiving assistance with cleaning is not an acceptable option because cleaning has been one of their life's occupations, but doing minimal cleaning may not be an acceptable option to others.

Case Scenario 2

Betty chose to adapt or synthesize the following task in a way that was meaningful to her. She knew that objects she had collected over the years needed cleaning periodically, but she did not like the thought of having others handle them. These objects were on high shelves and were out of reach without climbing on a ladder. She conducted her own analysis of the task. As a senior citizen, she was aware that climbing on a ladder was not an acceptable option because she feared falling, which could result in an injury. She hired someone to help her and was clear in defining this person's role. This person was to do the climbing to get the objects down from the shelf, and then Betty would wash them and direct the helper where to place the objects. This plan allowed Betty to have control over the task, handle the objects that were precious to her, and avoid the parts of the activity that could be potentially dangerous.

Activity Synthesis Within the Context of a Frame of Reference

How do occupational therapy practitioners use activity synthesis as part of their intervention? Where does activity synthesis fit into the overall intervention process? Activity synthesis is the reasoning process that guides us on how to use activities. When we use activity synthesis in an intervention, we should use it within a frame of reference.

Synthesis results from the practitioner's skills and abilities, his or her understanding of the client and his or her needs, the context in which the activity will occur, and the frame of reference that the therapist has determined to be the most appropriate for the client. Use of a frame of reference forces the synthesis to take place in the context of theoretical information. The theoretical information that underlies the frame of reference will guide what actually occurs. Thus, the actual synthesis occurs within the parameters of the frame of reference and how the frame of reference directs therapists to use, adapt, modify, or create the activity.

Case Scenario 3

Juan, a boy 8 years of age, was referred to occupational therapy for a handwriting problem. After a comprehensive evaluation, the occupational therapist referred Juan to an occupational therapy assistant to implement a program to develop hand coordination for writing on the basis of muscle strengthening by using the biomechanical frame of reference. The therapist selected this frame of reference because she determined that Juan has poor muscle strength and limited experience with fine motor activities. The intervention must take place within the context of Juan's school activities. After meeting Juan and reviewing the recommendations and discussing the frame of reference with the occupational therapist, the occupational therapy assistant, by using activity analysis and synthesis, determined that Juan should use an adapted pencil while writing and use paper with raised lines to give him more sensory feedback. Additionally, the occupational therapy assistant observed which activities in the classroom involved computer time. After careful analysis of what Juan does on the computer, the occupational therapy assistant decided to change the keyboard to one that provides more resistance and decided to raise the keyboard so that Juan must use his shoulders. If the occupational therapist had decided to use a developmental frame of reference outside of the classroom environment, the occupational therapy assistant would focus on Juan's personal interests, analyze those purposeful activities, and synthesize them as guided by the frame of reference. A developmental frame of reference suggests that a boy 8 years of age should relate to others in a competitive manner. Juan enjoys the game Connect Four.® The objective of this game is to pick up small checkers and put them into a vertical form and connect four in a row. The occupational therapy assistant involved Juan in creating a new competitive game. Guided by the developmental frame of reference, the occupational therapist assistant competed with Juan with the new rules that they developed together. To make the game address some of Juan's motor needs, they decided to place the checkers under various heavy objects around the room. Before putting the checker in the form board, Juan and the practitioner balanced themselves in prone position over a small ball by using the nondominant hand to balance and support weight. Additionally, a 2-lb. weight was placed on Juan's dominant hand.

All occupational therapy practice should involve theoretical information or rationales. Practitioners use activity synthesis within the context of that theoretical information. Activity synthesis is not separate or outside of the theoretical framework; rather, the theoretical framework guides activity synthesis.

Activity Synthesis as a Medium for Intervention

Typically, occupational therapy practitioners consider activity synthesis to be a medium to use when treating a client. Activity synthesis is generally a skill that practitioners use to improve function once they identify a deficit. Activity synthesis, however, is useful in many more creative ways and can assist in evaluating client performance, teaching new skills, refining a skill, and maintaining functional status or performance abilities. This section presents the use of activity synthesis for all of these purposes.

In synthesizing activities, the practitioner must be artful in developing or choosing an activity that suits the client's needs from a functional perspective and the client's interests from a personal perspective. If the activity does not meet both needs and interests, then the activity will not be successful in achieving its goal. The occupational therapy practitioner first takes the time to learn about the client by focusing on who he or she is as a person and his or her strengths and limitations. The practitioner identifies goals for the intervention and for the client with the client's input. This may involve analyzing the client's performance in particular activities and identifying performance components that are interfering with successful completion of the task. This process may involve some aspect of client education to increase the person's awareness of how he or she can improve performance or how performance in a particular area is affecting overall functioning. The practitioner then synthesizes activities with the client so that they are meaningful and beneficial.

Case Scenario 4

Janay has a weakness in her hands. She enjoys baking and has an interest in baking bread. This requires kneading the dough, which will strengthen the hands and provide Janay with an activity that is meaningful and pleasurable to her. This activity would meet her needs and interests. The therapist, when synthesizing activities for Janay, first considered using modeling clay as a therapeutic intervention, but Janay showed no interest in working with clay. This modality did not match her interest. Baking bread met her personal and therapeutic needs and may potentially lead to a more successful intervention.

Synthesis is not concrete. It does not follow a step-by-step process, and no one way is right or wrong. But several elements should be present for synthesis to be successful. First, the practitioner must develop an understanding of the client, including what is important to this person. Second, the practitioner must analyze activities to determine how deficits are interfering with performance. Third, the practitioner must identify a frame of reference that will help the client to overcome those deficits. And finally, together with the client, the practitioner must identify or devise activities that will help the client to overcome those deficits or develop the skills necessary for successful task performance.

Exercise 8

You have a new client, Malcolm. He has right hemiplegia secondary to a cerebral vascular hemorrhage. Before this trauma, Malcolm was an engineer working for the U.S. Navy. He held a very high-level position and designed equipment for ships. His hobbies included building things for his family and home by using many media (e.g., woodwork, electricity, mechanical devices). Synthesize several activities for this man by using clinical reasoning processes. Describe the steps you will use to develop the activities.

Exercise 9

Observe an intervention with a client. Identify the activities that the practitioner synthesized for the client. Try to identify the type of clinical reasoning that the practitioner used in this intervention. Did the practitioner synthesize the activities specifically for this particular client? Can you determine the client's investment in the intervention? Are you observing artful practice?

Evaluating Client Performance

Activity synthesis can be helpful in evaluating a client's performance within a context. The therapist may first determine whether a child can close a zipper on a doll or on an activities of daily living (ADL) board. He or she may then observe the child's ability to close a zipper on his or her own clothing. The child may easily close a zipper on an ADL board or on a doll, but the child must be able to close a zipper on his or her own coat. In this case, the therapist uses the synthesized activity to evaluate the child's performance within two different contexts. By observing the child's performance in these two contexts, the therapist can determine whether intervention is necessary and how to intervene.

Case Scenario 5

A therapist is working with Sam on developing social skills. In a group, Sam role-plays purchasing an item in a store. During role-playing, the therapist observes how Sam handles himself, whether his verbalizations are appropriate, and his ability to count out money to pay for the item. On the basis of Sam's ability to perform in the role-playing situation, the therapist can take Sam into a real store and observe his abilities in a real context rather than in a simulated situation. The therapist can use these observations to give feedback to Sam and to develop a plan for intervention.

Teaching New Skills

Synthesis can be helpful in teaching new skills. This is the type of intervention in which the practitioner typically thinks of activity synthesis. How does one devise a meaningful activity that will assist the client in developing new skills? By expanding on a previous example, when teaching a child to fasten clothing, one may first work on the skill in isolation on a doll and then make the task more complex by translating the same skill to fastening one's own clothing. In this situation, the therapist identifies the skills the client must develop and creates activities that will promote the development of that new skill.

Case Scenario 6

Ayisha has difficulties with money management skills. She does not watch how much money she gives to the store clerk and does not count her change. The therapist uses an acquisitional frame of reference and sets up a simulated store. Ayisha must pay for everything that she wants from the store, and the therapist works with her on management within this context. Periodically, the therapist plays the role of consumer and has Ayisha play the role of cashier. Through this activity, the therapist can teach Ayisha the basic skills necessary for developing the ability to manage her money.

Refining a Skill

Similarly, activity synthesis can be helpful in refining a skill. Once a client has attained a basic skill level, the therapist can enhance and embellish the activity to make the skill level more complex. When working on developing communication skills with a client with psychosocial dysfunction, the therapist may first work on having the client say "good morning" to others in a protected environment, such as a therapy group, and then work on how to conduct an entire conversation. Although the activity synthesis may begin in a protected environment, eventually the person must test the skills in the real world to determine their viability.

Case Scenario 7

Refer to the case scenario earlier in this chapter regarding Sam (Case Scenario 5). He is first developing social skills in a group by role-playing and then trying out the skills he has acquired in a real situation. The therapist can then work with Sam on refining his behavior in the real environment. Is he dressed appropriately to go out shopping? Does he make eye contact with store personnel? Can he ask questions appropriately if he needs to find an item that he wants to purchase? Can he handle money responsibly?

Maintaining Functional Status or Performance Abilities

Finally, synthesis can be helpful in maintaining one's functional status or performance ability. If a client has been working on strengthening her hands and has achieved an acceptable level of strength, then the therapist must work with the client to synthesize activities that would maintain that level of strength. Such activities must be of sufficient interest to the client so that she will want to continue doing them to maintain her hand strength. If the activities hold no interest for the client, she will have little incentive to continue with them. Therefore, the synthesized activities must incorporate purposeful and meaningful occupations for the client. Squeezing theraputty may not be a meaningful occupation, but molding clay into animals that she could give as gifts to a child may be more important to this person.

Case Scenario 8

Olivia has had difficulty with range of motion of the shoulder. She has received intervention and has been responsive to therapy. She can now raise her arms to 180° of shoulder flexion. The therapist initially suggested that Olivia do exercises to maintain this ability, but Olivia did not follow through on the exercise program. The therapist then made a home visit and suggested that Olivia place the dishes that she used most on the second shelf in her cabinets so that she would have to reach for them. Olivia was willing to do this, and the maintenance of her shoulder range became a part of her everyday life.

Artful Practice, Clinical Reasoning, and Activity Synthesis

Using activity synthesis requires artful practice on the part of the occupational therapy practitioner. Activity synthesis is not easy to teach because it is, in part, the product of experience. One does not start out as an artist. First, one learns how to use and play with materials, learns techniques, develops skill with the materials, and finally develops a personal style. These are the prerequisites to becoming an artist. Once a person has the basics, he or she may be able to develop into an artist, which takes time, practice, and experience. The same is true of the occupational therapy practitioner. Initially, the practitioner starts out as a novice with a technical or procedural understanding of what is going on with the client. Time and experience are necessary to develop into an expert who is able to be an artful practitioner. This requires considering not only the disability of the client and his or her functional level but also considering who the client is as a person.

Artful practice requires clinical reasoning skills. Fleming (1991) discussed three different types of reasoning that occupational therapy practitioners use: procedural, interactive, and conditional. Procedural reasoning involves making decisions on the basis of an understanding of the client's disease or disability. Interactive reasoning requires making intervention decisions with a focus on the person. Conditional reasoning is the most complex and advanced type of clinical reasoning. It requires the practitioner to consider the person and his or her condition or disability and to engage the person as an active participant in the intervention process. This requires a broad perspective related to the person, the disability, and the context combined with experience.

Schell and Cervero (1993) identified another type of clinical reasoning, pragmatic reasoning. This is a reasoning process in clinical practice that the context may influence both from a personal and organizational perspective. The economic, political, and organizational realities of practice affect the way that the therapist performs his or her interventions. Furthermore, the therapist's personal skills and ability to understand the practice environment and the needs of the client will affect what he or she does with the client. By using this type of reasoning, the therapist must have a thorough understanding of the setting, what is acceptable within this setting, what the payer will reimburse for this client, and what this client will accept. Then the therapist must match these factors with the his or her skills. Is the therapist capable of providing the intervention that will match the therapeutic environment and the needs of the client?

Experience contributes to the ability to be an artful practitioner. Researchers have studied the relationship between experience and practice with nurses, in particular the role of experience in decision making. Jones (1988) noted that experienced nurses tend to consider a broader range of possibilities than novice nurses when making decisions because of their prior experience and knowledge. In a comparison of experienced nurses and student nurses, Itano (1989) found that each group collected different types of data, with the more experienced professionals basing their data collection on their knowledge and experience.

All of these types of reasoning develop as the practitioner matures and gains experience. Artful practice requires an understanding of the person and must incorporate the person as an active participant in the process. Artful practice requires the therapist to have a high degree of self-awareness, to appraise his or her own skills and knowledge base realistically, and to choose interventions that resonate with the needs of the client and the realities of the setting. The practitioner does all of this within a theoretical context as well. The therapist should choose a theoretical framework or frame of reference that will fit the setting, the needs of the client, and his or her own knowledge base. The choice of a theoretical approach and therefore the choice or synthesis of activities should encompass all of these factors, and the practitioner should not make the choice on the basis of one area alone. Understanding personal, organizational, and client contexts is complex but critical to effective practice and activity synthesis.

Summary

Activity synthesis occurs in everyday life. Persons constantly develop occupations and activities that are meaningful to them. They modify and change activities so that they can perform them successfully. Activity synthesis appears simple because it is so common, but most persons do not synthesize activities in an organized and systematic manner. True activity synthesis is a complex skill, yet little research specifically discusses the topic of activity synthesis. Occupational therapy practitioners approach activity synthesis from an organized theoretical perspective, which requires an understanding of activity analysis, underlying performance components, the performance context, and of course the client. Furthermore, the frame of reference one selects for intervention, the ability to use clinical reasoning, and the artfulness of the practitioner strongly influence activity synthesis. Activity synthesis is a critical function of the occupational therapy practitioner in day-to-day interventions. ∎

References

Fleming, M. H. (1991). The therapist with the three track mind. *American Journal of Occupational Therapy, 45,* 1007–1014.

Itano, J. K. (1989). A comparison of the clinical judgment process in experienced registered nurses and student nurses. *Journal of Nursing Education, 28,* 120–126.

Jones, J. (1988). Clinical reasoning in nursing. *Journal of Advanced Nursing, 13,* 185–192.

Mosey, A. C. (1981). *Occupational therapy: Configuration of a profession.* New York: Raven.

Mosey, A. C. (1992). *Applied scientific inquiry in the health professions: An epistemological orientation.* Rockville, MD: American Occupational Therapy Association.

Mosey, A. C. (1996). *Applied scientific inquiry in the health professions: An epistemological orientation* (2nd ed.). Bethesda, MD: American Occupational Therapy Association.

Nelson, D. L. (1997). Why the profession of occupational therapy will flourish in the 21st century. 1996 Eleanor Clarke Slagle lecture. *American Journal of Occupational Therapy, 51,* 11–24.

Schell, B. A., & Cervero, R. M. (1993). Clinical reasoning in occupational therapy: An integrative review. *American Journal of Occupational Therapy, 47,* 605–610.

White, T. H. (1977). *The book of Merlin.* Austin, TX: University of Texas Press.

6

Activity Reasoning

Bernadette Mineo, PhD, OTR

In the course of actual practice, how do occupational therapists decide which activities they will use with their clients? This chapter offers some answers to that question. As you read the chapter, understand and appreciate that, as occupational therapists, we use activities for many reasons and reason about activities in many ways (in process, in the moment, and from a distance with hindsight and reflection). Time, experience, and reflective critical practice are necessary to develop expertise in the therapeutic use of activities.

Practice Reasoning for Occupational Therapists

The following is an example that depicts the sort of practice reasoning that occupational therapists use regarding purposeful activity and occupation. The example (Case Scenario 1) is from the text *Clinical Reasoning: Forms of Inquiry in a Therapeutic Practice* (Mattingly & Fleming, 1994). This case example alludes to the sort of judgments that occupational therapists make every day regarding using activities. The case example is a poignant and heart-wrenching illustration, one that leaves a lasting impression.

Case Scenario 1

Ann was a 26-year-old woman who had given birth, and had subsequently suffered a stroke. She was admitted to a rehab hospital with right hemiparesis. When I first met Ann, she was very depressed about being separated from her new baby and her main fear was that she would not be able to adequately care for the baby on her own. Adding to this fear was the knowledge that her insurance would not cover any in-home services. Her husband was her only family, he worked at construction every day, and they lived in a trailer park. In order to go home with the baby, she would need to be very independent.

The initial therapy sessions were centered around tone normalization, with an emphasis on mat activities, along with traditional [activities of daily living (ADL)] training in the mornings. Ann's husband visited daily and usually brought the baby with him. At first this was extremely frustrating to Ann, since she could not hold the baby unless she was sitting down with pillows supporting her right arm. She continued to voice anxiety around the issue of going home and being able to care for the baby. Her husband was also very worried about how this transformation would take place—the transformation from Ann as a patient to Ann as wife and mother. I spent a lot of time talking to Ann and her husband about the necessity of normalizing the tone and improving the movement of the upper extremity as a sort of foundation to the more complex functional skills Ann was so anxious to relearn.

Eventually it was time to spend the majority of the treatment time on functional skills. The two areas we focused on were homemaking and child-care. The homemaking sessions were fairly routine and traditional in nature. However, it proved to be a bit more difficult to simulate some of the child-care activities.

Our first obstacle was to find something that would be like a baby. We settled on borrowing a "recus-a-baby" from the nursing education department. We used this "baby" for the beginning skills such as feeding and diaper changing. Ann had progressed, but she still had slight weakness and a lack of coordination in the right arm and she was walking with a straight cane. The next step was to tackle walking with the baby. We, of course, practiced with a baby carrier. We also had to prepare for the event of carrying the baby without the carrier. I wrapped weights about the "baby" to equal the weight of the now 3-month-old infant at home. Ann would walk down the hall carrying the "baby," and I would be following behind jostling the "baby" to simulate squirming. (We became the talk of the hospital with our daily walks!!) Ann was becoming more and more comfortable and confident with these activities, so it was time to make arrangements to have the real baby spend his days in the rehab with his mother. This was not as easy as it might seem. The administration of the hospital was not used to such requests. But with the right cajoling in the right places this was eventually approved. The real baby now replaced "recus-a-baby" on our daily walks and in the clinic. While these successes were comforting to Ann and her husband, the fact remained that we were still in a very protective environment. The big question was yet unanswered—would these skills hold up under the stresses of everyday life, alone, in a trailer for 8 hours daily?

Never being one to hold to tradition, I decided to go to administration another time with one more request. I wanted to do a full-day "home visit" with Ann and her baby. This too was approved, and a week before Ann's scheduled discharge, she and I set out for a rigorous day at the home front. Once there, all did not go smoothly; Ann fell once and practically dropped the baby. She was very anxious and stressed, but we managed to get through the day. We talked and solved every little real or perceived difficulty. Both Ann and the baby survived the fall and the "almost" dropping. When we got back to the hospital, Ann, her husband, the social worker, and I sat down and realistically discussed and decided what kind of outside help was a necessity and what Ann could really accomplish in a day. Ann's husband adjusted his schedule, a teenage neighbor was brought in for 2 to 3 hours a day, and Ann was able to do the majority of the care for her baby.

Although this was not a story with a lot of pitfalls, I have been 5 years without my own patients; this was and is the most vivid of my clinical stories.

Note. From "A Commonsense Practice in an Uncommon World," by M. H. Fleming, in C. Mattingly and M. H. Fleming (Eds.), *Clinical Reasoning: Forms of Inquiry in a Therapeutic Practice* (pp. 94–115), 1994, Philadelphia: F. A. Davis. Copyright 1994 by F. A. Davis. Reprinted with permission.

Let us examine this example and think about some of the practice reasoning involved in the selection, progression, and grading of activity that the occupational therapist in this story, Maureen Freda, used during the intervention process with her client, Ann. Keep in mind, however, that the author did not interview Freda or engage in any other sort of additional written or spoken dialogue with her. Thus, this discussion of the case represents the author's interpretation as another occupational therapist and will reflect the author's reasoning about Freda's reasoning.

In addition, Freda's narrative account represents the telling of a clinical story long after it occurred. The way in which Freda told this story provides a kind of composite description of how she framed the problems to be solved and the activity decisions she needed to make in this case. Nevertheless, the case example is a narrative description of a course of events from the vantage point of hindsight. The picture ahead for Freda, because she was involved in the therapeutic process from moment to moment, may not have been quite so clear at the time. Finally, as this chapter discusses later when describing the importance of tacit knowing and the role tacit experience plays in the practice of using activities, while acting as a therapist involved in actual practice, one may not be able to give voice to all the reasons for proceeding as one does when one is actually engaged in "doing." The fact that even an expert clinician may not be able to articulate verbally a complete rationale does not, however, necessarily mean that the therapist does not know what he or she is doing and why.

In her initial description of Ann's case, notice that Freda considered what was going on in Ann's life (i.e., the realities that Ann would have to contend with that Freda would need to consider in developing a plan for intervention). Freda noted Ann's main fear—that she may not be able to adequately care for her new baby on her own. As the clinical story unfolds, this primary occupational concern of Ann's (i.e., her ability to care for her baby) becomes the guiding focus of occupational therapy. This concern does not merely become a goal that Freda sets for Ann; rather, Freda describes the concern throughout the story as Ann's main goal.

To get to this goal, however, Freda did not begin by having Ann engage in child care activities. She made the judgment that Ann needed a certain progression in the intervention. At first, Freda emphasized improving Ann's performance component skills (i.e., normalizing her tone and improving her right upper-extremity function). Freda noted that she explained to Ann and her husband that this emphasis was necessary as a foundation for Ann's relearning the more complex functional skills that she wanted to relearn (e.g., mat activities and basic ADL, dressing, hygiene). While in this early phase of the intervention process, Freda continued to bear in mind the occupational roles of wife and mother that Ann would need to assume once at home. Once into the second phase of intervention, Freda focused on what she referred to as "functional skills," that is, purposeful activities associated with the occupations (or occupational performance areas) of homemaking and child care.

Freda noted that child care activities were somewhat difficult to simulate. She attempted to find an activity solution to this problem and decided to use the recus-a-baby. The use of the recus-a-baby not only allowed her to simulate various child care activities but also allowed Freda to grade these activities, which provided opportunities to boost Ann's confidence while enabling Ann to practice safely and to test her skills without subjecting the real baby to any danger. Freda identified some of the basic activities that Ann would need to be able to do for and with the baby, but Freda additionally reasoned about which kinds of activity "experiences" she needed to add or incorporate while she and Ann were actively involved in these activities (e.g., jostling the baby to simulate the baby's movement and adding weights to represent the real weight of Ann's baby). Once Ann had opportunities to practice these simulated child care activities and acquired some beginning skills (and developed some measure of confidence), Freda then had Ann move on to the challenges (and fears) of handling her own baby.

After initiating all of these simulated and real-life activities in the safe, protected environment of the hospital, Freda recognized that practice in the real-life situation would be especially necessary for Ann because Ann will not be able to receive any home care services on her discharge from the hospital rehabilitation setting. This point marks the third phase of intervention in this case—practicing real-life activity in the real context in which it will take place. The all-day home visit with Ann that Freda arranged provided Ann with the opportunity to practice the skills she had learned in the hospital and provided a concrete test to determine how well Ann could maintain those skills. The mishaps and difficulties that occurred were probably just as important as Ann's successes in that they helped all the parties involved to come up with a plan for discharge that would more realistically support Ann. For example, the home visit provided crucial information that led to a more accurate evaluation of what would be necessary for Ann to return home so that the social worker could better assist Ann and her husband in finding the supports that they would need. Having a real test provided a kind of "reality check" for Ann and her husband. Thus, the home visit helped with the discharge plan in at least two ways: (a) It provided an evaluation of actual function in the real-life context, and (b) it provided a trial run in action rather than just discussing a hypothetical "Let's suppose this is the case. . . ." The plan for discharge additionally considered Ann's main goal—that she be able to do most of her baby's care. Having a teenage assistant in the home for a couple of hours a day will allow Ann to conserve energy (e.g., such a helper could assist Ann with homemaking tasks and child care support).

The case of Ann is a wonderful illustration of the sort of activity decisions and judgments occupational therapists must often make in their practices (e.g., determining how to work on child care activities). Nevertheless, some important information concerning this case is lacking. Given the brevity of Freda's presentation (as well the original circumstances surrounding its writing), much information is understandably absent (e.g., the subtleties and details of Freda's activity intervention with Ann), but some other types of omissions, information that practicing therapists would want and need to consider, would be helpful. For example, Freda made almost no mention of the roles that other members of the rehabilitation team played (e.g., the physical therapist, speech pathologist, psychologist, nurses), nor did she acknowledge their contribution in helping Ann to achieve her goals. Moreover, many of the activities Freda and Ann may have engaged in together as part of occupational therapy intervention may have been engaged in by other members of the rehabilitation team. For example, Ann's physical therapist could have had Ann practice walking with the recus-a-baby. Why raise these issues in the context of discussing this rather nebulous construct of activity reasoning?

As novices (or even as experienced therapists) reading Freda's story, we have the feeling that the occupational therapist played a pivotal role in Ann's progress and that the progression of activity intervention was so unique to occupational therapy. If you have that feeling, good! The illustration should not only be useful, but also it should inspire your future occupational therapy practice. Raising these other issues, however, helps one to understand that which is and is not unique about the way occupational therapy practitioners reason about activities and helps (in the long run) determine one's future identity as an occupational therapy practitioner and to understand the contribution of occupational therapy in relation to what other professionals have to offer. As occupational therapy practitioners, we do not "own the market" on activities. What we do own is the perspective we have regarding the therapeutic value and importance of purposeful activities and occupations, a rich perspective for which this text in its entirety offers a wide range of views.

Activity Reasoning

As evident from reading the various chapters of this text (and from the case example), numerous factors simultaneously play a role in the way an occupational therapist selects, structures, grades, and adapts activities to match the goals and needs of his or her clients. For example, in reasoning about activities and while engaging in activities with clients, an occupational therapy practitioner considers various properties or dimensions of activities (activity analysis); the strengths and weaknesses of the individual client and his or her interests, goals, and needs; the types of therapeutic approaches or frames of reference the therapist wants to implement; the meaning (and possible importance) of various activities to the particular client; the context in which clients perform activities (and how various aspects of that context can affect all the aforementioned factors); and the availability of and access to various activities.

All of the aforementioned factors pertain to activities and client functioning, but when engaged in the actual (not the theoretical) practice of occupational therapy, how do therapists put all these factors together? To address this question, we must consider other aspects of the equation, such as the sorts of clinical reasoning processes that occupational therapists may have to carry out during their actual practice and how the particular therapist's understandings, skills, and experience may contribute to his or her activity reasoning.

The Therapist With the Three-Track Mind

As noted earlier, the case example of Ann is from *Clinical Reasoning: Forms of Inquiry in a Therapeutic Practice* (Mattingly & Fleming, 1994). In this text, Mattingly and Fleming discussed the findings of a qualitative research study in which they focused on the forms of clinical reasoning that occupational therapists used in their thera- peutic intervention. On the basis of their interpretation of the data (through obser- vation of and in-depth interviews with the occupational therapists who participated in their study), Mattingly and Fleming proposed that, to address the entire problem complex of a particular client, occupational therapists make use of and must integrate multiple modes of reasoning. The authors identified and described three forms or types of reasoning strategies that therapists use to address different aspects of the problem complex.

1. Procedural reasoning

2. Interactive reasoning

3. Conditional reasoning

Procedural reasoning. Procedural reasoning is "the type of reasoning that thera- pists used when they tried to identify their patients' functional problems and to select the procedures that might be employed to help reduce the effects of the problems" (Mattingly & Fleming, 1994, p. 137). Mattingly and Fleming suggested that this type of reasoning is similar to the hypothetical or propositional reasoning advocated in the medical problem-solving literature. The occupational therapists who partici- pated in their study, however, used the words "problem identification, goal setting, and treatment planning" (Mattingly & Fleming, 1994, p. 121) as the words to describe the similar or equivalent sequence of diagnosis, prognosis, and prescription.

Although procedural reasoning is an important and crucial aspect of the clini- cal reasoning process, Mattingly and Fleming (1994) argued (as have many other authors) that clinical reasoning entails "much more than the identification of a prob- lem and the application of propositional logic to select a solution" (p. 34). If one studies the complex actions associated with expert practice, one will quickly realize that, in actual practice, a therapist must not only know what to do but also how to do it. In addition, a practitioner must determine what will work in a general or hypothetical case and what to do in the particular client's case in his or her particular circumstances.

Interactive reasoning. The second type of clinical reasoning that Mattingly and Fleming (1994) identified is interactive reasoning (i.e., reasoning about how to interact with clients). Mattingly and Fleming suggested that this is the form of reasoning we use during face-to-face encounters with clients and includes the strategies we use to enlist our clients in the process of intervention and change (i.e., how therapists collaborate with their clients and often with other members of their clients' lives, such as family members, caregivers, and teachers). Although other types of clinicians undoubtedly engage in a similar kind of complex "social reasoning" (e.g., a clinician's "bedside manner"), because of the nature of our role with clients, we often are involved not in "doing to" clients or "doing for" clients but rather are engaged in "doing with" them. Thus, having our clients participate in the intervention process is crucial; typically, without such participation, nothing much will or can happen during intervention. At times, we may not even appear to be doing much of anything except stepping back and allowing the client to do for himself or herself while making judgments about when and how to coach, encourage, support, and provide feedback about such endeavors and accomplishments.

Conditional reasoning. Conditional reasoning is the third type of reasoning. "We postulate that in using conditional reasoning the therapist reflects upon the success or failure of the clinical encounter from both the procedural and the interactive standpoints and attempts to integrate the two" (Mattingly & Fleming, 1994, p. 133). The authors described conditional reasoning as the "type of reasoning that therapists employed when they thought of the whole problem within the context of the person's past, present, and future; and within personal social, and cultural contexts" (Mattingly & Fleming, 1994, p. 121). Of all three types of reasoning, Mattingly and Fleming (1994) acknowledged that conditional reasoning is the most nebulous and difficult to define.

> We use the term "conditional" in three different ways. One is that therapists think about the whole condition; this includes the person, the illness, the meanings the illness has for the person, the family, and the social and physical contexts in which the person lives. A second is that therapists need to imagine how the condition could change and become a revised condition. The imagined new state is a conditional, that is, a proposed state, which may or may not be achieved. The third sense is that the success or failure of reaching a point in life that approximates that future image is very much contingent upon (or conditional upon) the patient's participation. (p. 133)

Reasoning is conditional because of the therapist's life experiences, knowledge, and understandings about the world, self, and others.

Activity Reasoning and Occupational Therapists' Use of Activities

In their clinical reasoning study, Mattingly and Fleming (1994) did not specifically focus on activity reasoning per se (i.e., they did not isolate how occupational therapists use activities); their focus was more general. What then does their proposed theory of the "three-track mind" have to do with how occupational therapists make judgments about using activities and the way in which therapists use activities? To begin to address this question, first consider what Mattingly and Fleming (1994) stated about occupational therapists' use of activities.

> Activities are not "prescribed" based on rules; rather they are selected based on sets of principles that guide the therapist to select activities that meet particular criteria. The criteria for activity choice are linked to the therapist's knowledge of the limitations that the clinical condition will place on the person's activity level, and on an understanding of the patient as a particular individual with particular interests and motives. (p. 202)

The chapters in this book represent the authors' and editors' attempts to elucidate some of these sets of principles and criteria for activity choice, including how the use of different types of clinical reasoning relates to the process of activity choice and the judgments therapists make about the activities in which they try to engage the client.

First, what role does procedural reasoning play in a therapist's selection of activities? Basically, procedural reasoning is the form of reasoning therapists probably use when considering the frames of reference or intervention approaches that they will use (given the sorts of problems the client presents). The knowledge, understanding, and skills we have developed that we associate with these frames of reference not only affect how we frame the problem complex the client presents but also suggest a set of principles for activity selection (e.g., structuring, grading, modification), principles that become some of the criteria that activities must meet. In other words, we try to devise an activity plan on the basis of the criteria for activity selection that a particular approach suggests, and we reason about using activities in a manner that fits (or meshes) with that approach. To determine which activities meet those criteria, we conduct quick or abbreviated activity analyses and syntheses and (on the basis of the kind of goals we want to address) consider whether we will use activities to promote performance component skills or performance areas and whether the process or the end product of the activity is more important. For example, consider some of the guidelines for activity selection when using a sensory integration approach. One would seek to provide activities rich in certain kinds of sensory input, typically tactile, proprioceptive, and vestibular input.

Although procedural reasoning about the use of activities pertains to developing and implementing an activity plan and the use of specific techniques (or procedures), interactional reasoning comes into play especially during our moment-to-moment interactions with clients (during our attempts to engage them in activities). Interactional reasoning involves the ways in which the therapist enlists the client in the process of intervention, how one collaborates with the client, how one actually intervenes (versus applying a set of procedures), how one attempts to engage the client in activity, and the judgments one makes in the moment during the actual therapeutic process while engaged in activities with the client. This form of reasoning additionally involves the strategies used to elicit performance, promote interest and motivation, and provide structure and feedback.

For example, in continuing the sensory integration illustration above, even though a traditional sensory integration approach tends to emphasize the importance of the activities while downplaying the importance of therapist–child interaction, a therapist using this approach still must consider how he or she will introduce various activities and enlist the child in the activity intervention process. For example, how does a therapist actually go about getting a child to try something that the child is reluctant to do? This situation may entail determining how best to introduce an activity so that a child is willing to try it (e.g., one may have the child observe another child attempting the activity or give a doll a ride on a piece of equipment or provide toys and equipment laid out in a particular arrangement and monitor how he or she reacts). Therapists must make moment-to-moment judgments, judgments about activity presentation, structuring, grading, progression, and modification as well as use of self on the basis of observations regarding how the child responds to the human and nonhuman environment and various activity situations. This additionally involves the actual practices, strategies, and behaviors in which the therapist engages (e.g., giving choices, monitoring tone of voice, and using body language [getting down to the child's eye level, whispering, ensuring the proximity of the therapist and child in relation to one another]).

But what about conditional reasoning? Conditional reasoning attempts to understand the individual person (client) from the context of his or her life world, to develop images of the future, and to assist the client to see these or other options. In other words, therapists envision how the "big picture" of the therapeutic process may come together and unfold over time and revise this vision in process as we intervene and interact with the client. In short, when we use conditional reasoning, we are taking the person's entire condition into account. In terms of activity selection, conditional reasoning is what leads us to choose particular activities over others; to tailor activities specifically according to the needs, goals, and interests of the individual client; to arrive at a more individualized course of action and activities; and to develop ever greater refinements to the activity–person match. For example, consider the kinds of activity refinements that Freda must have made during the course of her intervention with Ann on the basis of Ann's individual needs and circumstances.

In their study, Mattingly and Fleming (1994) found that conditional reasoning was not a type of clinical reasoning that new therapists used but rather was a type of reasoning that only more experienced therapists used. New graduates are in a position of having to struggle with the procedural and interactive forms of reasoning to combine what they have learned during their formal course of entry-level occupational therapy study with actual practice. Furthermore, the novice therapist cannot develop a full image because he or she does not yet have enough experience to do so. What role then does experience play in the development of clinical expertise in the use of activities?

The Role of Experience in Moving From Novice to Expert

While working on this section, I recalled an incident that occurred long ago when I was an occupational therapy student. At the time, I was completing a pediatric specialty fieldwork. Although I do not remember the particulars, I do remember that, despite the fact that I was doing well (according to the feedback I was receiving), I nevertheless was frustrated and disappointed when I compared my own skills as an aspiring occupational therapy student with the skills of the experienced occupational therapist who was my supervisor. When I shared these feelings with my supervisor, she responded in these words, "Do you think you're really being fair to yourself?" And, after a pause, she somewhat humorously added, "Do you think you're really being fair to me? I have almost 10 years experience as a therapist. If you expect your skills to be as good as mine are now after almost 10 years of practice, then I should be insulted!" I must have looked somewhat puzzled or perplexed, so she went on and explained that, if I expected to be as skillful as she was now, after only having had a couple of months experience, then I must not think too highly of her skills as a therapist.

This incident relates to several points in this section. First, a novice therapist cannot expect himself or herself (nor should others) to perform at the same level of clinical skill as that of a seasoned therapist. Second, experience does indeed play a crucial role in the development of clinical expertise and judgment. In other words, no substitute for experience exists; no amount of cookbook learning or calculative, analytical reasoning can substitute for the kind of tacit knowledge, understanding, and know-how that a therapist can only develop and improve over time through first-hand experience in real-life clinical situations. Third, "knowing that" and "knowing how" are very different concepts. As beginning therapists new to the practice of occupational therapy, you may *know that* you should do X,Y, Z, but you may not yet really *know how* to do X,Y, Z. Moreover, at the beginning of your career, your reasoning about activities may be somewhat slow, effortful, and deliberate as you try to incorporate and integrate all that you have learned about the practice of occupational therapy. You can, however, trust that, down the road, as you gain clinical experience, most of the information throughout this text regarding the use of activities in occupational therapy will make much more sense and in practice will probably become almost second nature to you.

Experience and the Development of Expertise

In response to claims made by researchers in the field of artificial intelligence (i.e., the idea that human intelligence can be programmed into computers), Hubert Dreyfus (a computer scientist) and his brother Stuart Dreyfus (a philosopher) (1986) argued that more is involved in human intelligence, judgment, and expertise than calculative, heuristic reasoning. To examine critically the claims that computer scientists could program computers to think like humans (e.g., design expert systems for tasks such as medical diagnosis or military defense), Dreyfus and Dreyfus developed a model of human skill acquisition that considered the role that tacit knowledge and firsthand experience play in the development of human expertise and judgment.

In their model, Dreyfus and Dreyfus (1986) described five stages or levels of human skill and judgment.

1. Novice

2. Advanced beginner

3. Competent

4. Proficient

5. Expert

They contended that each of these stages involves a changed perception of the task environment and mode of behavior. To move from novice to expert (in any sort of performance or task) requires not calculative reasoning but intuitive understanding and skill that one can only gain through experience and through the recognition and understanding of the similarities and differences of situations. The next several paragraphs discuss each of these stages and the processes of reasoning that are involved at each stage and illustrate how these stages relate to judgments made about and skill in using activities in occupational therapy.

Novice

According to Dreyfus and Dreyfus (1986), at the level of novice, the performer uses context-free rules to guide his or her actions. For example, the authors cited learning how to drive a car with a stick shift (manual transmission). At first, one typically learns to shift gears according to speed, which is a context-free rule. At this stage of learning and skill acquisition, the performer does not know yet that he or she should not follow the rule in all situations. He or she lacks a sense of the overall task and evaluates his or her own performance according to how well he or she follows the rules. The exercise of the skill requires much concentration to the point where one's capacity to attend to or do anything else (e.g., talking or listening to someone else) is limited. In other words, a high degree of focus is necessary, to the exclusion of everything else, to exercise or perform the skill.

Advanced Beginner

The second stage according to Dreyfus and Dreyfus (1986) is that of advanced beginner. After gaining some experience performing the skill or activity in real or concrete situations, the novice begins to learn meaningful features or elements and expands the "rules" to consider these new situational elements. For example, the person learning how to drive a car with a stick shift considers the sound of the engine (a situational element) and the context-free rule of changing gears according to the speed at which one is driving. At this stage, the performer is still following rules, but firsthand experience (i.e., tacit knowing) becomes more important than verbal description, and the rules one uses (to guide one's actions) now consider situational aspects as well as context-free components.

Competent

At both the novice and advanced beginner stages, a skill lacking is the sense of what is most important in the real-life situation. As one gains experience, the number of context-free and situational elements can be overwhelming. To cope, one either learns or is taught a hierarchical procedure of decision making (i.e., to choose a plan that becomes the perspective through which one organizes or frames the situation). "To perform at the competent level requires choosing an organizing plan" (Dreyfus & Dreyfus, 1986, p. 26). The person examines the situation by focusing only on those factors or elements that he or she considers to be crucial (given the organizing perspective or plan). The importance of elements may depend on the presence of other elements. Thus, as the performer becomes competent, he or she not only learns problem-solving but also learns the constellations or patterns of elements when he or she must make a certain decision.

For example, consider again driving with a stick shift. The competent driver, no longer hampered by the mechanics of operating the vehicle, drives with a goal in mind (e.g., getting from location A [home] to location B [work] as quickly as possible). He or she chooses the route according to distance and traffic considerations and ignores scenic possibilities. He or she may follow cars more closely than the usual rules for safety and may even violate traffic regulations.

Proficient

Another difference at the level of competent is that a new type of relationship between performer and environment emerges. In contrast to the novice or advanced beginner, the competent performer becomes involved in the outcome because of the organizing plan he or she developed. In other words, he or she becomes invested in the outcome because of the way he or she framed the situation.

Expert

Although problem solving and analytical decision making may lead to competence, Dreyfus and Dreyfus (1986) argued that the more rapid and fluid performance associated with human proficiency and expertise (the two highest levels of skill acquisition) requires the development of intuition. By intuition, the authors meant the sort of "understanding that effortlessly occurs upon seeing similarities with previous experience" (Dreyfus & Dreyfus, 1986, p. 28). They added, however, that

> Intuition must not be confused with irrational conformity, the reenactment of childhood trauma, and all other unconscious and noninferential means by which human beings come to decisions. Those all resist explanation in terms of facts and inferences, but only intuition is the product of deep situational involvement. . . . Intuition or know-how, as we understand it, is neither wild guessing nor supernatural inspiration, but the sort of ability we use all the time as we go about our everyday tasks. (pp. 28–29)

Central to such intuition is what the authors referred to as "holistic similarity recognition" or "the ability to use patterns without decomposing them into component features" (Dreyfus & Dreyfus, 1986, p. 28).

At the level of proficiency, the performer intuitively understands and organizes the task but still may need to think analytically about what to do (i.e., he or she goes through a process of detached decision making). However, at the level of expert, the performer intuitively understands and organizes the task and intuitively knows what to do (i.e., the expert does not make conscious, detached, deliberative choices). As Dreyfus and Dreyfus (1986) emphasized, "When things are proceeding normally, experts don't solve problems and don't make decisions; they do what normally works" (pp. 30–31).

Consider the example of driving again to illustrate these distinctions. As Dreyfus and Dreyfus (1986) noted, "On the basis of prior experience, the proficient driver, approaching a curve on a rainy day, may intuitively realize that he is driving too fast. He then consciously decides whether to apply the brakes or, remove his foot from the accelerator, or merely reduce pressure" (p. 29). At the level of expert, however, such detached, deliberate decision making would not be necessary. The expert driver would automatically do what was necessary (i.e., he would immediately react). "The expert driver becomes one with his car, and he experiences himself simply as driving, rather than as driving a car, just as at other times, he certainly experiences himself as walking and not, as a small child might, as consciously and deliberately propelling his body forward" (Dreyfus & Dreyfus, 1986, p. 30).

What Dreyfus and Dreyfus suggested (on the basis of this five-stage model of skill acquisition) is that, at the beginning stages of learning a skill or activity, rules are helpful in the sense that they "get us going" (i.e., they give us some general point of reference from which to begin). Continuation of this sort of "cookbook" approach, however, will not lead to higher levels of skill attainment. Continuing to follow only a set of rules, even if experience leads us to even more sophisticated rules, may actually hinder one's attainment of higher-level skills. Why? Because expertise, the authors contended, in the performance of almost any human skill (including the skills associated with being a professional) requires the development of involved intuitive understanding and judgment, not detached, calculative rationality. As we gain experience in performing a task, we build up a "library of distinguishable situations,"

situations that we remember as a whole and draw from to inform our future practice. As Dreyfus and Dreyfus (1986) pointed out,

> What should stand out is the progression from the analytic behavior of a detached subject, consciously decomposing his environment into recognizable elements, and following abstract rules, to involved skilled behavior based on an accumulation of concrete experiences and the conscious recognition of new situations as similar to whole remembered ones. The evolution from the abstract toward the concrete reverses what one observes in small children dealing with intellectual tasks; they initially understand only concrete examples and gradually learn abstract reasoning. Perhaps it is because of this well-known pattern seen in children, and because rule-following plays an important, early role in the learning of new skills by adults, that adult understanding and skill are so often misunderstood as abstract and rule-guided. (p. 35)

Occupational Therapists' Development of Expertise in Making Judgments About Activities

This section examines how skill acquisition may relate to occupational therapists' development of expertise in making judgments about activities and skill in using activities. For example, suppose that a specific goal is that a client be able to don his or her shoes independently. To address this goal, the occupational therapist must make some judgments about the client and how to structure the activity or task. For example, the therapist should consider what the client can do (and what he or she cannot do) physically, cognitively, and so forth. The therapist likewise considers the task and its requirements or characteristics. Then the therapist attempts to structure the activity, which involves making judgments about adaptations and modifications that may be necessary to enable that person to accomplish the task, such as the type of shoe, the position of the client when he or she performs the task, whether any adaptive aids might be useful, and so forth.

In another example, suppose that the client is someone who has had hip replacement surgery. How might the sort of judgments the therapist makes about the activity correspond to the therapist's level of skill attainment?

At the novice level, the therapist probably would try to follow some rules he or she has learned (e.g., some if-then statements learned during academic coursework that purportedly apply to the type of clinical condition the client has). For example, in the case of a hip replacement, the novice recalls the rule that the therapist should instruct the client to observe hip precautions. To this end, the therapist may examine how the client positions her body, give the client a shoehorn with a long extended handle, and use elasticized laces in the client's sneakers. Basically, at the level of novice, the therapist would advise the client regarding what to do according to the set of rules (or protocol) he or she has learned regarding the general case of a hip replacement. The therapist would likewise probably gauge his or her own performance as a therapist according to whether he or she recalled all the rules and whether the client adhered to them. The therapist at this stage is more likely to be somewhat rigid about following this protocol, perhaps even to the exclusion of noticing other aspects of the client and the client's concerns. This therapist would probably treat all clients with hip replacements in the same fashion.

At the level of advanced beginner, what may be some of the situational cues that the therapist adds? As the novice gains experience working with clients who have hip replacements, he or she may notice, for example, that certain client characteristics such as weight, height, gender, age, and the presence of other clinical conditions may influence how clients are able to don a shoe while observing hip precautions. At this stage, the therapist would probably be a bit more comfortable with what those hip precautions are and may begin to recognize the similarities and differences in the performance of donning shoes among clients with hip replacements. The therapist may then begin to modify the activity to fit the characteristics of the client better (e.g., to decide when during a session he or she will have the client practice donning shoes).

Suppose that the therapist encounters a hip replacement client who, after several sessions of training, is not following the hip precautions, absolutely refuses to try to don her shoes, and wants nothing to do with any adaptive aids the therapist has to offer. At the competent level, the therapist, instead of simply viewing the client as uncooperative, may try to problem solve the reasons for the client's response to the activity. For example, instead of walking away and coming back at another time or persisting with encouraging the client to do the activity in the prescribed manner, the therapist may recognize that some sort of modification of the activity protocol will be necessary to address this particular client's needs and concerns. Even though the aim of intervention is for the client to be able to don her shoes independently while observing hip precautions, the therapist at the competent level is able to incorporate other considerations into the activity reasoning process (i.e., to frame or reframe the situation to devise alternative activity solutions). For example, the therapist may understand that he or she must first find out what is bothering this client and then devise some other tactics to try in the interim (e.g., talking to the client, talking to the staff members, trying to introduce an alternative activity).

In using the same example, the therapist at the level of proficiency may have a more immediate understanding of what the problem is (i.e., the sense not only that something is bothering the client but also what that something may be). For example, on the basis of previous experience with other clients and with this client, the proficient therapist may recognize and understand that this client was not only angry and frustrated but also that the anger and frustration were in part related to difficulties with short-term memory (i.e., what the client learns or hears one day, she tends to forget the next). Given this almost immediate and intuitive understanding, the therapist would then attempt to address these other issues. In other words, the therapist would formulate a plan on the basis of the understanding (or perspective) of the problem in this particular case.

At the highest level of skill and understanding, that of expert, the therapist would not only recognize and understand the problem almost immediately but also would be able to institute a course of action just as intuitively. The therapist would have a repertoire of strategies that he or she has tried in the past (with clients who have had hip replacements and with those who have had other sorts of conditions) that he or she could attempt to use in the present situation. The therapist would be able to react and respond in a rapid and fluid manner rather than having to pause to think, reason, and formulate what to do next. For example, the therapist would know just what to say to the client and how to restructure the situation to enlist the client in activity.

This section's aim is not to categorize therapist behavior and responses but rather is to illustrate that a progression exists in the development of skill and know-how. The above example illustrates how Dreyfus and Dreyfus' model of skill acquisition may relate to the development of expertise in reasoning about and using activities. That you are able to fit your own (or your colleagues') behavior and performance into the five levels of skill acquisition is not important; rather, you should come away with a sense that a developmental progression exists. We all follow this progression but at different rates and depths of progress. Moreover, our skills will vary along the continuum of development (i.e., we may become expert in some techniques or procedures while becoming only marginally competent in others on the basis of our practice experience and our own innate abilities, personalities, temperament, and style). Just as not everyone who learns to play chess will progress to the level of expert, not every therapist will become an expert, certainly not in all areas of occupational therapy practice. In addition, each time a therapist learns a new set of techniques or a new approach or explores the use of newer, less familiar activities, he or she will again follow these stages of skill acquisition. Furthermore, as therapists, we must consider that our clients likewise experience similar processes of skill acquisition. Just as therapists should not expect themselves to be able to go from novice to expert immediately, therapists should not expect that of their clients.

Becoming a Reflective Practitioner

Even if a therapist is functioning at the level of expert, this does not mean that the therapist never consciously critically reflects on what he or she is doing. As Dreyfus and Dreyfus (1986) noted,

> While most expert performance is ongoing and nonreflective, when time permits and outcomes are crucial, an expert will deliberate before acting. But . . . this deliberation does not require calculative problem solving, but rather involves critically reflecting on one's intuitions. And even after critical reflection, experts' decisions don't always work out. (pp. 31–32)

Schon (1983, 1987) described the form of reflective inquiry that he believed supports highly competent professional practice. He offered a model and proposed an epistemology of practice that addresses the art of professional practice (not just the science of it) that he formulated on the basis of his observation and in-depth analysis of how highly competent practitioners deal with the uncertainty, indeterminacy, and uniqueness that typically characterize the situations they encounter in actual professional practice.

Schon (1983) argued that the epistemology of practice that has long dominated the professions developed from a foundation that assumes the supremacy of technical rationality. From the perspective of technical rationality, professional knowledge and skill are nothing more than the application of scientific theory and technique to the instrumental problems of practice.

Such a view of professional practice relates to the split that has traditionally occurred between practice and research in the professions: the professions give their practical problems to the university (the source of research), and the university gives back scientific knowledge that they expect the professionals to apply and test. This split promotes a kind of division of labor, and the split reflects and fosters a hierarchy of knowledge (i.e., that those supposedly creating the professional knowledge are above the level of those applying it, that practical knowledge and know-how are not as important or "lofty" as theoretical knowledge).

The problem with an epistemology of practice that uses technical rationality as its base (a perspective that evolved out of the positivist tradition in science) is that it fosters a gap between professional knowledge and the demands of real-world practice, in which the situations are "messy," and the ends are not always fixed and clear. An epistemology of practice that involves technical rationality does not consider how professionals actually deal with what Schon (1987) referred to as "the indeterminate zones of practice" (i.e., situations of uncertainty, uniqueness, or value conflict), nor does this epistemology acknowledge the important role that craft and artistry play in professional practice.

In contrast to the objectivist view of knowledge inherent to technical rationality, Schon proposed an alternative epistemology of professional practice, one with a constructionist view. Although Schon (1983) was concerned with how professionals solve problems, he maintained that "the situations of practice are not problems to be solved but problematic situations characterized by uncertainty, disorder and indeterminacy" (pp. 15–16). When making decisions and judgments about what to do, the practitioner must "set" the problems to be solved, (i.e., he or she constructs a theory of this particular case on the basis of his understanding and appreciation of it, and, in turn, he or she shapes the situation according to this appreciation). Schon (1983) argued that

> Although problem setting is a necessary condition for technical problem solving, it is not itself a technical problem. When we set the problem, we select what we will treat as the "things" of the situation, we set the boundaries of our attention to it, and we impose upon it a coherence which allows us to say what is wrong and in what directions the situation needs to be changed. Problem setting is a process in which, interactively, we name the things to which we will attend and frame the context in which we will attend to them. . . . It is the work of naming and framing that creates the conditions necessary to the exercise of technical expertise. (pp. 40–42)

Schon thus placed technical problem solving and problem setting within the context of a broader form of reflective inquiry. In addition, he contended that the best practitioners in any professional field are typically artful in some way, that virtuoso practitioners do not make judgments and decisions on the basis of formulas or rules, and that expert professional practice entails a kind of "improvisation." Such improvisation, he stated, involves ways of knowing and reasoning associated with a process that he referred to as *reflection in action* and takes on the underlying structure of "a reflective conversation with a unique and uncertain situation" (Schon, 1983, p. 130).

According to Schon, *knowing in action* is the characteristic mode of ordinary practical knowledge, for example, the sort of knowledge shown when someone knows how to dress himself or pitch a baseball to a hitter. With such tacit knowing in action, the action reveals the knowing (i.e., the knowing is implicit to the action itself and is only evident through that action [judgment, decision, or performance]). Not only does the person come to do the action spontaneously, but also he or she characteristically knows more than he or she can describe in words. (This idea is not unlike what Dreyfus and Dreyfus discussed concerning the development of expertise in any skill.)

In Schon's view, knowing in action is not only essential to the skillful performance of every day activities, but also it is just as essential to professional practice. As he explained,

> The workaday life of the professional depends on tacit knowing-in-action. Every competent practitioner can recognize phenomena—families of symptoms associated with a particular disease, peculiarities of a certain kind of building site, irregularities of materials or structures—for which he cannot give a reasonably accurate or complete description. In his day-to-day practice he makes innumerable judgments of quality for which he cannot state adequate criteria, and he displays skills for which he cannot state the rules and procedures. Even when he makes conscious use of research-based theories and techniques, he is dependent on tacit recognitions, judgments, and skillful performances. (Schon, 1983, pp. 49–50)

Through observing and reflecting on one's actions, one may be able to describe the tacit knowing implicit to those actions. However, stated Schon (1987), such

> descriptions of knowing-in-action are always constructions. They are always attempts to put into explicit, symbolic form a kind of intelligence that begins by being tacit and spontaneous. Our descriptions are conjectures that need to be tested against observation of their originals—which, in at least one respect, they are bound to distort. For knowing-in-action is dynamic, and "facts," "procedures," "rules," and "theories" are static. (p. 25)

For example, as Schon (1987) further explained,

> When we know how to catch a ball, for example, we anticipate the ball's coming by the way we extend and cup our hands and by the on-line adjustments we make as the ball approaches. Catching a ball is a continuous activity in which

> awareness, appreciation, and adjustment play their parts . . . it is this on-line anticipation and adjustment, this continuous detection and correction of error, that leads us, in the first place, to call activity "intelligent." Knowing suggests the dynamic quality of knowing-in-action, which, when we describe it, we convert to knowledge-in-action. (pp. 25–26)

Moreover, our descriptions, no matter how detailed, will always be incomplete because capturing every nuance of every action in words is impossible.

Although Schon acknowledged the vital role that knowing in action plays in the ongoing performance of professional activities (as well as ordinary daily life tasks), he emphasized that inevitably situations occur in which our actions (e.g., familiar routines or procedures) produce unexpected outcomes that can be positive or negative (i.e., when what happens fails to meet our expectations or in some other way surprises us). We may respond to such surprise (or uncertainty, uniqueness, or value conflict) by casting it aside or ignoring it, or we may respond to it by reflecting. Such reflecting, stated Schon, comes in two forms: reflection on action and reflection in action.

Reflection on action is what we do when we step back to think about what we did that may have resulted in the outcome. We may do this sometime after the fact, or we may reflect while in the midst of the action by pausing to "stop and think." In reflection on action, the reflection "has no direct connection to present action" (Schon, 1987, p. 26). In other words, our reflection does not lead to our reshaping of this particular situation or our actions related to it. We may, however, reflect or think in action.

> We may reflect in the midst of action without interrupting it. In an action-present—a period of time, variable with the context, during which we can still make a difference to the situation at hand—our thinking serves to reshape what we are doing while we are doing it. . . . We might call such a process "trial and error." But the trials are not randomly related to one another; reflection on each trial and its results set the stage for the next trial. Such a pattern of inquiry is better described as a sequence of "moments" in a process of reflection-in-action. (Schon, 1987, pp. 26–27)

The distinction then is that, when we reflect in action, our reflection and actions are one in the service of each other (i.e., our reflections influence our actions, which in turn influence our further reflections and actions regarding some present situation, one in which our reflections and action can still bring about change).

To illustrate the difference between reflection on action and reflection in action, consider again Freda's case example regarding Ann. Freda's presentation represents her reflection on action. Such reflection, although it may influence Freda's (and our) future actions in future situations, in no way could have any bearing on the interchanges that actually transpired between Freda and Ann (because all such interchanges occurred in the distant past). Some of the actions or judgments Freda made (e.g., using the recus-a-baby, jostling the recus-a-baby while Ann was holding it and walking with it, adding weights to the recus-a-baby) may have resulted from a process of reflection in action.

Let us next examine what the structure of such a reflective conversation looks like and discuss the stance toward inquiry in such a process. According to Schon, the practitioner must first frame the problematic situation to create a manageable problem that he or she can deal with (i.e., he or she must set the problem). How the practitioner frames the situation suggests a way of shaping the situation to intervene to solve the problem that he or she has constructed. As he or she frames and begins to shape the situation, he or she steps into the situation and makes himself or herself a part of it. To test the frame, the practitioner conducts an experiment in which he or she adapts the situation through a "web of moves." Each move elicits "back talk" from the situation. As the situation talks back, the practitioner listens and reflects. His or her reflection on the situation's back talk invites new response, further back talk, further reflection, and so on. Key to the transactional nature of this sort of reflective conversation with the situation is that the practitioner remains open to the situation's back talk, including remaining open to one's failure to change the situation. The practitioner must see the problem as a "moving target" because, as a phenomenon, the problem will continuously be changing, and any further actions will hinge on changes brought about by earlier actions.

How the practitioner frames the problem does not only result from theoretical and technical knowledge but also results from past experience. How does past experience have a bearing on practice? Schon believed that, through experience, the practitioner builds up a repertoire of "exemplars" to use as a basis for composing new variations. Practitioners do not use exemplars to create generalizations; instead, exemplars serve as metaphors for recognizing this as that (i.e., exemplars promote recognition of similarities and differences to past situations without necessarily being able to say how one is similar to the other at first). Such recognition is not enough. Schon contended that the practitioner must test the frame he or she imposes (i.e., he or she must conduct an experiment that will test the frame).

The sort of experimentation that the reflective practitioner engages in is similar to yet different from that of the researcher. To understand and appreciate the distinctive character of experimentation in the practice sense, Schon stated that we must consider that different types of experimentation exist and that these serve different kinds of functions. He identified and described three types: exploratory, move testing, and hypothesis testing.

When a practitioner undertakes an action to see what might happen without making predictions or having any expectations regarding what the outcome might be, he or she is engaging in exploratory experimentation. Such "What if?" experimentation serves the function of probing, which helps the practitioner to have a better understanding of the situation and to obtain additional information. This type of experimentation is successful when it leads to the discovery of something new.

A practitioner is conducting a move-testing experiment when he or she takes an action to produce an intended change. In the simplest cases, if the action produces the intended outcome, the move is affirmed; if the action does not produce the intended outcome, the move is negated. In more complicated cases, the action is likely to produce other effects beyond those intended that may or may not be predictable and or desirable. In these cases, the practitioner affirms the move when he or she approves of the consequences as a whole and negates the move when he or she does not approve of the consequences.

Hypothesis testing is the third type of experimentation. This type is the one practitioners tend to associate with the word *research* (although research may involve exploratory and move-testing experiments). When conducting a hypothesis testing experiment, the experimenter aims to produce or specify the conditions under which this hypothesis and competing hypotheses would be disconfirmed. The hypothesis that most strongly resists refutation is accepted (i.e., a process of elimination discriminates among competing hypotheses). (Although the one that resists refutation is accepted, the acceptance is tentative, such as discovering some other contributing factor in the future that could lead to its refutation.)

What is different about hypothesis testing experimentation in practice compared with research? In research, the aim is to understand a phenomenon. In practice, the aim likewise involves understanding a phenomenon but only in the service of change (i.e., the primary emphasis is on changing the situation). The practitioner thus cannot remain distant and objective; he or she must violate these canons of a controlled experiment. The situation a practitioner creates is in part of his or her own making. He or she must be in the situation (i.e., be a part of it), which means that the practitioner influences the totality of the object of the study. Furthermore, the practitioner tries to confirm and not refute the hypothesis. The practitioner engages in moves that change the phenomenon to make the hypothesis fit (i.e., he or she tries to make the situation conform to the hypothesis). Thus, if the practitioner ignores resistance to change, then he or she falls into self-fulfilling prophecy. To avoid self-fulfilling prophecy, he or she must remain open to failure. In other words, he or she must listen to the findings associated with his or her moves (i.e., remain open to the situation's back talk), and if he or she does not find sufficient evidence that supports the hypothesis, then the practitioner must consider the possibility that he or she cannot support his or her hypothesis and may need to entertain alternative hypotheses. In addition, in the practice context, the practitioner continues to experiment only to the point where his or her moves are affirmed or yield a new appreciation of the situation.

Although Schon (1983) separated the types of experimentation to describe each, he argued that experimenting as one reflects in action all at once entails exploration, move testing, and hypothesis testing, that "the three functions are fulfilled by the very same actions" (p. 147). This, he says, is what gives experimentation in practice its distinctive character.

Becoming a reflective practitioner and developing a stance toward practice along the lines that Schon suggested are important, especially regarding the use of and reasoning about activities. Why? First, as you gain clinical experience, you will find that you cannot merely apply a standardized protocol of activities. Not all situations will be exactly the same. Nor will you be able to predict with certainty what the outcomes of your actions (and the activities selected) will be. How are you going to deal with the surprises you encounter? Schon's conceptualization of professional practice and the stance toward inquiry that he suggested may better enable you to appreciate and cope with the uniqueness and uncertainties you will encounter.

Second, as Schon noted, as one's practice becomes increasingly spontaneous (i.e., tacit and intuitive), a certain amount of overlearning may occur (i.e., you may begin to do things over and over again without questioning what you are doing, without considering alternatives, and so forth). When overlearning occurs, a practitioner may not only miss some important facets and fail to recognize features that warrant addressing or that he or she should consider, but also he or she is likely to experience burnout and boredom. Developing a stance toward practice (and the use of activities) that appreciates the importance of reflection in action may provide an antidote to overlearning and help to prevent burnout.

Third, engaging in reflection in action can help a practitioner to appreciate and remain open to multiple perspectives (i.e., to try on different "thinking caps" rather than adhering to only one, to select from competing perspectives that seem to best fit the situation at hand, and to choose alternative approaches to reframe and address a problem when the frame first selected and the ensuing actions undertaken fail to produce the outcome desired).

Finally, reflection in action is a process that is akin to what Mattingly and Fleming (1994) referred to as conditional reasoning. What Schon offered is a way of conceptualizing professional practice and a stance toward inquiry in practice that may help to promote its development.

Summary

This chapter concerns the reasoning process that leads occupational therapists to select activities appropriately with and for their clients. The work of Mattingly and Fleming (1994) involves an example of activity reasoning with a review of steps in the reasoning process. These steps move from preparatory activities to simulation of valued activities to activities based in real life. Exploring the contrasting types of reasoning of new and experienced occupational therapists is a major thrust of the chapter. The work of Dreyfus and Dreyfus (1986) described stages of the development of reasoning skills. Finally, the work of Schon (1983, 1987) completed the picture with an emphasis on reasoning techniques and their rationales in practice. Because Schon was particularly interested in how practitioners apply reasoning in day-to-day intervention, he emphasized the processes of clinical reasoning engaged in while directly involved in practice. Schon (1987) presented his approach with three types of experimentation: exploratory, move testing, and hypothesis testing. All of these consistent and complementary approaches to clinical reasoning assist the reader in better understanding the process of selecting appropriate activities for and with clients. ■

References

Dreyfus, H., & Dreyfus, S. (1986). *Mind over machine: The power of human intuition and expertise in the era of the computer.* New York: Free Press.

Fleming, M. H. (1994). A commonsense practice in an uncommon world. In *Clinical reasoning: Forms of inquiry in a therapeutic practice* (pp. 94–115). Philadelphia: F. A. Davis.

Mattingly, C., & Fleming, M. H. (1994). *Clinical reasoning: Forms of inquiry in a therapeutic practice.* Philadelphia: F. A. Davis.

Schon, D. A. (1983). *The reflective practitioner: How professionals think in action.* New York: Basic Books.

Schon, D. A. (1987). *Educating the reflective practitioner: Toward a new design for teaching and learning in the professions.* San Francisco: Jossey-Bass.

7

The Application of
Activities to Practice

Ann Burkhardt, MA, OTR/L, BCN

A sign posted at Ellis Island, NY, includes a statement from a young woman who immigrated to the United States as a child.

> The whole experience was very frightening. . . . They brought me up to a room. . . . They put a pegboard before me with little sticks of different shapes and little holes. . . . I had to put them in place, the round ones and the square ones . . . and I did it perfectly, "Oh, we must have made a mistake. This little girl . . . naturally she doesn't know English, but she's very bright, intelligent." So they took the cross (chalkmark) off me so we were cleared. (Victoria Scarfatti Fernandez, a Macedonian Jewish immigrant in 1916, interviewed in 1985)

Clearly, the puzzle the examiners gave this child had neither context nor meaning for her. The puzzle was an ineffective tool to measure her intellect, but it was the best tool available to the examiners at the time. Time changes, humans change and grow, but the underlying concept that activities have meaning when they are in context and perspective for the person endures.

Value and Use of Activities

Occupational therapy practice and beliefs support the value of activity as an effective tool in the process of change. The practice of occupational therapy values the use of activities in the context of the concept of occupation. How each of us occupies our time relates to many variables and values. Current thinking in the field supports the belief that spirituality is one key to the meaning and value of activities. Two key concepts of spirituality are existentialism and metaphysics.

Existentialism is the symbolic meaning persons experience through the performance of or engagement in daily life tasks. For example, whenever I put my earrings in my ears, I remember my grandmother's statement to me when I was 15 years of age: "Earrings make you look so girlish. They give us each that little something extra, don't you see?" Existentially, putting on my earrings is a spiritual activity for me. I valued my grandmother's opinion and words. The activity has personal, spiritual meaning for me because I remember my grandmother as I do it, and I loved her deeply.

Metaphysics is the perception that participation in activities in the earthly plane somehow correlates to our relationship to a higher power, such as God, a Great Spirit, or angels, or that life has a higher purpose. Metaphysical activities may include religious activities, but they may additionally include nonreligious activities that have deep spiritual meaning. For example, doing activities to support one's church or spiritual community (e.g., stewardship activities) may have metaphysical meaning. Engaging in rituals (e.g., the symbolism of exchanging vows and rings in a wedding ceremony) likewise has a metaphysical basis. The ceremony is spiritually symbolic for the persons who marry each other and represents a commitment to each other in the eyes of God and humankind. In addition, the act of praying may be metaphysical. One could argue that seeing the glories of nature in person can make persons feel connected to the universe. Many persons who have see the Grand Canyon can attest to this. Being among a large number of persons for an event, such as being in Central Park after John Lennon died, can be a metaphysical experience. Pilgrims who go to Mecca each year and Christians and Jews who travel to Jerusalem all experience a heightened sense of connectedness to the universe in metaphysical terms when they make these journeys.

Occupational therapy practitioners use activities in a proper context in relation to the person they are treating to bring about change and to restore meaning in life. Practitioners are agents of change. Occupational therapy practitioners promote change through the use of purposeful activities in the context of real life and spiritual meaning as a catalyst in the process of change. Purpose in doing the activity must be inherent for activity participation to be effective as a treatment modality. Using activities out of context or using tasks that have no personal meaning to a client is futile and purposeless because those types of tasks are rote and repetitive and do not translate well to everyday existence. These activities do not improve the quality of life.

Several (Neistadt, 1994; Trombly, 1995) have studied the outcomes of activity use with clients. Separately, they have found that clients perform tasks with greater ability when a task is in context for them. Reaching for an object one wants to use, for example, results in better reaching ability than reaching for an object in a simulated circumstance. Clearly, using activities involves more than the physical subcomponents of the task. Persons perform better under normal, contextually applied circumstances.

This concept may seem revolutionary to some occupational therapy practitioners. In the 1970 and 1980s, many occupational therapy practitioners used activities to transfer subcomponents of activities into a later, greater functional purposes. At that time, using cones, blocks, puzzles, and other therapeutic activities to try to develop subcomponent skills became popular. This concept is part of a "bottom–up" approach to treatment. Practitioners used subcomponents of activities (specific tasks) rather than the functional activities themselves to promote change. Some motor learning frames of reference still promote this approach to a certain degree. These frames of reference propose that using subcomponents of activities can promote the acquisition of the skill necessary to engage in occupational performance. Other occupational therapy practitioners who use a motor learning frame of reference focus treatment on tasks that promote the actual acquisition of the desired skill in context (e.g., forming a fist with one's hand on the handgrip of a walker rather than gripping a cone). The act of gripping in context should promote a better functional outcome.

In the 1990s, a movement began to use actual participation in activities of daily living (ADL) therapeutically rather than focusing on subcomponents as a first line of action in treatment. This "top–down" approach to treatment relies on having clients do their daily life tasks as the evaluation and treatment focus. The clients perform the tasks in as close to a natural setting as possible. Neistadt's (1994) and Trombly's (1993, 1995) works have demonstrated that using a top–down approach to intervention is more effective than using a transfer training approach. Development of client-centered assessments has had an effect on how clients choose to focus their occupational therapy to improve their ability to care for themselves and to participate in activities that they personally value.

Reasoning in the Selection of Activities

As discussed in chapter 6, the choice of activities must result from logic and sound reasoning. In occupational therapy, clinical reasoning is the process that underlies the logical, contextual choice of activities. Clinical reasoning involves several types of reasoning: procedural reasoning, contextual reasoning, conditional reasoning, and narrative reasoning (Mattingly & Fleming, 1994). Outcomes of procedural reasoning, contextual reasoning, and conditional reasoning form the basis for the narrative reasoning or storytelling process that guides the selection of the right activity for the client. Narrative reasoning in process tells a story about the person receiving occupational therapy and his or her activity history. The story takes shape as rapport builds between the practitioner and the person and as the factors that declare the need for change in how the person lives his or her life emerge or declare themselves in full view of life (past, present, and future).

Procedural reasoning is a process through which the therapist gathers data about the person receiving intervention: What was the event in the person's life that led the person to require services? What were the medical issues (in a medical model) or reasons for occupational therapy intervention (in a community-based context), and what were the psychological issues and the social issues or concerns affecting the person's general health and well-being? Procedural reasoning generally involves more time for a novice practitioner than it does for a skilled practitioner. Once a practitioner gains competence in evaluation and intervention, he or she has greater proficiency in deductive reasoning on the basis of familiar practice trends. A novice practitioner seeks evidence to build an understanding of the underlying issues. An experienced, competent practitioner sums up the factors surrounding a case with greater implicit insight and greater speed. The experienced practitioner anticipates a clinical context more rapidly on the basis of experience and skill. For example, a novice practitioner will review a medical chart and need time to process the meaning of tests and the findings of scans and X rays. An experienced practitioner will read and process that material more rapidly and will seek clues to limitations the person may encounter as he or she attempts to engage in normal life tasks and activities.

Contextual reasoning occurs through gaining insight and perspective into how the events that the client has experienced may affect his or her ability to resume life roles. Conditional reasoning involves shaping the occupational therapy process context to the client's perceived need for change and desire to work with the practitioner toward change. Practitioners gain insight into the person's perception of his or her functional ability and the issues he or she personally wants to address in intervention.

Sometimes, a therapist may have potential goals for a client that the client does not have for himself or herself. For example, if a male client has had a hip replacement and has met his goals in therapy but continues to require his wife's assistance to don socks, then the occupational therapist should determine whether the patient's personal goal is to be able to don socks. Although the therapist may know that the client could don socks independently with a sock aide, if the client wants his wife to continue to do this for him, and the wife is satisfied with this, then intervention relative to donning socks would not be necessary for this client. The client may instead identify other goals that are a higher priority for him. This client may be more concerned about how to resume his sex life. This is a common area of concern for many clients that surgery and rehabilitation staff members often overlook. Sex education may be a more pertinent and appropriate area of client intervention than donning socks. Perhaps the client seeks both interventions. The practitioner should personalize the actual application of activities case by case and person by person.

Case Scenario 1

Joe Brown is a man 63 years of age. He is married to his high school sweetheart and is the father of three adult children. Mr. Brown is a self-employed freelance news photographer. He recently had his right hip replaced. Mr. Brown can participate in all of his self-care activities independently, but he continues to rely on his wife for assistance with his right sock. Mr. Brown likes having his wife assist him with his sock. He says having her put on his sock allows them a few quiet moments together at the beginning of the day. He is happy with this system and does not want to do this task independently. Mr. Brown is a landscape photographer. He frequently stands for long periods because he specializes in time-lapse photography. He would like to work with the therapist to develop a system that would allow him to sit while he uses his tripod so that he can take pressure off his right leg when he works for long periods of time. In addition to photography, the Browns enjoy ballroom dancing. Mr. Brown wants to conserve his energy during the day so that he can begin ballroom dancing again with his wife.

The focus of intervention for Mr. Brown thus changes from a focus on self-care activities to a vocational context and its related activities. Mr. Brown is a photographer and wants to go on photographic expeditions. The focus of treatment is to modify or adapt the activity so that Mr. Brown can engage in his photographic occupation. Because landscape photography requires that Mr. Brown change his positioning, the practitioner and Mr. Brown explore the use of a portable seat to allow him to develop greater endurance. Because intervention in this case is limited to the hospital setting, the occupational therapy practitioner may provide simulated opportunities for Mr. Brown to practice the various tasks involved in taking photographs. On the other hand, if the occupational therapy practitioner examined Mr. Brown in home care, private practice, or community-based practice, then the practitioner may have an opportunity to go with him into the field and to observe his actual, in-context participation in the modified activity.

Activities Selection and Application in the Real World

In the context of occupational therapy, intervention attempts to help someone to function within the performance areas of self-care, work, play or leisure, and rest. A balanced lifestyle is one in which a person is able to function across these domains while maintaining a balance among physical, psychological, emotional, and social contexts. Occupational therapy promotes holism and a balanced lifestyle for all persons across the life span. The context of the application of occupational therapy is vast and diverse. Occupational therapy practitioners may use their skills of activity analysis and synthesis to focus on the person's ability to participate in the roles that form his or her occupational roles. This section of the chapter provides some guidance and suggestions on how to apply activities in the real world of practice.

Occupational therapy practitioners' use of activities in the real world involves creating the "just-right" match among the client, the context, the activity, and the service delivery model. The ultimate goal of an occupational therapy intervention is for the client to engage in occupations. As stated throughout this book, one valuable tool is purposeful activity. All purposeful activities involve two goals, the goals of the client a nd the goals of the occupational therapy practitioner. Many factors influence the selection and use of activities, including the different abilities, needs, desires, and motivation of the clients; the practice site in which the intervention takes place; the service delivery model; the resources that are available to support the intervention; and the knowledge and skills of the practitioner. The following sections discuss activities within the circumstances of real-life practice that occupational therapy practitioners confront daily.

Purposeful Activities That Address the Client's Unique Needs

Occupational therapy practitioners select and use purposeful activities that address the unique developmental needs of the client. Thus, the practitioner always considers a person's unique needs when selecting activities for intervention. Beginning with the client's needs, the occupational therapy practitioner learns from the client which activities are appropriate. By working with the client, the occupational therapy practitioner matches the specific purposeful activities to the client's needs.

Newborns and young children's purposeful activities. Purposeful activities for a newborn usually involve activities in response to the child's specific needs (e.g., feeding, changing a diaper). These activities taking place between infant and adult provide the infant with necessary sensory stimulation. Playful sensory stimulation activities provide opportunities for infant–caregiver interaction. Occupational therapy practitioners use their knowledge of normal growth and development and the nature of sensory input to guide the selection of specific activities.

Case Scenario 2

A child who is born prematurely or one who requires hospitalization in a neonatal intensive care unit (NICU) requires special attention. These children receive stimulation passively, and special caregiver and infant activities are necessary. The intervention may involve developmental stimulation from the therapist or a trained caregiver such as swaddling, holding, gently rocking, and supporting the premature infant in a positional device within the controlled atmosphere of the incubator amid monitor wires, pulse oximeters, and respirators. The baby may benefit from being held and feeling the heartbeat of another warm-blooded human being as well. Newborns who are born prematurely may not be neurologically ready to receive a bombardment of activity. Often, these babies have not had time for their nervous systems to mature to the level of a full-term newborn. Feeding can require skill and knowledge regarding the baby's ability to suck and swallow, and the therapist can assist and facilitate learning these concepts with the parents or other caregivers. Some recent studies in aromatherapy have indicated that an infant in the NICU may be less stressed if he or she smells lavender or vanilla (Dunn, Sleep, & Collett,1995).

Case Scenario 3

If premature infants in an NICU cannot swallow, both breast-feeding and bottle-feeding are inappropriate because the babies would aspirate into their lungs anything fed to them by mouth. This could result in a life-threatening circumstance, aspiration pneumonia. An occupational therapist who works in an NICU, however, knows that these infants may have developmental problems if they do not receive oral stimulation, such as that resulting from sucking on a nipple. The therapist in an NICU contextually knows how to use a pacifier to stimulate the mouth as normally as possible. The occupational therapist likewise knows which pacifier is best for the neonate in this context. For example, some neonates use orthodontic nipples. This may be the nipple of choice for infants who have metabolic disorders and who may have abnormalities in the development of their hard palate related to nutritional issues.

Activity for the infant is often embedded in the care and attention they receive from caregivers. Infants need periods of being held and require someone else's help to sustain their nutritional needs. Someone else must address their elimination of waste. Interaction at first may involve turning one's head toward a rattle or making eye contact or face-to-face contact. Over time and as the nervous system and body develop, infants become more interactive by seeking eye contact or verbally expressing their needs. Infants cannot speak, so making noise, cooing, or crying are the ways that infants attempt to address their needs. Activity participation depends greatly on responses from others.

Case Scenario 4

Developmentally mature infants who are born addicted to substances such as cocaine may have neurological reactions to the withdrawal of the drugs. They may require more handling, positioning, and developmental stimulation than full-term infants or other premature infants who were not exposed to chemical substances. Activity for these infants is passively introduced. They respond to the input as they receive and perceive it. Infant massage can promote relaxation and offset gastrointestinal discomfort that many infants experience while withdrawing from substances.

Newborns quickly learn to respond to movement, feelings, and sounds generated by their own movement or action. Gradually, activities of the infant begin to become purposeful or self-directed as the infant interacts and responds to his or her world. Objects in the environment, including all kinds of people, become important as the newborn responds to them. Infants develop an awareness of their bodies as they repeatedly move and repeat actions over and over. Wearing a wrist rattle gives auditory feedback that results from active movement. Newborns generally see only the colors black, white, and red. Often newborns are drawn visually to corners of rooms or to patterns that include straight and rounded lines. They begin to track visually. Placing black and white drawings of faces around the crib can provide various choices of objects to track visually and maintains infants' interest in their environment for longer periods of time. The sound of a human voice conveys information about the human environment. The sound of a parent's voice and the quality and degree of tactile stimulation influence the interactive environment for the infant.

Infants require another person's assistance to set up and initiate play. Infants passively play but learn to track visually and fix on objects of interest. Moving objects, such as spinning tops, can be intriguing. Playful activities for infants include using rattles and other toys (e.g., stuffed animals, rattles, activity centers, cloth books, cloth balls, tops).

Feeding is an important purposeful activity for infants and young children. Children who cannot suck require oral stimulation and manual facilitation to reinforce attempts at sucking. Sucking and swallowing are vital functions. One needs these functions to swallow secretions (e.g., saliva). To draw nutrition normally through breast-feeding, an infant must be able to suckle a breast. Others must introduce activity to the infants, but the activity requires a response from the infant to have a successful outcome. Sometimes infants need help in encouraging the development of a skill to overcome developmental delays under abnormal circumstances. Infants respond to the input as they receive and perceive it. Repetition shapes behavior and the ability to respond.

Case Scenario 5

Parents may require assistance to learn when to discontinue a child's use of a pacifier. Tears and emotional adjustment may be necessary to assist the toddler to stop drinking from a bottle in favor of a covered drinking cup. Finger foods can stimulate early self-feeding behaviors. For example, children usually learn to finger feed before trying to feed themselves with a spoon. Learning to adjust or modulate the position of the spoon through the fingers results in less spillage and mess during feeding. Some one-to-one time with a skilled care provider, such as an occupational therapy practitioner, can assist parents in making the right choices for the baby while stimulating and facilitating skill development.

Case Scenario 6

Occupational therapy practitioners frequently work with older children who have developed food aversions because they could not eat by mouth for a time because of metabolic disturbances. When older children begin to eat after years of not eating, a slow-paced, consistent motivational strategy to gain their interest and participation may be necessary. Children with food aversions may need encouragement to explore textures in their mouths. Creamy is quite different from crunchy or bubbly (like soda pop). Spices and herbs alter taste. Salty is quite different from sweet. One strategy may be to create a "clean plate club." When everyone involved in the child's care is aware of the intervention, these persons can provide a lot of positive reinforcement whenever the child eats all of the food on his or her plate. Over time, children eat because of the reinforcement and because of their eventual pleasure in eating and actively receiving nourishment.

Initial interactions between human beings, children, other more mature persons, and the nonhuman environment shape one's response to life.

Adolescents' purposeful activities. Because of their developmental needs, adolescents often take part in activities that are physically demanding and involve other persons of their own age. Social groups of peers often strongly influence adolescents' activity preferences. Purposeful activities for adolescents involve a wide range of activities that vary on the basis of communities, the person's culture, and the person's skills and abilities. When selecting an activity with an adolescent, occupational therapy practitioners must use careful reasoning to guide the adolescent toward an activity that he or she can perform with some competence. Adolescents often fear that peers and adults are watching and judging them when they engage in activities. Furthermore, the adolescent should not perceive the chosen activities to be infantile, immature, or useless. When engaged in a purposeful activity, the practitioner must address the overlying psychological issues that may arise as the adolescent participates.

Selection of activities with adolescents must carefully consider the limited attention span and concentration of many teenagers in any or all settings. If an adolescent has attention and cognitive impairments, the occupational therapy practitioner can work with him or her to improve and maximize study habits, memory skills, sequencing of life skill activities (e.g., instrumental activities of daily living [IADL] in context), ordering of activity participation, and limit setting and redirecting behaviors that are potentially self-destructive. Additionally, many adolescents are self-conscious during attempts to practice self-care activities, especially tasks that are more intimate in nature, such as toileting or skin inspection. In partnership with the adolescent, occupational therapy practitioners can select activities that are acceptable to the client and are therapeutic.

Adults' purposeful activities. Adults have an extensive range of activity needs depending on their personal circumstances, such as health status, disability status, developmental skills, life circumstances, or personal desire. As when working with adolescents, occupational therapy practitioners should strive to work in partnership with adult clients and their significant others to verify that the therapeutic activities are acceptable to clients and meet their needs.

When selecting activities with adults, occupational therapy practitioners often begin with the presenting problem or the condition. On the basis of the problem or area of difficulty and knowledge of the client and his or her needs, the occupational therapist begins by suggesting to the client various activities that are appropriate for the goals of therapy. By working in collaboration with the client and, in some cases, his or her significant others, the occupational therapist develops an intervention plan that includes those activities that the adult finds acceptable, challenging, and gratifying. The adult client must understand the relationship between participation in the activity and long-term therapeutic goals.

When working with adults, adapting activities to address therapeutic goals may be necessary. For example, clients with orthopedic conditions, traumatic conditions, or burns may commonly need to execute specific actions. When this is the case, the occupational therapist creatively adapts one of the client-selected activities to include the specific actions necessary for therapeutic purposes. When adapting or modifying activities, involving the client is again important (e.g., when activities become too contrived, they may become meaningless and thus not therapeutic). Choice of activities and ability to participate in an activity program will depend on the client's interest, ability, and needs. A balance of self-care activities, socialization, and avocational activities may be useful with adults who do not have cognitive impairments.

Most adults value their independence in completing self-care activities such as personal hygiene and grooming tasks. When adults have immobilized limbs or wounds, common objects may require adaptation to allow participation in basic self-care tasks. For other disabilities, occupational therapy practitioners may need to adjust the method the person normally uses so that he or she may be successful in completing self-care tasks. If a person cannot bathe or groom himself or herself in the manner to which he or she is accustomed, the occupational therapy practitioner may need to simulate the environment that is closest to home as possible and have the person practice adapting bathing or a grooming routine. If feasible, the occupational therapy practitioner may practice the actual adaptation with the person during a home visit before his or her discharge to the community. If adults have mobility problems, training in adapted techniques and training in and provision of adapted equipment may be the focus of activity participation.

Purposeful Activities That Are Selected Because of Distinctive Characteristics

Occupational therapy practitioners often select activities for intervention because of the distinctive characteristics of the activity. Practitioners use an activity analysis of the activity to match the activity and its inherent characteristics to the needs of the client.

Choosing purposeful activities for children. For children, the choice of activities depends on chronological and developmental age and the child's intact abilities. Children who are ill still seek interaction with persons and toys. Adapting toys to encourage and enable participatory play can be a focus of intervention. Furthermore, technological devices and equipment allow children to interact actively with their environment.

Case Scenario 7

Children with impairments may benefit from special adaptations to encourage and allow their participation in activities. Children with cancer, such as leukemia, may develop peripheral neuropathy as a result of chemotherapy. Adding switch activation to wind-up toys, for example, may provide opportunities to play actively and to manipulate toys despite impairment. Children with heightened sensory awareness and poor sensory modulation may benefit from activities that encourage sensory integration such as parachutes, therapy balls, swings (if the children do not have seizure precautions), rocking chairs, bubbles, and balloons.

Children who cannot interact well with their environment as a result of disease or disability can sometimes gain control through environmental adaptations such as the use of environmental control units or computerization. A child with progressive muscular dystrophy, for example, can still gain mobility in the appropriate powered mobility device and under the right circumstances. The child may operate computers by using adaptive switches, mouth sticks, head controls, joysticks, or sip-and-puff mechanisms. Games may assist the child in mastering the adaptive devices during the training process. Connecting successful outcomes with rewards can build self-esteem and a comfort level for the child in the use of the adaptation. One colleague who worked with a young child with C6 quadriplegia shared the following story of how she built a docking station for various mouth sticks for the child (J. W. Shoenhaupt, personal communication, January 16, 1999).

Case Scenario 8

Joe gained mastery over the mouth sticks by playing a game of fish. The therapist placed various objects within his reach. The child had a few shapes for each adapted terminal end of a mouth stick in the docking station. Joe had to retrieve and replace each stick as needed to fish for all of the objects. The therapist had a matching set of mouth sticks, and she fished for the objects with the boy. Once they had retrieved all of the objects, the player with the most objects won the game. This is one example of how a game can be a training activity for adjusting to the use of adaptive devices.

Most activities have a specific performance component that is a key aspect of the activity. Accordingly, some activities are fine motor, gross motor, or perceptual depending on what the key performance component of the activity is. All activities require skills in more than one performance component. When occupational therapy practitioners select activities, however, they often group them according to the dominant performance component. These activities then become associated with a specific goal. As part of daily practice, occupational therapy practitioners select activities because of the dominant performance component.

Case Scenario 9

A major area for occupational therapy practitioners in school-based practice involves handwriting ability. Children develop hand skills by various means. One occupational therapist who has studied, written, and presented on handwriting skills is Mary Benbow (1995). A child must have good control of the entire extremity before he or she can achieve skilled writing. A child must first receive proprioceptive input to his or her shoulder to develop body sense of the arm in space. Activities that Benbow (1995) recommended include writing in overhead planes on a blackboard, an easel, or paper taped to a wall. The overhead positioning of the arm provides stimulation to the rest of the body, and the child develops skilled use of the arm in overhead planes. The child's balance is stimulated, and this gives him or her an ability to develop the use of his or her arms in multiple contexts. A MagnaDoodle® writing toy may provide proprioceptive feedback to the arm. Activities with proprioceptive and kinesthetic feedback assist the child in developing coordinated movement and skill development.

Children learn and enhance hand skill development and foster concentration and prevocational skill through the use of craft activities. Arts and craft activities were once a primary focus of occupational therapy. Over time and with an increasing emphasis on working in the medical model, many occupational therapy practitioners abandoned or deemphasized the use of arts and crafts. Engagement in arts and craft activities reinforces hand skill development, increases the ability to concentrate and follow written directions, and fosters creativity and effective use of leisure time. Arts and crafts is a mechanism for building a child's self-esteem through the completion of a finished project to keep for oneself or to give as a gift.

Case Scenario 10

Occupational therapy practitioners often select activities that focus on a child's development of psychosocial skills. Children who may have learning disabilities (e.g., dyslexia) or who may be dealing with a difficult psychosocial adjustment (e.g., the divorce of their parents) may act out and physically attack others. These children often lack self-esteem and may feel guilty about or responsibility for the divorce. When they are experiencing the loss of one parent from the home, these children may glorify the parent who has left, and they may act out and strike out at the parent who continues as their caregiver. An occupational therapy practitioner can work with the child to find more productive ways to express his or her feelings and to develop better interaction with the custodial parent and others under controlled circumstances. If the child is having a problem writing or reading and becomes frustrated, sometimes by 7 years of age the child can begin to work with a computer to substitute for the frustrating activity (such as writing). Seeing words in a composition may be less threatening. With a computer, the child can macrocode words, group words together in frequently used phrases, and store words that give the child difficulty.

Having children participate in controlled play activities one on one with the practitioner can improve their interpersonal skills and their ability to engage in parallel and cooperative play in various situations with others. Therapists may need to set goals for the activities with the child, and practitioners may need to set limits on acting-out behaviors during the session. Sometimes a practitioner has an advantage over a parent in encouraging children to discuss their feelings. A rapport with an impartial third party who works with the child, like an occupational therapy practitioner, may be less fearful and threatening to the child. Truthful sharing with family members may generate fear of rejection or reprisal.

Choosing activities for adolescents. For adolescents, selecting activities requires an artful match with the activity and the client's personality, social skills, and motivation. Adolescents may have various physical, psychological, and emotional impairments. Problems that occupational therapy practitioners may encounter include dyslexia, vision impairment, physical impairment, and acting-out behaviors associated with anxiety, depression, poor coping ability, personality disorders, or schizophrenia. Adolescents with dyslexia may be involved in delinquent behavior. Many adolescents convicted of crimes in their teenage years have learning impairments. Computer-based programs can be valuable with this population. The child's attention skills may benefit from computer games and access to the Internet; the child can achieve success through use of a fun format to achieve successful participation with the written word and media.

Adolescents often need to develop life skills. Life skills programs are currently a topic area targeted for federal and philanthropic funding. Various media are available for life skills training. One group of graduate students in a management and supervision class at Columbia University in New York recently proposed a computer-based life skills program in a drug and alcohol treatment setting for adolescents. They suggested using key words as target phrases for search engines to locate the program source, which promoted acceptance and a sense of belonging. In a hospital setting, a life skills program may have information on how to perform IADL and basic ADL tasks when living with various impairments.

Adolescents often develop positive behaviors when they are role models for others. Making adolescents responsible and contributing participants in systems works extremely well in positively facilitating behavioral change. Some important topics for adolescents include safe sex, prevention of smoking and drug abuse, and proactive development of good eating and physical activity habits. Individual activities with a counselor, participation in a group activity in which participants take turns at leadership, and use of multimedia activities involving film, slide presentations, rap sessions, graphic arts, and performing arts are all media that practitioners can use to develop activities for adolescents.

Teens with impairments still may seek out opportunities to be role models to younger siblings. Role modeling can enhance self-esteem. The perception of feeling valued or admired for one's skill, wisdom, and contribution is self-affirming and valuable to both the role model and the protégé. An occupational therapy practitioner can coach a teenager through this process or assist the teenager with skill development if the practitioner is skilled in the activity.

Choosing activities for adults. For adults, selecting activities requires matching the adult's specific performance deficit with an activity that has performance requirements that address the deficit. Although most children learn by repeating activities over and over in the same contextual relationship before they modify the activity or tire of the core activity, adult learners generally learn best when they have various tasks and activities from which to choose or alternate. Adults tend to do well with repetitive tasks only when the tasks involve improving mobility, such as exercise machines or a desire and focus on the ability to walk. Many commercially available types of therapeutic exercise equipment for home use are rote and repetitive, and many adults use them as clothing collectors rather than to get in shape. Adult learners require different types of learning challenges. In inpatient rehabilitation settings, adult activities often closely relate to self-care, the ability to function in the home or community, or the return to work. To vary skill acquisition methods, many inpatient rehabilitation settings use group activities to foster choice and diversity into the recovery process and to retain the client's active interest in participation. Some examples of groups in inpatient settings include movement groups, strengthening groups, upright mobility groups (focusing on standing ability and mobility in standing or walking), cooking groups, and specific diagnostic category groups (e.g., hemi group or amputee group). Some groups may contain a psychosocial adjustment activity, such as sharing questions and concerns about their conditions and their anticipated degree of recovery.

When mobility impairments are severe or accompanied by communication impairments, occupational therapists may use technological resources to assist adults. Use of environmental control units, powered mobility, or computerized adaptations are examples of high-technology resource equipment. In the training phase, once the client obtains technology for personal use, the occupational therapy practitioner can use games or other fun activities in the training process as a way to assist the client in acquiring the agility and skill to substitute the function of the technology for his or her own impaired functional ability. The person can play games alone such as computerized solitaire, or the person can play games competitively with the therapist, a volunteer, or a friend.

When occupational therapy practitioners treat adults who work, practitioners may select activities that directly relate to the client's employment. Adults who work full-time spend an average of 7 1/2 hr a day, 37 1/2 hr a week, at work. Work-related activities generally focus on the activities that describe the position the person fills. In work environments, the focus of intervention may involve doing a work task in a modified way. Persons who use strong postural sets to accomplish tasks may be prone to injury because their muscle activity is maximized. Relearning less stressful ways of doing work tasks can be one focus of work-related occupational therapy practice.

Case Scenario 11

The most common injury in a work setting is back injury (Nassau, 1999). Placing objects in the environment to improve the ergonomics of task performance, sometimes by using trial and error and sometimes by using commercially or custom adaptations, can be a focus of activity. One factor that influences recovery from back injury is smoking. Workers who sustain a back injury and smoke are less likely to return to work.

Case Scenario 12

The second most common work-related injury is cumulative trauma disorder (CTD; Feuerstein, Miller, Burrell, & Berger, 1998). Carpal tunnel syndrome can develop from a CTD of the carpal tunnel. Changing the heights of monitors, the ergonomic demands of the keyboard, the amount of time spent at computer terminals between rest breaks, the position of the keyboard, or adequate ergonomic seating support may be necessary. Occupational therapy practitioners can teach workers to keep schedules of rest and stretch breaks. Fun activities that encourage changes in posture and gross mobility rather than concentrated use of the hands may provide a balance between concentrated clerical activity and a healthy amount of break activity.

Activities may help to develop new skills. When clients are adjusting to life with impairments, sometimes they are unable to resume all of their previous life roles. Learning new activities can assist in their adjustment to a lifestyle after becoming disabled. The old cliché is that a client will say, "Will I ever play the piano?" With experience, the therapist learns to retort, "Well, did you ever play before?" A few years ago, a young man with bilateral hand burns and an interest in jazz asked me this question. Initially we chuckled at our dialogue. Several years after his hospitalization, he came back to visit. He sat at the piano in our clinic and proceeded to play an absolutely amazing rendition of Scott Joplin's "Maple Leaf Rag." In retrospect, trying to play the piano as a part of his inpatient therapy could have been appropriate for this gentleman. The activity, although new to him and potentially disappointing to him, could have been meaningful and motivating. Whenever a patient asks this question these days, my answer is different than it once was. Activity choice is individualized and unique in each case. Being an active listener can be ultimately the best strategy for problem solving and activity choice.

Influence of Context on the Selection and Use of Purposeful Activities

Practitioners select activities relative to the context in which the client will use them. Occupational therapy practitioners work in various practice settings and with various age-groups. Settings include the home, schools, hospitals, long-term care facilities, day treatment, business and industry, community settings, and institutions of higher learning. Occupational therapy practitioners work with all age-groups across the life span: infants, children, adolescents, young adults, middle-aged adults, and elderly persons. The use of activities in context in occupational therapy will vary case by case and setting by setting. One age-group may value certain activities in one context, whereas another age-group may consider the same activities meaningless in another context.

In all treatment settings, use of clinical reasoning assists the therapist in prioritizing the focus of treatment across physical and skilled movement, psychological and emotional, and cognitive and social domains within the context of self-care (e.g.,

removing one's own bandage, establishing a sense of control, washing one's face, donning one's clothes, eating one's meal, age-appropriate toileting), work (e.g., studying
or writing in the hospital school or with a tutor, using a computer for a school-aged
child), and leisure or play (e.g., testing physical limits, role playing and pretending,
discussing or sharing feelings, expressing fears, coping with fears and pain, gaining a
sense of self and privacy and self-esteem, experiencing success through activities in all
levels of developmental groups, making friends, exploring and developing continuing relationships with family, experiencing moments of joy and pleasure, learning
cause-and-effect relationships, learning to accept and test social limits, developing
coping skills and strategies to manage the effect of illness on life, and instilling day-
to-day living with a sense of hope so that change can occur to improve quality of life
and to work toward the best outcome in treatment). Rest is likewise something one
learns. As children, we rely on the adults in our lives to structure our naps and rest
periods and to determine bedtime for us. Our bodies and minds require rest to assist
with processing all that has happened in our lives each day. Without rest, our thought
processes become adversely affected. We are less able to concentrate, and our social
behaviors deteriorate. Rest is an ADL.

Settings for services for children. Occupational therapy practitioners provide services to
children and their family members in a wide range of environments, including
NICUs, acute hospital settings, early intervention programs, home care settings,
school-based practice, inpatient psychiatry, and wellness-based practice.

Case Scenario 13

Children who may be at risk developmentally or have developmental delays are
eligible for early intervention services. Occupational therapy practitioners usually
treat children receiving early intervention either at home or in a community-
based clinic setting. Children receiving care in this category are from birth to
3 years of age. Activities for infants and young children who are at risk for developmental impairments should focus on parent–child interactions. Much of the
context of interaction between the occupational therapy practitioner and family
members revolves around hands-on demonstration and working with the parents
and other caregivers on their interactions with their child. Activities include
showing parents how to hold the child and how to promote the child's motor
abilities along a developmental continuum. Parents receive education regarding
how to recognize developmental milestones and how to promote the child's ability to grow and develop.

Children in the hospital have a role; they are pediatric clients. Play is too often
lacking in their day-to-day hospital routine. These children lack stimulating activity;
they become isolated and may developmentally regress. A child who is hospitalized
may seek time and opportunity to play with toys that he or she should have outgrown
in a chronological sense. This developmental regression is not necessarily pathologi-
cal in context. Reverting back to a remembered level of mastery with a toy can be
comforting. Occupational therapy practitioners learn to adapt to the child's needs for

developmental stimulation by introducing challenges throughout play to progress the child toward a more appropriate level for her or his age and the sophistication of the child's nervous system at any given moment. Recently, I met a boy 6 years of age who wanted to play with Teletubbies™ toys rather than with his model trains and Lego® blocks. The Teletubbies fascination resolved when he began to develop trust in the situation and in his caregivers. Fear and an illness contributed to his regression.

Case Scenario 14

Activities that promote self-care for children may all be available within the environment of the hospital room. Most children have their clothes and socks and shoes, implements to wash their face or brush their teeth, cups or bottles to practice feeding, and some toys (e.g., pull toys, favorite stuffed animals or dolls, books, crayons, and coloring books or pads). Therapy balls may be readily available. Therapy balls can provide balance stimulation. Play rooms or childlife departments may have other toys or experiential learning tools, including computer technology. Several disciplines may use the same or similar equipment with children for noncompeting treatment goals. Practitioners may observe interaction with parents or others during play. Children often offer insights into their understanding of their illness by revealing confidences as rapport evolves into trust. Engaging parents in treatment can assist with carryover of therapy goals.

Case Scenario 15

Children in acute hospitals are often admitted for medical or surgical intervention. Children in occupational therapy have many medical or surgical conditions. The conditions vary according to the specialty departments within the setting. Often children who are hospitalized regress developmentally. Illness may preclude engagement in play. Children normally and naturally test limits and explore new behaviors during play. In a hospital setting, all rehabilitation recovery from a child's perspective occurs through play activity. If a child has a burn, for example, he or she may need to maintain range of motion at the joints over which the burn extends. Having the child reach for a stuffed animal, pull a pull toy, or ride a bike can assist with the child's willingness to move and demonstrate active range of motion within the context of an activity and participate in play. This strategy will have the dual purpose of using activities to encourage movement and participation to produce a successful recovery outcome. The therapist must have a dual agenda to accomplish effective treatment with hospitalized children. Providing the opportunity to play while working to prevent possible side effects of the medical or surgical treatment that could affect their future ability to succeed is the goal. The possible problems vary according to the child's condition and its treatment.

Case Scenario 16

Not all children regress during hospitalization. Some children, despite illness, adjust well and seek out opportunities for age-appropriate developmental play participation. One therapist treated a girl 7 years of age who experienced smoke inhalation and exacerbation of her asthma when her family home caught fire. She had learning disabilities before her smoke inhalation but was experiencing some new balance problems. Despite hospitalization and a need for intermittent oxygen through a nasal canula, when her older brother and sister visited her in the unit, she wanted to go to the play area for a physically challenging game of Twister®. She played, tolerated the play well, and enjoyed the challenge. The game was not simple for her, but she did perceive it as fun and therefore was willing to challenge herself in the attempt to participate in the game activity.

Case Scenario 17

Occupational therapy practitioners have increased their visibility and standing in schools during the past 20 years. One issue in school systems is the mainstreaming of children with impairments into regular classrooms. Practitioners in school-based practice may participate in classroom activities with the children they treat. These practitioners may determine whether adaptations in the classroom could facilitate participation and assist a child in meeting his or her learning objectives in an individualized education program (IEP). Sometimes where the child is seated in the classroom can be important. If a child has a visual impairment and needs to be closer to the chalkboard, the occupational therapist may recommend a modification of this positioning in the classroom. If the child has difficulty responding verbally, the occupational therapy practitioner can work with the child and educational team to enable communication through the use of augmented communication technology, such as a speak-and-spell board or computerized assistance.

Case Scenario 18

Children who are inpatients in a psychiatric setting may have several issues that have so severely impaired their activity participation that they are hospitalized and separated from mainstream society. Childhood schizophrenia is one problem in this setting. Children who have hallucinations from an early age may not respond well to either their own human environment or to external environments, both human and nonhuman. Children with schizophrenia may not initiate play or peer interaction. Activities may assist the child in skill development, including basic self-care activities. Learning to wash and dress oneself and gaining a sense of pride from the ability to demonstrate age-appropriate self-care accomplishments may benefit the child. Learning to concentrate and to do activities from single to multiple steps is another way of teaching skill acquisition and grading activities with increasing difficulty to dually support establishment of self-esteem, work- and school-related behaviors, and socially acceptable emotional and behavioral interactions. Crafts and games can be useful tools in this setting. Sensory integration activities that challenge mobility and coordination skills are useful. Activities should be pleasing and fun for the children to encourage willing participation and age-appropriate skill development. Whether skipping rope, playing hopscotch, or playing team games or board games, children in all settings must learn to play and relate well to others and have a sense of participation and accomplishment.

————————

Working with parents and caregivers on strategies to achieve successful participation in play, age-appropriate developmental self-care activities, and self-esteem building can be a focus of treatment. Parents and caregivers may need to learn how to hold a child, how to position a child, or how to engage a child in play. Parents may need guidance and encouragement to let children participate and repeat attempts or fail in the process of trying. Many children acquire passive behaviors. They do not seek out opportunities to play or participate in their self-care. Occupational therapy practitioners who work in home care often must practice limit setting with caregivers so that the child takes the lead in self-care, schoolwork, and fun activities.

Settings for services for adolescents. Adolescents receive occupational therapy services in various settings, including hospitals, homes, and the community. Adolescents may be hospitalized in acute care settings for many reasons. Some of the leading causes of hospitalization related to trauma in adolescents are motor vehicle crashes and sports-related injuries. High-risk behaviors are one causal factor leading to the propensity for these injuries. The injuries may involve head trauma (e.g., concussion, head injury with central nervous system involvement, contusions), spinal cord injuries (at all levels including cervical, thoracic, lumbar, and sacral regions), and fractures (e.g., long bones, pelvis, spine, joints, small bones of the face, hands, and feet). Recovery depends on the constellation of the activities and the ability of involved organs and structures to heal. When adolescents are hospitalized for long periods, they may not be able to attend school and may need tutoring. If the child has sustained head injuries, he or she may have impaired cognitive abilities and may need to relearn many life relationships from a low level of cognitive skill. The occupational therapy practitioner may use graded task activities to increase attention skills and may work together with the educational staff members at the hospital and with the parents to adjust educational programming to the child's new appropriate skill level. Often, adolescents who have head injuries and cognitive impairments have impaired attention and social skills but may be aware of inappropriately presented activities that may seem infantile to them. Attempting to pace the learning experience from a skill acquisition approach may require the unique participation of an occupational therapy practitioner. Many other educational and health care providers do not have knowledge about cognitive and perceptual impairments in relation to their influence on neurobehavior and performance of activities. Developing a new personality and new socially acceptable behaviors requires plenty of opportunities to try out new skills as the child develops them. The practitioner may develop activities by tapping into the adolescent's interests to assist him or her in new role development. For example, being a collector can be a role. Acquiring a collection can be a challenge to one's memory (knowing what one has as well as thinking about what one would like to acquire), the ability to sequence or organize the collection, the ability to seek out new information by problem solving about how to find resources, the ability to communicate with those resources, the ability to negotiate acquisition terms for new items to add to the collection, the ability to manage money, the ability to recognize financial constraints, and the ability to budget money to meet the goals of building the collection. The collection can be highly individualized. Some suggestions are autographs, postcards, e-mail messages, letters from near and far, baseball cards, and memorabilia.

Adolescents are hospitalized for other general medical and surgical problems. Cancers of the bone occur mostly during adolescence. Amputations as a result of cancer greatly affect adolescents. While at a developmental stage at which persons are most sensitive and aware of appearance, the ability to sustain their lives and to get their cancer to enter a stage of remission depends on their losing a body part. Activities to promote acceptance of their modified body image can be useful.

Case Scenario 19

Finding role models who have had amputations and providing an opportunity to meet someone else who has had an amputation from cancer and who has survived and gone on to live well are possibilities. One program that may involve occupational therapists is the Achilles Track Club. In New York, the Achilles Track Club sends representatives to some hospitals to work with adolescents with impairments who have a desire to participate in track and field activities. Participants in the Achilles Track Club have participated in and completed marathons, including the New York City Marathon. An adolescent need not have been a runner before becoming an amputee to participate in the Achilles Track Club.

Adolescents in home care settings are often in a transitional stage between the hospital and the community. If they are recovering from an illness or injury, home care may provide them with time to explore community integration. Community mobility involves more than leaving one's apartment; it involves crossing streets and entering and leaving buildings (e.g., businesses, churches, social clubs, theaters, housing units, open air settings, parks, and fields). If the adolescent has impaired mobility, then obstacle courses to learn to operate or navigate a wheelchair or ambulatory device may be a focus. With wheelchairs, learning to pop up the wheels, use public or private transportation, and participate in team wheelchair sports are all possible activities. Ambulatory adolescents may require adaptations to enable participation in a particular sport. Sometimes reinventing roles may involve exploring possible activities through searching the Internet and participating in interest surveys or interviews to determine or explore interests.

Adolescents in community settings may be coping with social risk situations. Single parents today head many families. Afterschool programs often contain activities to teach adolescents effective study habits. An adolescent can develop job skills through volunteering at a neighborhood center or through volunteering in the community in jobs such as Meals on Wheels, which delivers food to ill or elderly persons. Volunteering in the spiritual community (e.g., ritual activities such as serving as an altar assistant) is a metaphysical spiritual activity and may be instrumental in the ado-lescent's worship of a higher power and community-sustaining values and beliefs. Volunteering in community projects can instill citizenship and influence value devel-opment toward the need to sustain and support the community.

Settings for services for adults. Adults receive occupational therapy services in homes, hospitals, clinics, work sites, and the community. In home settings, reimbursement mechanisms often severely limit activities. Activity choices usually relate to basic self-care or the ability to accomplish household tasks. By definition, to qualify for home care services, a person must be confined to home. Once a person has gained commu-nity mobility, he or she often must transfer his or her care to an outpatient setting. Activities in home care may focus on making the environment as accessible as possi-ble. Home-based occupational therapy often concerns self-care IADL, such as kitchen-related activities. A client at home may need to participate in meal prepara-tion activities. The practitioner makes activity choices on the basis of what the client reports is his or her habit (the way he or she ordinarily does things at home). If the practitioner chooses activities in collaboration with clients that are within the scope of standardized occupational therapy scales or measures, then outcome data can support the validity of the process of occupational therapy. The ability to engage in activities that a client chooses and that are directly applicable to his or her daily life is valuable to the client and to the other customer in this interaction, the insurer or third-party payer. Focusing on participation in ADL and enabling clients to participate again in their own care make sense from both personal and financial perspectives.

When intervening with adults who work, occupational therapy practitioners may use activities beyond concentrating on the specific work activities to include activities that facilitate skills to improve the work social environment and the work-ing context. These interventions go beyond changing, adapting, or modifying one activity to enhancing the entire work situation. Practitioners can suggest creating competitions for workers to determine how job tasks could be modified. Sometimes workers, the persons closest to job tasks, have greater insight into needed change. An occupational therapy practitioner can use employee competitions to encourage cre-ative problem solving and sharing concerning the job tasks. Group activities and dis-cussion groups are useful and encourage new ideas. Allowing staff members to perceive that they are partners in the work safety process can be a successful strategy to empower workers to appreciate their role in preserving their personal health and the overall health of their workplace.

Money-related activities are crucial to adults who want to return to the com-munity with a low level of supervision. Budgeting, writing checks, paying bills, counting change, and using bank machines are all activities that can be useful for this population. Some professionals may overlook postoperative cognitive impairments. Adults who have had general anesthesia may have mild cognitive impairments that alter their clarity of thought and memory, sequencing abilities, and higher executive functions.

Communication activities are likewise important. Can the person recall what to do in an emergency? Does the person know how to call 911? Does the person have vision or auditory impairments that affect the ability to use a standard telephone? Can the person express his or her needs? Using activities or scenarios to encourage function in various circumstances is crucial to safety and the ability to return to the community. Persons with cognitive impairments often need caregivers present in the home all of the time. The occupational therapy practitioner and the interdisciplinary treatment team must come to a consensus on a case-by-case basis concerning these issues.

Traditional purposeful activities in subacute care include basic self-care and individual or group participation in some IADL that the client must do to some degree to return to the community, such as cooking activities. An improvement in ability can move a person closer to discharge or change her or his status to a higher functional physical unit or a setting in assisted living if the person will remain within the community in which he or she received subacute care. If adult clients in subacute settings will not be returning home and may be in the setting for a longer period, practitioners can use activities that assist clients with their adjustment to institutional living. For example, reviving avocational interests that the client may have lost over time, planning and selecting objects from the client's home to decorate new living quarters, creating memory books, retrospectively organizing old photographs into a meaningful storylike context, and developing a new style are all strategies to direct activity choices for occupational therapy in context.

Purposeful Activities Support Health and Wellness

Children develop health habits by 7 years of age. Children additionally hear health messages from other children more so than from adults. Adolescents and older siblings, in particular, have a strong influence on the development of health habits. Stress can affect children and adults. One technique that is reassuring and stress reducing for children is massage. The confusion for children concerning touch is in learning to distinguish between appropriate and inappropriate touch. Having a health professional such as an occupational therapy practitioner trained in infant or child massage is one vehicle for children to learn tolerance of appropriate touch and to learn about reducing stress from an early age. If we teach stress management as part of habilitation rather than as rehabilitation in adulthood, then perhaps more children in our society would be better adjusted and less stressed. Some ways that children can receive wellness messages are through activities with their parents. Parents can learn massage techniques, such as infant massage. Aromatherapy may reduce stress. Relaxing music associated with time to slow down and cool down can support the need for relaxation.

The American Medical Association (AMA) recently held a press briefing regarding the increasing problem of childhood obesity (Gortmaker et al., 1999). The AMA's overall message was that children need to learn earlier to be more physically active. We are too sedentary in our society; thus, many children are too sedentary. A correlation exists between the number of hours that children watch television per day and their propensity to be obese. Occupational therapy practitioners work with children to develop activity schedules and prospectively to learn balanced lifestyle concepts as they grow and develop. Mapping out times for physical play (team or individual sports) such as martial arts, swimming, paired team sports (e.g., tennis), walking, running, and climbing can all be invaluable in preventing obesity. If children develop good health behaviors, they may carry over these habits into adulthood, live healthier lives, and perform at their own personal best.

Good nutritional behaviors are essential for school-aged children. In our society, many children only eat one meal at home each day. Children can hear messages about balancing nutritional choices and recognizing when to eat as well as what to eat. Occupational therapy practitioners who work in wellness programs with children teach them to select proper foods and to prepare the foods. An occupational therapy practitioner may work with a nutritionist and parents toward the goal of developing good nutritional habits in children of preschool age through graduate school. One component of this program is to assist children to learn to love their bodies as they are. Early detection of food and eating disorders may occur prospectively. Additionally, pro bono participation in children's sports teams may serve to reinforce good eating habits and serve to thwart misconceptions about starving or purging oneself to participate in one-to-one contact sports that overly focus on weight control.

Adolescents often engage in risk behaviors and test the rules for life and living. Adolescents, however, can at times accept the challenge of being role models for younger children. Adolescents can be effective communicators and role models if they have information to use to influence younger siblings or friends. This is a proactive application of information and a therapeutic and educational strategy from a health promotion perspective. Some of the activities that create risk of injury, and about which one can give health messages, are sports activities such as bicycling, in-line skating, and water sports, in which the use of helmets and protective gear can prevent death or injury. The use of helmets is controversial. Helmets protect the cranium and may lessen traumatic impact to the skull. Bicycle helmets are constructed of firm foam but do not cover the face. Motorcycle helmets engulf the head and protect the face but terminate at the cervical spine. Surviving a motorcycle crash may result in traumatic brain injury or spinal cord injury. Prevention of injuries through safety messages and instilling safety as a value can be of lifelong benefit.

Adolescents may develop maladaptive behaviors through peer pressure, ineffective socialization, or demoralizing impoverished experiences. Occupational therapy practitioners can act as positive role models and assist teenagers in developing life skills. Life skills with mentally impaired chemically addicted populations are one of the primary priorities in philanthropic funding for behavioral disorders. Creating positively oriented Web pages that teenagers can access to learn everything from doing laundry, to budgeting funds, to developing realistic and affordable leisure activities in the community can be part of life skills programming. With the dissolution of extended families, adolescents have fewer closely related and accessible adults after whom to model themselves and their behaviors.

In addition to helmets, when in-line skating, additional protective gear for the limbs is necessary to prevent blunt trauma to the arms and legs. Awareness of the surroundings in which one plans to skate and taking time to inspect the scene for possible injury hazards can be helpful in preventing an injury. Adolescents can take a leadership role to prepare and deliver safety messages while gaining value for these messages in their own lives.

Preparation and participation in sports activities have become so closely aligned with the need for medical intervention that sports medicine has become a specialty area of practice. Contact sports have a great potential for injury. Occupational therapists may specialize in sports medicine. Activities related to sports may include strengthening and coordination and strengthening tasks before playing a sport during the actual sporting season. In addition, designing and implementing the use of protective strategies can avert potential injury while engaging in the sport. Occupational therapists can design programs and strategies for prevention of injury during sports activities. Design of adapted devices and fabrication of devices from composite materials are part of occupational therapy practice. Use of visualization and guided imagery has been effective with scuba divers and other athletes (Blumenstein, Bar-Eli, & Tenenbaum, 1995; Morgan, 1995). These tools are complementary medical techniques and require further training for occupational therapy practitioners beyond the basic education and training received in professional education.

Occupational therapy practitioners can coach adolescents and their parents or guardians to explore the resource opportunities relative to these initiatives. Coaching implies acting in a capacity through which persons learn to set goals and identify or explore potential opportunities. Coaching does not require expert skill or knowledge attainment but merely the skills necessary to problem solve and provide resource opportunities. Activity analysis and synthesis and an awareness of social and cultural context are necessary in this process.

Water sports can result in spinal cord injuries, thermal injuries, and drowning or near-drowning incidents. Safety messages concerning proper methods to use when diving, boating, and swimming can be straightforward and useful. Again, adoption of principles concerning safety can influence value development for the adolescent.

In addition to sports activities, adolescents tend to abuse substances such as tobacco, alcohol, and drugs (e.g., prescription, over the counter, and illegal). A program in Boston in which adolescents received positive messages to prevent tobacco use resulted in a decrease in the incidence of children starting to smoke in that neighborhood. Some health promotion groups such as SADD [Students Against Drunk

Driving] and DARE [Drug Abuse Resistance Education] teach adolescents positive refusal behaviors so that adolescents will not succumb to peer pressure to use illicit substances. The "Just Say No" campaigns of the federal government have been effective in this regard. The media and advertising strongly influence values in American society. Antitobacco advertising has been effective in helping persons to quit smoking. As health educators, occupational therapy practitioners can use health-promoting activities with groups and persons to promote positive health choices.

Finally, teenagers can respond positively to speaking about psychological and social stress that they experience. Adults who are positive role models for teenagers may encourage them to discuss stress individually and in support group settings, such as exam or test stress. Sometimes the experience of this stress is related to other issues such as undetected dyslexia, which is a learning disability. Often, however, stress relates to irrational or rational fears. Adolescents can manage fear and stress well with stress reduction techniques such as guided imagery and visualization, hypnosis, or conscious relaxation. In addition, knowing that others will listen to your fears and support you through resolution of your problems can change feelings of belonging and value as a member of a social group or family. When adolescents do not develop skills for effective and active management of their stress, they act out. Acting out can result in violent behaviors, such as suicidal ideation, attempts to commit violence, or abuse directed toward family members and others.

As life patterns emerge and responsibilities broaden, adults often overlook their own needs in favor of meeting the needs of their family members. Adults who are parents often are so invested in supporting their children's efforts in activities (by acting as chauffeur as well as cheerleader and financier) that they do not plan or participate in physical activity for their own benefit. Adults in middle age often develop conditions that result from the development of later-life pathology.

One common condition that responds well to wellness initiatives is hypertension. Adults with hypertension can often control their condition through diet and exercise. Occupational therapists work with at-risk populations, such as well adults who want to improve their health. Setting up a schedule that encourages personal investment in one's own health can be a focus of occupational therapy. Configuring time to encourage a balance of self-care, work, play or leisure, and rest is the definition of balanced lifestyle in occupational therapy terms. Occupational therapy embraces the value that a balanced lifestyle promotes health. Working toward the achievement of successful participation in meaningful activities is the method through which humans occupy their time within the constraints of their life roles and responsibilities.

Changing habits to promote better health is a part of wellness strategies. One of the habits occupational therapists can assist adults to change is smoking. Changing habitual routines in which one may experience a desire to smoke is one strategy. At the 1999 Representative Assembly of the American Occupational Therapy Association (AOTA), the Commission on Practice recommended that AOTA support the Agency for Healthcare Policy Research *Guidelines on Smoking Cessation for*

Healthcare Professionals on the basis of a 1998 resolution ("RA '99 Action Items and Summary," 1999). The four-step process has been effective, and its application is straightforward in an occupational therapy context.

Finally, decreasing stress is a major wellness initiative. Stress can influence the development of cardiovascular disease. Occupational therapists can use mind–body techniques to promote conscious awareness in preparation for activities. Occupational therapists use some movement techniques (yoga, tai chi, qi gong, Alexander technique), meditation (e.g., guided imagery, transcendental technique, neurolinguistic programming, prayer), and other miscellaneous techniques (e.g., aromatherapy, massage, acupuncture, traditional medicine techniques). Use of these techniques requires additional training beyond the basic level of occupational therapy education. Clients may be interested in techniques that are congruent with their socialization and are in an appropriate cultural context.

Culturally based mind–body techniques can be meaningful and more comforting for some clients. One recent trend in the United States is the move toward traditional Native American ceremonial activities. Ceremonial drumming and dancing are spiritually meaningful and draw on both existential and metaphysical aspects of spirituality through participation. These activities are occupationally based and are in a context that occupational therapy practice can embrace.

Adults often are referred to as "weekend warriors," which refers to participation in sports. A high potential for injury exists when adults attempt to push their performance to the limits. Without the advantage of consistent training in preparation for such a demand on the body, these participants are prone to injury. Activities can include exploration of interests that the person has concerning sports and, after evaluation, opportunities for the person to do warm-up exercises or train for the sport.

If an occupational therapy practitioner is not competent in a sport, he or she can coach clients through the process of identifying training centers through resources such as the Internet, local newspapers, or networking in communities. The occupational therapy practitioner can assist adults who want to do more physical activity to choose sports that are challenging but within the realm of possibility. If the person has a physical condition that warrants protection, the occupational therapy practitioner can work with the client to develop a system of protective strategies or devices to allow participation with consideration for safety and injury prevention.

Selecting Purposeful Activities for a Client's Therapeutic Needs

Sometimes the circumstances of the client's or the child's condition define the choice of activities. When this is the case, the occupational therapist develops an intervention plan that includes activities that are therapeutic but may not be within the acceptable or usual (culturally) appropriate criteria that occupational therapists most often use to achieve the ultimate goal of client engagement in occupations.

Case Scenario 20

In pregnancy, some women are restricted to bed rest for months before giving birth. Healthy adults have difficulty accepting this confinement. Occupational therapists can use activity interest inventories with this group of healthy adults and design an activity program for effective time use while on bed rest. Participation in craft activities, reading, and paperwork activities can fill leisure time. When dealing with mobility restrictions, mothers on bed rest benefit from adaptive devices for ADL that require reaching one's feet or retrieving items off the floor. Avoiding excessive strain on the pelvic floor can assist with sustaining an at-risk pregnancy.

Case Scenario 21

Children who have cancer may have visible appearance issues and precautions for activity involvement. Alopecia (loss of hair) and peripheral neuropathy (both of which are chemotherapy-associated side effects) are transient, resolvable problems. When a child experiences these problems at school, other children may tease him or her and not support the child psychosocially. Children who are receiving chemotherapy on an ongoing basis may have indwelling intravenous lines, catheters, or ports. Having any trauma or contact with the lines can be dangerous for the child because the lines could dislodge and cause complications or could place the child at increased risk for infection through the line. Social isolation can make a child less willing to be in school and less willing to participate. Occupational therapy practitioners can work with these children in the classroom to adapt activities as necessary to allow participation in class. In addition, occupational therapy practitioners can assist the child in the situation to experience success at activities and to ease social reintegration with peers. Again, occupational therapy practitioners are skilled in both the medical model and in school-based practice. They are aware of and can collaborate with other professionals to determine adaptations to allow participation. Practitioners are potentially invaluable in school-based practice because of their ability to treat children holistically and to use activities that are challenging and fun to achieve the goals of classroom reintegration, even in the face of impairment or disability.

Case Scenario 22

A boy 6 years of age who received chemotherapy for his leukemia and had hair loss and peripheral neuropathy may, through working with an occupational therapist, find a new personality for himself in the classroom. He finds a cool hat. His splints that support his wrists during classroom activities are a neon color. He covered his splints with Star Trek™ stickers. He invents a Star Trek personality for himself. He writes with a special multicolor pen grip. Maybe he has a laptop computer that allows him to share information about what the class is learning each day with the mainframe computer of the *USS Enterprise.* Using play and reestablishing a special role in a familiar situation are activities that can build self-esteem and peer acceptance of someone who is different but wants to belong.

Case Scenario 23

Some occupational therapy practitioners work with children who are recovering from trauma or illnesses and who may need some follow-up care relative to their medical or postsurgical conditions. One group of children who may deal with issues of resocialization in the classroom are children who are recovering from burns. Burns may result from various situations, such as children playing with matches, house fires, accidents near hot water sources and kitchen activities, and crimes in which fire, hot substances, or chemicals are used as weapons. Often health care professionals use dolls, such as The Kids on the Block (North Sound, Everett, WA), to demonstrate the appearance of the pressure garments that the child will wear while recovering from the burn to control scarring. In addition, children may view pictures of burn scars and may ask questions concerning whether the scars will ever go away, whether the child will experience physical pain, and so forth. Once the child returns to school, he or she may require assistance from the school-based practitioner for range of motion and exercise activities to encourage mobility and redevelop coordination or dexterity. School-based practitioners may be involved with compliance in wearing pressure garments and other scar management devices or splints. Facial and hand burns can be particularly difficult for children. Peers may not like to look at these children or touch their hands as children usually do in play, or the other children may be too curious to touch. Touch in the remodeling phase of a scar can be painful. Additionally, some games may involve too much risk relative to contact of graft sites and healed sites. The occupational therapy practitioner, as the service provider in the setting who has the most experience in the medical model, may need to work with physical education teachers regarding choice of appropriate activities or modifications of activities to allow the student to participate in gym class.

Case Scenario 24

Adults who have acute medical problems may be too ill to move around well and may become physically deconditioned. Fatigue is a major limiting factor related to activity tolerance. Many hospitals have fatigue committees that strategize about how to keep adult medical inpatients active in an effort to overcome deconditioning that may result from inactivity. Some of the medical issues affecting average-aged adults include heart disease, cancer, kidney disease, hematological conditions, impaired immunity (immune deficiency syndromes), and infectious disease (e.g., hepatitis, tuberculosis, malaria, severe bacterial or viral infections). Pacing activities and developing daily activity schedules and self-care routines can be beneficial to configuring activity to avoid fatigue. Occupational therapy practitioners can be valuable team members on fatigue committees because occupational therapy includes logical graded application of activity to enhance daily life.

When persons are febrile (feverish), they may have decreased tolerance for activity. Occupational therapists can work with the person or caregivers to arrange the environment better and to provide education concerning energy conservation and work simplification. Additionally, coaching clients to maintain their abilities by doing their daily self-care can be an issue. Fatigue is a side effect of many medical conditions and is costly to remediate. Prospective intervention to prevent long-term deconditioning resulting from avoiding activity as a result of fatigue can save money and support the need to decrease the length of inpatient hospital stays.

How Activities Are Therapeutic in the Long Term

Activities are a means to motivate persons to participate in the process of living. To do activities, one interacts with others (human environment) and other things (non-human environment). Within the context of occupational therapy, activities are the tools that the client uses to acquire skills, to complete tasks, to resume participation in meaningful occupations, and to fulfill life roles. The number of possible tools is as vast as the known universe and goes beyond that to the unknown areas of life we have yet to explore or create.

In choosing activities to use in practice settings, the occupational therapist must collaborate with the client and caregivers. Through an appreciation of the person who will take part in the occupational therapy process, activity choices are meaningful in the context of each client's life, experiences, hopes, and dreams. The challenge for occupational therapists is to grow and to continue to learn about activities while remaining mindful of the client's role in choosing activities to work toward personal goals in the therapeutic process.

Through analysis of each activity and synthesis concerning how the client can perform the activity in a context appropriate to his or her life, an occupational therapist can assist the client in acquiring the skills she or he will need to live life to its fullest. Some activities are old and familiar and have great personal meaning either privately or publicly. Other activities are newly acquired and produce new meaning and life satisfaction as the client's life roles shift and he or she explores new occupations. Being occupied is generally life satisfying and life supporting. The more personally valuable and meaningful the role is that the person fulfills through his or her occupations and activities, the greater the value of the therapeutic intervention will be that enables living life to its fullest.

Summary

Activities are part of everyday life. As a rule, we all engage in activities we choose or must do to take care of ourselves, our family members, the groups of which we are members, and the populations in which we live. In real life, we only break activities into component parts when we learn them as novices or when we teach them to others. Most of us never stop to think about how what we do day in and day out frames the ways in which we spend our time. Although occupation is originally a 19th- and early 20th-century concept, as our society technologically advances, occupation will become more precious to us. Through occupation, our lives become meaningful.

Interaction with life and with others, through the process of doing and sharing, supports our feelings of connectedness to a whole. We do not need to feel isolated or inept. Regardless of handicaps, disabilities, or impairments, we can do activities, participate, and have an effect on the process of life and living. ■

References

Benbow, M. (1995). *Kinesthetic fine motor activities* [Videotape]. (Available from Clinician's View, 6007 Osuna Road NE, Albuquerque, NM 87109)

Blumenstein, B., Bar-Eli, M., & Tenenbaum, G. (1995). The augmenting role of biofeedback: Effects of autogenic, imagery and music training on physiological indices and athletic performance. *Journal of Sports Sciences, 13*, 343–354.

Dunn, S. C., Sleep, J., & Collett, D. (1995). Sensing and improving: An experimental study to evaluate the use of aromatherapy, massage and periods of rest in an intensive care unit. *Journal of Advanced Nursing, 21*, 34–40.

Feuerstein, M., Miller, V. L., Burrell, L. M., & Berger, R. (1998). Occupational upper extremity disorders in the workforce: Prevalence, healthcare expenditures, and patterns of work disability. *Journal of Environmental Medicine, 40*, 545–555.

Gortmaker, S. L., Peterson, K., Weicha, J., Sobol, A. M., Dixit, S., Fox, M. K., & Laird, N. (1999). Reducing obesity via a school-based interdisciplinary intervention among youth: Planet Health. *Archives of Pediatric and Adolescent Medicine, 153*, 409–418.

Mattingly, C., & Fleming, M. H. (1994). *Clinical reasoning: Forms of inquiry in a therapeutic practice.* Philadelphia: F. A. Davis.

Morgan, W. P. (1995). Anxiety and panic in recreational scuba divers. *Sports Medicine, 20*, 398–421.

Nassau, D. W. (1999). The effects of prework functional screening on lowering an employer's injury rate, medical costs, and lost work days. *Spine, 24*, 269–274.

Neistadt, M. E. (1994). The effect of different treatment activities on functional fine motor coordination in adults with brain injury. *American Journal of Occupational Therapy, 48*, 877–882.

RA '99 action items and summaries. (1999, February 4). *OT Week, 13*, RA13–RA19.

Trombly, C. A. (1993). Observations of improvements of reaching in subjects with left hemiparesis. *Journal of Neurology, Neurosurgery and Psychiatry, 56*, 40–45.

Trombly, C. A. (1995). Occupation: Purposefulness and meaningfulness as therapeutic mechanisms, 1995 Eleanor Clark Slagle lecture. *American Journal of Occupational Therapy, 49*, 960–972.

8

Designing Group Activities To Meet Individual and Group Goals

Mary V. Donohue, PhD, OT, FAOTA
Ellen Greer, MA, OT, CPsyA

The challenge for the occupational therapy practitioner in designing group activities is to target the needs of the person and the needs of the group. The therapeutic skill of the master clinician's activity interventions involves balancing these needs in developing individual and group goals. This chapter describes how the activity group therapist identifies individual and group needs, goals, and activities and describes the dynamic nature of the person and groups as they interact around activities. The chapter highlights therapeutic actions of the practitioners and adaptation of the group activities and discusses the role of occupational therapy practitioners in assisting clients to use their developing social skills as they transition into community settings.

Activity Contexts in Occupational Therapy Groups

Humans by nature function within groups from birth: in the family, in school, in religious centers, in sports, in clubs, and in volunteer or professional organizations. A group is a gathering of three or more persons who band together for a joint purpose for a continuous period of time. Group activities consist of tasks of work or actions of play in which individual members jointly engage. The earliest group activities for infants and toddlers include family meals and family play. Later, children participate in family food preparation, travel, and cleaning as a group.

Occupational therapy practitioners' use of activities in groups is unique. We use activities to create contexts or environments that will produce change in occupational therapy groups. The activity is a therapeutic intervention. Occupational therapy practitioners use four major curative interventions in groups.

1.   The activity

2.   The occupational therapy practitioner's use of self

3.   The group members as persons

4.   The group's process or interactions

The combination of these interventions enables occupational therapy groups to offer a unique, reality-based treatment opportunity. We discuss aspects of these interventions throughout this chapter.

First, we focus on occupational therapy practitioners' use of activities in groups. The unique expertise of the occupational therapy practitioner is to design and adapt each activity so that it meets the therapeutic needs of each client and the group. For example, if the activity is a joint all-group mural with everyone performing the same task side by side, the design or format of the mural can foster cooperative interaction across the group. If the joint activity is making brownies and involves shelling walnuts, measuring sugar, sifting flour, grinding walnuts, cracking eggs, greasing a pan, turning on an oven, pouring batter, and setting a timer, group members assume and can learn various roles to work together as a team. The group interactions in the making of the food and the end product itself can be enjoyable for all members.

Another unique dimension is the way practitioners use materials in activities. If the clients draw a mural with markers, then the occupational therapy practitioner can deliberately distribute a minimum number of boxes of markers to foster sharing, thus further enhancing an atmosphere of group interaction. If group members and the occupational therapy practitioner discuss brownie baking ahead of time, then members can volunteer for jobs that they might like to do or that they do best, thus highlighting individual skills and contributions within the group environment. Likewise, if a discussion regarding who should be assertive or who should try other behaviors precedes the role-playing activity with which members will practice listening, then the occupational therapy practitioners can modify the activity, materials, or the environment to ensure that the role-playing activity addresses these needs. By modifying activities or the methods of engaging in activities, individual members and groups as a whole can achieve therapeutic goals jointly.

Persons Participating in Purposeful Activities Within the Group Context

The social aspects of a group support a person's learning of new skills and behaviors. Learning as a group allows persons to support each other's learning styles and can foster a cooperative learning environment. Group leaders play an important role in helping group members to support and motivate each other. Role modeling and camaraderie develop from seeing others carry out and participate in the activity.

Characteristics and Contexts of Activities

In thinking about selecting group activities, occupational therapy practitioners plan for group members' needs and goals, the activity's characteristics, and the context of the group. First, we consider the group members' individual and group needs and goals. We describe this process in detail later in this chapter. Simultaneously, practitioners consider specific characteristics of the activities themselves to decide whether the activities are appropriate to meet individual and group needs and goals. Some characteristics of an activity are the length of time for completion; the degree of structure, creativity, and flexibility in the activity; the objectives of the activity; and the levels of cognitive ability, social interaction, and manual dexterity necessary to perform the activity. Finally, we consider the context in terms of where the group will take place. The context of the group includes the location of the activity's usual venue, its simulation in a center's setting, its time of day, the length of time for completion, and its emotional atmosphere of work, play, relaxation, study, and discussion. The environmental context may require physical movement, provide musical or other auditory stimulation, expose members to sensory food or chemical aromas, engage members in psychosocial interaction, or challenge their cognitive abilities.

Referral to an Activity Group

Many methods exist by which persons become participants in activity groups: by assignment to a required group, by request of the person to belong to a particular group, or by recommendation of a staff member on the basis of an evaluation of a need or strength.

At the outset, defining an activity group will differentiate it from verbal groups and general community or unit groups. An activity group in a hospital or treatment center is a group whose primary modality or therapeutic intervention focuses on activities. In occupational therapy activity groups, the ongoing discussion or processing of the interactions around the activity is an important aspect. Additionally, at the end of each activity group, the practitioner leads a verbal discussion of group members' interactions and feelings.

Required Groups

Sometimes in a hospital unit, as soon as a person is able to focus on an activity or to tolerate the presence of others in a group, the occupational therapy practitioner places him or her in a generic unit group for observation and evaluation. Persons who are not yet ready for a group may need individual intervention until they are ready to participate. In these group sessions, the occupational therapy practitioner must operate within the existing structure of the activity group program, which involves evaluating the individual needs, goals, abilities, and experiences of the members. The practitioner must treat the clients in the group as much as possible by adapting the activity to most of the group, by providing accommodations in selecting the activity, and by using methods to involve the persons attending that day. In some units, the activity group setting is a room with cupboards containing general supplies for games and arts and crafts. In this type of setting, the practitioner may invite each person to select an activity for one of the sessions that day.

Another setting in which we may expect universal attendance is in a group in a classroom. In classrooms, practitioners often assign children to groups on the basis of their skill levels or specific tasks that the children need to do. In some cases, children may need to attend special groups according to their specific deficits. In clinics, practitioners may assign adults to a group on the basis of the clients' disabilities (e.g., a cognitive skill group), on the basis of their therapeutic needs (e.g., a cooking skills group), or because one specialized practitioner is treating clients in the same area (i.e., all the clients with arthritis may be working at the same table). To maintain an interactive dynamic in these required groups, the occupational therapy practitioner must elicit the cooperation and motivation of the members through individual intervention and must discuss the goals of the group with all members present. Another strategy for involving the members of a required group is, as mentioned earlier, to incorporate the members in the selection of the activity or to ask them for their ideas for activities. In a school setting, the practitioner can ask the child about preferences for reading topics or types of games during remediation for arithmetic skills. Similar circumstances may apply in required adult literacy groups or nursing home geriatric groups. Sometimes practitioners attempt to meet the needs and goals of the group of persons by providing several activities that change daily to maintain interest and to encourage exploration of new activities.

Groups naturally influence the dynamic of interaction among the practitioner, the activity, and the other members of the group because clients must attend the groups. The activity selection in groups with required attendance may need to come initially from the practitioner. By the end of the group session for the day, the practitioner may ask the group members how they liked that activity and which activities they would like to select for the rest of the week. Client participation improves when we offer the group members choices within the group so that required attendance is not a burden.

Personal Methods of Referral

Some persons choose to join certain groups for personal reasons related to their needs or goals. They may select these activity groups from a list on a brochure or a handout provided by the center or hospital. Persons join these groups for various reasons and often have predetermined personal goals. When conducting these kinds of groups, the participants may have a greater role in determining the activities and the focus of the group.

Personal contact through conversation and friendly interviews with prospective group members is one approach to evaluating membership for any type of activity group. Even after a person joins a group as a result of some type of general attendance or screening, the activity group leader can ascertain if this group assignment is appropriate via an interview or a conversation with the person.

Conversations with other unit, school, or team professionals are personal methods through which one can make a referral to a group. Professionals can make these personal referrals on a one-to-one basis or in a group team meeting through joint discussion of what the person has requested or appears to need in terms of a specific activity group designed to achieve some individual goal. When persons are unable to speak for themselves, as in some cases of depression, stroke, dementia, or autism, family members can sometimes provide information regarding which activities have been appealing to the person in the past that would relate to some group offered on the unit, at the school, or in the community center.

Group membership criteria for self-selected groups must be clear so that potential members and professionals can understand them. Protocols and handouts explaining group goals, activities, and methods must be specific regarding criteria for group membership. Professionals often refer persons to groups with expectations about what the group can offer. When the group is an activity group, the referring professional should either speak to the occupational therapy group leader or fill out a referral form from the occupational therapy program that indicates goals for the person. In mental health settings in which attendance at groups is not a requirement, a practitioner may need to use personal contact through conversation and friendly interviews with prospective group members to influence them to attend appropriate activity groups.

Referral to Activity Groups on the Basis of a Specific Assessment

A practitioner may base a referral to a particular group on the results of an assessment. For example, the Allen Cognitive Levels test (Allen, Earhart, & Blue, 1992) leather task assessment or the Contextual Memory Test (Toglia, 1993) may assist in indicating the cognitive group performance level of a person. Allen's Routine Task Inventory (Allen et al., 1992) may point out the cluster of activities of daily living (ADL) skills that require a specific group for independent living skill training. A lack of balance in a person's time use results on Barth's Time Configuration (Barth, 1978) could indicate a need for a time management group. The Coping Skills Inventory (Zeitlin, Williamson, & Szczepanski, 1988) may assist in determining the individual social interaction abilities of preschool children. The Group Level of Function Scale (Donohue, 1998; Donohue, Blount, & Swarbrick, 1996) can assist in answering the questions "At what level of group performance is this person?" and "At what level of group performance is this group as a group?" This scale, which the authors developed from Mosey's (1986) five levels of group interaction, can evaluate whether the person and the groups available are at a parallel, project or associative, egocentric cooperative, cooperative, or mature level of group interaction skill (Table 1). Seven major factors of group structure (Johnson & Johnson, 1991) may ascertain the level of group

Table 1
Factors of the Group Level of Function Scale (Donohue, 1998)

Mosey's Five Levels of Group Interaction	*Seven Factors of Group Interactive Behavior*
1. Parallel level group	1. Cooperation
2. Project level group	2. Norms
3. Egocentric cooperative level group	3. Goals
4. Cooperative level group	4. Communication
5. Mature level group	5. Activity behaviors
	6. Power
	7. Attraction

performance: cooperation, norms, goals, activity behaviors, power, attraction, and communication. This assessment can assist in referring persons to specific social skill training groups and assertiveness training groups.

Goal Setting and the Activity Group

Before developing goals, occupational therapists evaluate clients through interviews and performance of specific activities to ascertain functional abilities and skills. After evaluating the client's performance and determining probable needs, the person and the therapist together establish therapeutic goals. When establishing therapeutic goals related to participation in an activity in a group, several goals may be necessary. Therapeutic goals may address the person's goals to work on in a group, general group goals, goals of the activity, goals set by the practitioner, and goals of the other group members. These goals are interrelated. Sometimes one goal takes priority over another depending on circumstances and disabilities. This section discusses these types of goals and interrelationships in this section, along with the process of goal setting (Table 2).

Table 2
Five Categories of Goals in Activity Group Work

1. Person's goals within the group

2. General group goals

3. Goals of the activity

4. Goals set by the practitioner

5. Goals of other group members

Process of Goal Setting in Groups

The process of goal setting and clarification of goals is ongoing before, during, and after the activity group sessions and involves an understanding of the various types of goals that exist among the members of the group: goals of the person, goals of the other persons in the group, joint group goals, goals of the activity, and goals of the practitioner for the group. Members of the group have goals for each other that they believe another member needs to pursue and that they hope the other member will pursue. The practitioner must balance all of these goals. How can clients achieve the goals through the activities? The work of the members of the group and the practitioner jointly is to inform the group of their goals and to discuss their perceptions of all of the goals to enable each other to work on and to achieve these goals through the activities. The members and the practitioner can jointly select activities that will provide members with an opportunity to practice their goals within the group. The group members and the practitioner then allow others to use them "therapeutically" as a social mirror or partner for various types of psychosocial and cognitive interactions.

In addition to individual goals that the person and the occupational therapist set before participating in groups, the practitioner routinely asks each group member "What are your personal goals in the activities of this group?" This repetition is necessary so that the person states a commitment to the goals to the group as a public contract of intention. If the client's goals are unrealistic, then the group will respond by asking the client how he or she intends to achieve that goal. Other common occupational therapy practitioners' questions are "What activities can you work on this week to accomplish your goals?" or "What do you think would be the first activity to achieve your goal?" In both questions (interventions), the occupational therapy practitioner asks the client to set a more manageable, realistic short-term goal. Through this process, the client continually refines goals by examining whether his or her goals are "do-able" in the group through the activities available.

As a client enters the group and begins participating in the activities, the other members and the practitioner can provide the client with constructive feedback about the appropriateness of the client's goals. Problems in working on the activity or with members of the group suggest other necessary goals or other goals that are more essential. At this point, the client, the group members, and the practitioner may jointly "go back to the drawing board" to reexamine the goals of the members and of the group. Previously unstated goals may now come forth, and the group members may jointly agree on these goals as important to the individual clients in the group. What applies to one client may apply to several members of a group, especially particular activities; such an activity would become a group goal for all.

Just as persons reveal their usual interpersonal styles with their family members or friends through their manner of approaching group members, persons may reveal a nonproductive activity achievement pattern that is dysfunctional when engaged in an activity. The occupational therapy practitioner is responsible for pointing out to clients when they need new goals to deal with ineffective social interaction or dysfunctional activity efforts. The artful practitioner points out to the client how the new activity goals relate to previous goals.

Personal Goals Within the Group Context

No two persons have the same configuration of needs and goals to maintain health, prevent disability, recover from disability, or adapt to limitations of disability. Occupational therapists evaluate a client's abilities and performance of functional activities, including evaluating the client's ability to perform activities in groups. The evaluation may involve examining performance areas, performance components, and performance contexts (American Occupational Therapy Association [AOTA], 1994b). Occupational therapists use various assessments to determine a client's needs, abilities, and limitations related to his or her engagement in purposeful activities and occupations (Asher, 1996; Christiansen & Baum, 1997; Hemphill, 1988).

Two important methods of collecting relevant data are interviews and activity performance. A conversational interview provides in-depth information about the client's values, beliefs, and view of the world. Therapists encourage clients to discuss their preferred activities and those in which they do not like to engage. Becoming acquainted with the person as a whole, with his or her spectrum of activities, is essential in occupational therapy. Ascertaining the person's preferences is necessary to establish rapport and a therapeutic relationship (Yalom, 1985). Occupational therapists ask clients to engage in specific activities to evaluate clients' performance skills and abilities. The actual performance of activities alone and in a group provides valuable information. Performance in a wide range of activities provides a holistic picture of the person and his or her needs and abilities. An occupational therapist, after completing a comprehensive evaluation, works with the client and other group members to establish appropriate goals for all members. Finally, the occupational therapist guides the group in selecting appropriate therapeutic activities that meet the goals.

Culture

Occupational therapy practitioners must respect and acknowledge their clients' values and beliefs. Shaping self-awareness of one's culture, beliefs, assumptions, and biases regarding other cultures and lifestyles is an essential aspect of developing a therapeutic use of self and in bringing about change in self and others. Increasing self-awareness provides practitioners with the knowledge and skills necessary to work with persons of varying backgrounds. Cultural competence provides insight that is necessary for an effective goal setting process. Cultural competence provides a knowledge base with which a practitioner can select activities that meet the cultural needs of a group. When practitioners view their own culture from a multicultural model (Locke, 1992), they have a fuller appreciation and respect for a wide diversity of cultural experiences and can relate this knowledge to activities for members of a group.

Case Scenario 1

Wanda, an occupational therapy assistant, accepted a position at a local long-term care facility with a diverse population. During a supervisory session, she discussed with her supervisor how insensitive members of the group were to cultural differences. She observed members of one cultural group making ethnic slurs toward persons of other cultures. She was upset that, by not intervening, group members may have perceived her to be condoning this behavior. She decided to implement a multicultural holiday group and to integrate new activities from different cultures. The group goal was for members to become sensitive to the culture of others and to be able to describe and share their own culture with each other. Holiday songs, videotapes of ethnic dances, and storytelling were the activities she chose to heighten self-awareness, challenge old beliefs, and bring about new knowledge of each other's cultures.

What is culture and how does it relate to collaborative goal setting with the client and to the activity group process? Culture is the result of socially acquired and transmitted patterns of behaviors. Culture is grounded in symbols, customs, beliefs, institutions, and objects (Locke, 1992). A person's culture specifies a person's activities, social relationships, motivations, perceptions of the world, and perceptions of the self (Steward, 1972). These components are important to consider when determining which goals are appropriate for the client and when selecting activities. Some questions to consider are: How does the person approach activity? How important are goals in life? How do we define roles? What is the achievement orientation of the culture? What is the predominant world view? How do we define "self"? What kinds of persons do we value and respect? All of these questions can be part of the open-ended interview.

When practitioners are aware of and are responsive to the cultural background of group members, they can create activities that move the group toward defining its own group culture. Thus, the collaboratively established norms of the new group incorporate each client's cultural norms. When clients begin to care about belonging to a group, they may set aside their cultural patterns to cooperate with the new group. Each client and the practitioner must give up some cultural behavior to create new norms that will meet the needs of everyone in the group (e.g., experiment with degrees of disclosure with cultural others, start work tasks on time).

Client Goals

Clients come to activity groups with their individual goals in mind. They may be thinking, "What is in this for me?" "How can I receive treatment along with others at the same time?" "Will I like the activities here?" "Will my goals fit into the group goals?" These questions are all legitimate. The practitioner group leader must keep in mind that some persons are not comfortable in groups. One way to create an environment in which clients feel welcome is to ask clients to state their individual goals for the group. A discussion can help clarify how participation in joint activities and group members' interactions can help clients achieve their goals. The client may need guidance in selecting the goals most suitable for group activity interventions and may need assistance in omitting goals that are not appropriate for this particular group. For example, a group member in a prevocational group who says that he or she would like to be an attorney needs help examining what preparatory steps are necessary to become an attorney by way of admissions, education, and examinations. Group members and the practitioner may suggest more appropriate goals such as volunteering at a law office. The group may discuss goals related to developing the skills necessary to complete the tasks of filing, operating a copy machine, or computer data entry. During these goal setting discussions, a practitioner must be careful not to criticize the client's aspirations and demoralize the client. Setting realistic and achievable short-term goals related to the client's desires often assists in this situation.

Exercise 1

Adolescents find goal setting particularly difficult. Perhaps they find goal setting too abstract, perhaps they cannot think in terms of the future, perhaps they associate the goals with what adults want for them, or perhaps their peers jointly devalue goals in groups in which attendance is mandatory. In any of these cases, writing a contract with adolescents jointly with the team of professionals and parents is helpful. This strategy may be essential to counteract the strong influence of their general peer group. Working with a group of adolescents who have signed contracts to achieve certain activity goals strengthens the likelihood of their adopting the norms of their new group. Answer the following questions: What are the favorite group activities of adolescents? Typical activities? Unique activities?

Group Goals

Before joining a group, each client needs information about the purpose and goals of the group. The practitioner may handle the orientation to the goals of the group verbally or with a brief handout. A written statement of goals for an activity group can provide details about the cognitive, motor, sensory, psychological, and social aims of the group. A written handout, which has the advantage of visual effect, acts as a semi-contract and has the added value of serving as a permanent reminder of the therapeutic activity goals of the group. When a client first joins a group, the group leader must orient the client to the group and explain the general goals of the group. General goals are each client's expected level of interaction within the group and the expected level of participation in the group activities. Joint group activity goals may not be obvious to group members, so the practitioner should clearly establish these goals when a new member enters the group.

In occupational therapy groups, the practitioner reminds the group of the activity goals. At each session, the practitioner states the daily goals of the group and relates them to the client's daily life. When the goals are abstract, such as in cognitive skills training, the practitioner must connect the activities regarding improvement of memory to the particular daily skill of list making and eventual greater independent living. In another example, a negotiation group devoted to assertiveness training by its nature involves defining what assertive behavior is versus aggressive or passive behavior so that all members understand the stated goal of the group.

The practitioner working in activity groups must balance the goals of individual clients with the goals of the group. As the group member enters the activity group, the practitioner routinely asks, "What are your personal goals for the activities of this group?" In this way, the practitioner connects the client's goals to the group's activity goals. After the group has completed each activity, the practitioner leads a follow-up discussion to review the group goals. During this discussion, the practitioner should ask members to reflect and examine how they addressed their individual and group goals during the activity.

Goals of the Activity

Some goals are inherent to the context of the specific activity group. For example, the major group goal for an assertiveness training group is clear from its title. In another example, a prevocational work habits group may imply a focus on the goals of daily attendance, arriving on time, and keeping to a schedule. A group involving ADL social skills implies a goal of learning how and when to greet neighbors, friends, storekeepers, waiters, doormen, and bus drivers.

During participation in the activities, the practitioner reinforces each client's goals by encouraging his or her optimal performance of each task and the completion of the activity itself. The practitioner facilitates positive behavior by using therapeutic use of self and the group process. Should a client have difficulty joining in the group's activity, the practitioner must adapt the expectations of the group or the activity to ensure that the client can participate at his or her level of functioning. Sometimes, the client's reaction to the activity may be resistance, which the practitioner can resolve through exploration during the group processing discussion. At other times, the practitioner may determine that a particular group is not therapeutic for a client and may refer the client to a more appropriate group.

Case Scenario 2

A practitioner may observe within a group that one member must temper his or her aggressive style of interaction with others because he or she intrudes on other members' space by taking their materials. The practitioner can encourage other members who passively permit the person to take their supplies without objection to work on the goal of assertiveness with persons who ignore their rights. By setting up an activity such as making a brochure or decoupage by using shared magazines, the practitioner gives all persons an opportunity to practice their goals in this activity therapy group. In another session, the practitioner can plan to engage the group in the activity of role-playing appropriately assertive behavior by asking which persons need to practice which roles. In a group that goes on a weekly outing, the practitioner can foster a discussion in an advance meeting for members to speak up to negotiate for their choice of a destination for the trip that week. If a passive member complains to the practitioner that he or she wants to go to a certain place next week, he or she can negotiate to choose the community activity location (e.g., zoo, museum, pet shop) at the planning meeting the next week.

After the client enters an activity group and begins to indicate a need either to change behaviors or to practice another level of activity performance, group members and practitioners adjust their goals. These adjustments are a natural part of the dynamic nature of goal setting. Changes in goals accommodate the contextual factors and daily dynamic needs of the group. While engaged in activities, group members' performances and behaviors may reveal other necessary goals. At this point, the client and practitioner may jointly reexamine the priorities of all of the goals.

Realistic Activity Goals

Questions arise in the minds of beginning practitioners such as, "What process can I use when group members set unrealistic or inappropriate activity goals?" A wide range of groups exists for members at various stages of cognitive or psychosocial readiness. Some groups involve persons with specific conditions (e.g., developmental disabilities, cerebral palsy, schizophrenia, depression) or specific disabilities (e.g., motor impairments, attention deficits, learning disabilities). Practitioners select activities for all of these groups with attention to the client's needs and the group goals. Both the clients and the group can achieve their goals if the activity is relevant and planned well. When presenting activities, the practitioner must be continually aware of the goals that each client has for others in the group because these expectations can foster or impede achievement of activity in the group.

A common problem in working on a group goal is client resistance. Once the practitioner understands what the resistance to treatment is, he or she works on giving the unmotivated client an opportunity to address these issues during the group activities. Occupational therapy practitioners believe that, when we expose a client with resistance to other group members engaged in activities, the client will join in as he or she sits with others engaged in the activity. At times, the practitioner pairs experienced and inexperienced group members. This satisfies a client's expertise through recognition of strengths or skills and supports the client who needs encouragement to undertake an activity.

Activity Group Intervention

Purposeful activities per se are a major tool in occupational therapy. Another equally important tool is the use of activity group process. Often in occupational therapy, activities and group process work together to meet the specific needs of clients.

Group activities are essential for learning social, play, and psychological inter-actions of a developmental nature. The occupational therapy practitioner selects play activities because of their learning potential for the individual child as well as for a group of children. Many activities are necessary in a group for the children to achieve their therapeutic goals of imitating positive role models. Aspects of the activity address each child's personal and social needs to varying degrees (as much as each child can make use of the activity).

Most work settings require that persons work in groups. Persons with and without disabilities must be able to function in groups. In groups in which persons perform the same activities such as working a fast food restaurant, working in a computer office pool, stocking supermarket shelves, or recording and filing medical records in a large medical office, persons must know the social work skills appropriate to the setting, office policy, and a particular supervisor. These skills include learning the tone of the group regarding work information, exchange of banter, and the time acceptable to talk to others around the task without disturbing the demands of the work. Persons involved in rehabilitation must learn or relearn these skills so that they are not misfits by engaging in inappropriate greetings and do not interpret remarks in a paranoid manner or remain silently aloof. Many clients who receive occupational therapy need activity group process intervention to assist them in developing their social skills.

Selecting Group Activities To Meet Goals

What are the preferred activities that occupational therapy groups use for interventions today? A survey of mental health practitioners conducted by the AOTA Mental Health Special Interest Section (Bair, 1998) indicated that the most regularly used activities in groups were training in ADL, assertiveness, behavior management, coping skills, self-awareness exercises, social skills, and time management. These activities are both realistically related to goals for persons with psychosocial learning needs and are attractive because they provide an opportunity for growth in these areas. Many of these group activities fall into the category of psychoeducational activities, and current texts about activity groups in occupational therapy discuss these activities (Bruce & Borg, 1993; Cole, 1998; Early, 1993; Posthuma, 1996). A study by Duncombe and Howe (1985) indicated that the 10 types of groups that occupational therapy practitioners most frequently offer in their treatment of group members are exercise, cooking, task, ADL, arts and crafts, self-expression, reality-oriented discussion, sensorimotor, and educational groups.

Table 3
Surveys of Major Preferred Activities in Activity Therapy Groups

AOTA Survey (Bair, 1998)	*Duncombe and Howe (1985) Survey*
Training in daily living skills	Exercise
Assertiveness training	Cooking
Behavior management	Tasks
Coping skills	ADL
	Arts and crafts
Self-awareness exercises	Self-expression
Social skills training	Sensorimotor
Time management	Reality-oriented discussion

Satisfying and practical group activities provide beginners with examples of some common group activities (Table 3). As often as possible, the skilled practitioner, in selecting group activities, combines the element of enjoyable, appealing activities to what the goals of the persons in the group require. As an approach to therapeutic intervention, therapists such as King (1974) and Allen and colleagues (1992) emphasized the need for activities that attract the group members and even distract them from the treatment aspects of their involvement.

Food-Related Group Activities: An ADL and Social Skills Training Activity

Over the years, food selection, food preparation, and sharing of food have been time-honored activity favorites of many clients and practitioners. Many clients are eager to join a food-related group. Purposeful goals of food selection include learning to make economical food choices that are easy to prepare. This goal demands the cognitive ability to know what is available, to compare prices, and to evaluate ease of preparation. Other purposeful goals of food-sharing activities include the psychological readiness to cooperate with others and the social skills to relate to others during a meal, snack, or party.

The group members may enhance the enjoyment of the food with music, decorations, and placemats. Conversations while planning, preparing, and consuming the end product can provide important therapeutic opportunities. The cognitive aspects of food selection can incorporate educational group sessions devoted to the activity goal of learning what type of diet is nourishing and appealing.

Self-Esteem Building Activity: A Self-Awareness Activity

Many versions of this activity exist, all of which build self-esteem for persons in a group, thus meeting a basic psychological goal of mutual respect for other group members. In some cultural groups, being "dissed," or being disrespected or put down by others, is a great concern. Many persons have low self-esteem while in rehabilitation and are discouraged and depressed because of their disability. In one version of this activity, the occupational therapy practitioner requests that all group members write three positive characteristics about themselves, one on each of three index cards, without giving their name. By way of introduction, the therapist can encourage the group to overcome tendencies to think modestly of themselves. The practitioner guides the group to think positively and to write down traits that they believe are their strengths. The group leader then instructs the members to place their three cards in a box. Someone mixes the cards, and another member can pick out one card at a time. The member reads the trait aloud, and the practitioner says, "Who in this group do you think has this trait?" A good follow-up question is, "Why do you believe that this person has this trait?" Then the practitioner asks, "Who else has this trait in this group?" After the group has identified several members with this trait, the group leader then says, "Who originally wrote this trait about themselves?" If the group members had not identified that person as having this trait, the practitioner says, "Why do you think that you have this trait?" In this way, answering questions becomes a group activity. This procedure continues for as long as time allows and ends with a discussion of positive traits and strengths in general, how persons perceive themselves, how we can all think more positive thoughts about ourselves, how members felt about members identifying them as having a positive trait, and how this activity changed the climate of the group. Although the major "activity" of this group is discussion, the activity meets cognitive, social, and psychological goals for the group, and persons usually leave the group with a warm, positive regard for each other.

Sensory Relaxation Group Activity: A Coping Skill Activity

Learning how to relax and relaxing in a group are other favorite activities. Some group members must learn how to relax. Group instruction in meditation to follow the breath and movement of the lungs is a revitalizing experience that persons in the group can ponder and begin to feel the rhythmic regulation of breathing by the diaphragm. In another relaxation activity, cognitive control of muscles through behavioral regulation of arm, leg, stomach, back, and facial muscles gives members a sense of mastery over feelings of tension and anxiety.

Activities that involve identifying scents and associating them with memories incorporate cognitive and sensory performance components. Such activities may involve first wrapping the bottles or cans of spices, colognes, or perfumes in paper and then having group members explain what they associate with that scent. After most of the members have talked about their memories, they can then identify the scent.

The Challenge of Work-Related Activity: A Daily Living Skill Activity

Many group members are ready to take on the challenge of work-related activities and find these activities gratifying because they meet the person's esteem needs. Completing tasks in computer, clerical, wood, greenhouse, ceramics, food preparation, and other work skills builds habits of timeliness, attendance, and cooperation. Task groups enable members to learn how to relate to a boss, how to relate to others in the task, and how to carry a project through to completion. Vocational skill groups are popular because they permit the members to experience feelings of competence in a job situation.

Music-Based Group Activity: A Semisocial Activity

A favorite activity of many group members is listening to music. Occupational therapy practitioners can structure this activity in many ways. The practitioner must take the lead in providing initial audiotapes or compact discs if the group is in an inpatient unit. In a day hospital or outpatient setting, having group members bring in their favorite audiotapes or compact discs is preferable. When this is not feasible, a preliminary discussion about the types of music members like adds an aspect of negotiation and collaboration before the practitioner brings in music.

Music can be the basis for combinations of group activities that involve listening, movement, and discussion. Art projects performed to music are two-dimensional activities that combine two enjoyable spheres to enrich and distract the group members from serious concerns. Group members can share and describe feelings that arise while listening to music. Thus, music can incorporate factors of social interaction through discussion and observation of others enjoying the music, the psychological experience of relaxation and stimulation of moods, the motoric expression of rhythmic movement, the cognitive recognition of music development and performance, and the sensory activity of listening pleasure.

Group Process and Participation in Purposeful Activities

During a group session in which practitioners use purposeful activities, the "doing" of activities may need adjustment, adaptation, or change. Perhaps the group needs a longer warm-up, a more detailed explanation of directions for the activity, or a step-by-step demonstration of the activity. Perhaps only some persons in the group need this extra attention. The occupational therapy practitioner must be flexible in carrying out the activity if the abilities of the group or persons demand flexibility. The practitioner may have underestimated the length of time to complete the activity. The activity may then need to continue on a subsequent day. Even more difficult is the need to slow down the pace of a group that wants to rush through an activity rather than relish its performance. In this case, if a group has a low attention span or tolerance for sustaining an activity, the practitioner may need to suggest to the group members how to elaborate on the activity to obtain full benefit from it. On the other hand, if an activity completely falls apart (e.g., if it rains on an outdoor ball game, or if the van for the trip is out of service), the practitioner must role model the expression of some disappointment while providing ideas for an alternative plan for the day. If some unforeseen occurrence happens, such as an emergency or the sudden illness or death of a group member, the practitioner must set aside the planned activity and address the issue in a discussion appropriate to the level and interest of the group. The group can discuss this process later by reflecting on how members dealt with the issue.

Practitioner's Role as Clients Participate in Group Activities

Occupational therapy practitioners plan their actions to ensure the best outcome for group members. Once the practitioner has verified the group's goals and has identified client goals, the practitioner selects the frame of reference most appropriate to guide the selection of activities. The specific frame of reference describes the approach the practitioner will use in presenting the activity, responding to the clients, and managing the group process. Common frames of reference occupational therapy practitioners use when working with groups include those of Bruce and Borg (1993), Cole (1998), Howe and Schwartzberg (1995), and Posthuma (1996).

The expectations of the beginning practitioner may be unrealistic for some group members. Practitioners' projections for the group members could range anywhere from optimism to bias regarding the potential ability of group therapy to bring about change. Practitioners must be aware that low expectations for group members could impose a barrier to progress in rehabilitation. Another caution for practitioners is not to become too attached to "star" clients who are successful in using group activity therapy and want to remain group members. Unconsciously, a practitioner may inhibit the growth of the client and give nonproductive messages to the group.

A major challenge of the occupational therapy practitioner is to balance his or her own expectations for the end product of the activity with achieving the therapeutic goals for the group. Poorly produced art and crafts, slipshod food preparation, and inattention to skills in games undermine the value of the activity. Practitioners who avoid intervention or omit discussion of the goals and meaning of the activities deprive the group members of the full therapeutic benefit of the activity. Both performance and the process of awareness of the group's interaction with each other and with the nonhuman environment are rich sources of recovery and human growth potential. Both performance and process should be intertwined, not on even basis every session, but over time with some proportional balance of product and process. In attaining a balance between product and process in activity groups, practicality is important. Perfectionism in the performance of the activity or the end product is counterproductive to the group therapeutic process if the group member never completes a goal. This is a lesson that the activity goals can engender, and the need for practicality serves as an opportunity to address a member's tendency to be obsessive, which is a quality of many persons who need therapy.

Nature of Interventions in Groups

As with all aspects of treatment in occupational therapy, evaluating incremental or graded aspects of an intervention is essential. First, intervention should use an approach appropriate to the activity context. In general, if an activity is work oriented, then the interventions or guidance can be of a businesslike nature. In fact, although some humor is always helpful in relaxing group members, too much humor in a prevocational group may teach behavior that may distract members from their tasks.

The occupational therapy practitioner frequently reminds the group members of the group goals and the goals inherent in the activity. For example, if the activity is a type of sport, dance, or movement, then the practitioner can remind the group of the benefits of physical activity for building muscles, increasing lung capacity, and stimulating endorphins. During a movement activity, the practitioner can remind group members of how the coordination of movement is achieving the goal of a more cohesive group through awareness of the parallel movement of others.

When a client's behavior conflicts with his or her individual goals, the intensity of the intervention must be proportional to the negative behavior and the therapeutic goals. When a practitioner has repeatedly reminded a client of the therapeutic goals, the practitioner may need to adjust group interventions in a graded manner (Table 4). For example, in a group, if two members always pair up and never mix with other persons in the group as they engage in their activities, the practitioner may need to set a goal for and with the pair to interact more with others. If the pair sits together as the group assembles on a given day, then the practitioner would initially ask them to sit near others in a direct behavioral intervention. If during the activity the pair spends long periods of time together, then the practitioner can remind them

Table 4
Practitioner Interventions in Activity Groups in Graded Order of Use

1. Ask a question about the behavior.

2. Use humor if appropriate.

3. Remind the member of his or her goal.

4. Give a direct instruction.

5. Increase observations of behavior in the processing period.

6. Set up a contract with written goals.

Carry out all the above in a caring manner. Be yourself. Use your own style.

that their goal is to build social skills with many members. Finally, in the discussion section of the group, if the pair offers to carry out the group's goal of preparing a meal the next day by volunteering to shop together, the practitioner again would remind them that one goal of the group is social interaction. This reinforces the pair's goal by linking it to the group's goal. Furthermore, the practitioner may remind the pair that being together too frequently could weaken the group's cohesion and represent the loss of an opportunity to try out new behaviors.

When interventions are not effective for a member, a contract may be necessary that outlines the specific changes in behavior that the client must demonstrate. When a more serious, personal intervention for one group member is necessary, the practitioner may need to speak with the client outside of the group.

Processing in Activity Groups

Group process is always happening whether the group and practitioner choose to focus on it or not. The elements of group process include the goals of the group and the goals of persons in the group; attraction toward the activity and the members of the group; power assigned and assumed; roles of task organization, maintenance of the group, or individual resistance to the group; the cooperation or climate of the group regarding goals of the group and members; the communication patterns of quality, quantity, and direction of speech; the norms of the group's members individually and as a whole; and the nature of long-range and daily activities. Many books have focused on the factors of process in groups (Bruce & Borg, 1993; Cole, 1998; Howe & Schwartzberg, 1995; Kaplan, 1988; Posthuma, 1996; Ross, 1997; Yalom, 1985).

Processing is the heart of the therapeutic nature of activity group process. Without processing, the group would be a social club, a team, or a class but not a therapeutic group. Good things may happen in these other groups, but the groups are not focused therapy. Processing takes time and can be emotionally challenging and scary to some, but if practitioners carry out processing as we and other authors have described, the result should be the emergence of the curative growth process (Yalom, 1985). For occupational therapy practitioners, understanding the structure and the key components of processing is fundamental to leading a therapeutic group. The processes of the group's session make the leader a reflective practitioner engaged with the group in a meaningful activity. Practitioners must be comfortable asking the following questions.

- How do you feel about what happened today?

- How do you feel about the nature of the activity?

- How do you feel about the exchange of emotion?

- How do you feel about the time you devoted to each part of the activity?

- How do you feel about the effort to achieve the goal?

- How do you feel about how the cultural norms manifested themselves?

The practitioner can ask the following questions.

- Did you (we) achieve our goals through this activity?

- What emotions did you see in the group here today?

- Can you tell the group why you wanted to leave?

The judgment of the occupational therapy practitioner is necessary to evaluate which questions are most pertinent by first asking himself or herself the following questions.

- How much can the group absorb today?

- What is the group ready to handle?

- Do the group members need a gentle or direct push in a particular direction?

- How much time do we have?

- What should have first priority among the interactions or factors today?

- Which issue relates to the largest number of members or the neediest subgroup?

- What was the strongest emotion evident today?

In engaging group members in processing, the occupational therapy practitioner should expect some resistance as indicated above. Certain groups with limited cognitive skills, such as children or persons with dementia, may need a modified expression at their level of vocabulary. Group members with limited emotional capacity, such as persons with chronic schizophrenia, need examples regarding what a basic level of emotion is. Thus, the person's unique needs and abilities influence the degree of processing of any group member.

The best way for a practitioner to learn about group processing is by doing it and by discussing the process in supervision. In supervision, the practitioner examines the group process factors, the segments of processing, his or her resistance and transferences, and the resistance and transferences of the group. Like any therapeutic skill, the more the practitioner does it, analyzes it, and works at it, the better he or she becomes at using group processing as a therapeutic tool. When a practitioner enjoys the skill, the practitioner then knows that he or she has learned it (see Box 1).

Collaboration

Collaboration is the process of persons working together on an endeavor. In individual and activity group therapy, one may view the collaborative process through a therapeutic lens to set therapy goals. Practitioners' expectations for collaborative

Box 1
Teaching and Learning Activity Group Process Membership and Leadership Skills

Teaching group process through experiential and emotional learning prepares and empowers students to experience the dual roles of group member and group leader. Instructors plan experiences in a progressive sequence that the didactic information reinforces. Instructors provide an emotional learning experience by requiring students to examine their own process, feelings, and responses to the group experience.

Learning about groups begins with the students' previous experience with groups and their biases, assumptions, and beliefs about group therapy. Students must discuss their prior experiences in groups, including taking a previous course, leading a group at work or in the community, or being a group member in therapy. Learning about therapy groups requires that students be involved in groups. Therefore, groups of students should meet on a regular basis to develop group process skills. Students should keep written logs of their thoughts and feelings. In these logs, students should reveal their true opinions about their group experiences.

Laboratory instructors are powerful role models for students. In class, instructors should model behaviors that students can imitate, expand, and change to their own style. Each class begins with the instructor evaluating the "emotional temperature" in the room to get a sense of the feeling, tone, and emerging resistance patterns (Kirman, 1982). If the instructor senses discomfort, confusion, or giddiness, then he or she should work with those feelings as the students begin their collaborative journey. Should resistance patterns emerge that interfere with the function of the class such as lateness or absence, the instructor must resolve those issues for everyone to learn (Kirman, 1982; Yalof, 1996). Every group is different and will develop unique transferences and resistances to their groups and to the instructor.

Students are usually eager to understand how to be a good group member. They want to support their fellow students, and they want to find a way to express their own individuality. A conflict may arise when the instructor works with the students to establish their own goals and the group goals. At this time, the instructor makes the shift to an observer and requires the students to plan and implement activities to meet specific goals. The way that the instructor interacts with the group changes as he or she becomes an observer who provides ongoing supervision to facilitate the students' development of group leadership skills.

Training therapy groups are not therapy groups; however, sessions offer possibilities for some members to do therapeutic work. No member of the group is expected to do extensive therapeutic work, yet some members who take advantage of the opportunity have a valuable therapeutic experience (Yalom, 1985). Activity group process courses emphasize the cognitive aspects of understanding group interactive theory in lecture-style classes that

(continued)

Box 1 (*continued*)

additionally incorporate experiential elements. Occupational therapy students should carry the language of the course into the laboratories. Students learn that, although the basic goal of the laboratories is educational, the process may develop clinical and therapeutic skills. In fact, the laboratories in activity group process will facilitate the growth of professional skills and relationships in occupational therapy students. This growth can occur if students are open to sharing and to receiving genuine responses from their peers.

The experience of being an instructor in activity group process is an exciting and challenging undertaking. Although instructors may organize and plan the learning activities in the laboratory for and with the students, instructors must be ready for any issue, any interaction, and any emotion to arise. Being open to such occurrences is part of being an instructor in an experiential course. The occupational therapy practitioner leading a therapeutic group has a similar experience. Within the parameters of the activities planned and the limits of good judgment in keeping goals of the group in mind, the occupational therapy practitioner must be open and ready to listen and to allow interactions to happen. Some students and practitioners are uncomfortable with this unknown, unstructured, and artistic nature of activity group process. The abstract nature of the course and of activity groups intimidates some learners and practitioners who are more comfortable with structured interventions. In activity group process, understanding the evaluation of group factors and individual goals as applied through creative activities provides the structure necessary for therapeutic intervention.

For the students' learning process, observing the leadership of others in the laboratory and understanding which interventions are most suitable and effective assist in building a reservoir of good therapeutic judgment necessary for the ongoing evaluation of all group situations. Leading a group activity with peers to meet their expressed learning needs of assertiveness, stress reduction, or confidence likewise adds to the reservoir of good judgment. Discussing what one sees, hears, and feels as the group processes the activity of the day together expands the cognitive and emotional contributions to the reservoir of good therapeutic judgment. Within any activity group session with patients, so much demands good judgment: timing of activity length, timing of responses, deciding whether an intervention should be made now or later, and deciding whether another intervention that day would be "badgering" the group members. The activity group process course laboratory involves the expectation that integrating the group factors during class will provide prototypes of various sample experiences that are "good enough" to accomplish reasonable goals for the day.

Instructors should encourage students at the beginning of the course and during the process not to allow the opportunity to take advantage of learning through experience in the group laboratories to "slip through their hands" because a semester is a short time in which to lay the foundation for group leadership skills. Students should hear the experience of previous students who expressed regrets at the end of the course that they approached this course in an academic manner only. An opportunity during fieldwork to co-lead or lead activity groups is essential in consolidating the group leadership skills of evaluation, intervention, and processing around activity goals in treatment or quality-of-life expansion groups.

goal setting must consider the clients' and group's levels of function. When the beginning relationship is fragile or ambivalent, establishing a therapeutic rela-tionship will be most successful when the practitioner can foster a cooperative environment on the basis of the needs of the person or group. How does this occur, and what tools must the practitioner use to establish a cooperative goal setting environment?

First, every practitioner must be aware of transference (Yalom, 1985). When a client or a group as a whole experiences a transference to the practitioner, the client experiences feelings, reactions, and processes in relation to important persons in early life, and these feelings transfer to the practitioner (Bollas, 1987; Freud, 1912; Yalom, 1985). Transference is important because clients cannot always tell practi-tioners about their pasts, but they can communicate their history through transfer-ence (Bollas, 1987; Yalom, 1985). How does the beginning practitioner know transference is occurring? Sometimes the practitioner becomes aware of a particular feeling, a pattern of interaction, or nonverbal communication coming from a person or the group.

Case Scenario 3

Celia, a practitioner in a geriatric setting, noticed that, whenever she worked with Mr. Brown (who had a reputation for being taciturn and withdrawn), he seemed to respond to her like a loved one, with tenderness and warmth. No objective rea-son for his reaction to Celia was evident because they were just getting to know each other. Celia learned during a group activity when residents were sharing their reminiscences that she resembled the woman he loved in his young adulthood.

In response to the person, the practitioner will have feelings and attitudes related to the person's transference, which is called a countertransference (Sandler, Dare, & Holder, 1995). Celia, in her collaborative goal setting sessions, was aware that she looked forward to working with Mr. Brown, whereas her colleagues all com-plained about his behavior. This contrast indicated to Celia that her unique feelings were important in getting to know Mr. Brown. Her countertransference feelings were critical in establishing a collaborative therapeutic relationship. The positive transfer-ence and countertransference condition would ultimately empower Mr. Brown to work toward his therapeutic goal of developing interpersonal skills in a hobby explo-ration activity group at the nursing home.

When occupational therapy practitioners are aware of countertransference in relation to the person or group, they have a rich source of data to assist them in facil-itating the growth of the client while he or she engages in purposeful activity. Staying close to the intuitive and countertransference feelings that emerge in the therapeutic collaboration assists practitioners in choosing the frames of reference that best serve the process of goal setting and creating contexts for the attainment of goals.

Case Scenario 4

Timmy, an energetic and impulsive boy 9 years of age, was having difficulty concentrating and focusing in the classroom. Mina, his school-based occupational therapist, was aware that Timmy wanted to please her, although he could not control his behavior when working with her. By using her intuition that Timmy needed structure, modeling, and positive reinforcement, Mina was aware of her countertransference of wanting to play with Timmy and just have fun together. When reflecting on this awareness with her supervisor, Mina chose frames of reference from sensory, interpersonal, and behavioral theory to develop a treatment plan to help Timmy gain mastery over the impulses that interfered with learning. Consistent with the frames of reference, Mina selected activities for Timmy that allowed him to discharge energy constructively, such as bean bag throws from a swing apparatus, trampoline jumping, and obstacle course play. Mina helped Timmy select specific activities as part of the goal setting process. As part of the plan, Mina and Timmy agreed that she would reward him with a star on his score sheet whenever he achieved a goal.

The successful implementation of a frame of reference relies on the occupational therapy practitioner's therapeutic use of the self (Mosey, 1996; Posthuma, 1996; Yalom, 1985). Therapeutic use of self, finely tuned, enables practitioners to understand what the client or group wants and ultimately leads to the necessary questions that help the client and the group identify personal and group goals. When Mina recognized that she wanted to "horse around" with Timmy, she was able to use this insight to redirect herself. Through the therapeutic use of self, Mina was able to ask Timmy questions about which kinds of activities were satisfying for him and what constituted a structured environment that was therapeutic and not recreational. When clients feel understood, they can tell the practitioner what they need.

Beginning practitioners require ongoing supervision and a group of peers to discuss their own reactions and feelings toward what happens during group activities. This supervision and peer support facilitates the practitioner's development of skills that are essential to the therapeutic use of self. With increased experience and self-reflection, practitioners develop skills that meet the specific and unique needs of clients. Mina, for example, was able to express in supervision how overwhelmed she felt when working with Timmy. She realized that she just wanted to throw away the rules and play with him. She knew from her professional education that Timmy needed a structured environment to control his impulses and that she was an important aspect of the therapeutic environment. Mina and her supervisor explored the pros and cons of various frames of reference and, through dialogue, collaborated and decided on a plan to use a frame of reference involving behavioral theories. Even the master clinician who is quite comfortable working in multiple frames of reference uses collaborative supervision to sort out and constructively use the web of feelings that results from complex therapeutic interactions.

Transference and Resistance

This section describes how transference and resistance emerge and how practitioners use them in the dyad or activity group. Resistance "embraces all of the forces that prevent the patient from functioning…in an emotionally mature way. It is the main form of communication of the patient's conflicts, life history and character structure" (Rosenthal, 1985, p. 167). Often, beginning occupational therapy practitioners have personal beliefs and assumptions that support a philosophy of practice that aims to empower clients to find meaning in engaging in occupations. When collaborating in a new therapeutic relationship, both the practitioner and the client bring their own unique character and patterns of response to the therapy process.

Case Scenario 5

Drew, a recently graduated occupational therapist, wants to empower his new client John to identify therapy goals independently to prepare to enter a problem-solving group at a day hospital. In the first goal setting session with Drew, John could not verbalize what he wanted or needed in group treatment. John's history suggested that he allows others to think and make decisions for him about his activities. Drew found himself becoming irritated by John's passivity. Drew realized that he was creating goals and leading John to think from Drew's perspective. In supervision, Drew discussed the pattern that was emerging, which included John's resistance to think and his attempt to try to have Drew think for him. Drew reflected on John's and his own behavior in the problem-solving group. John passively sat in group with Drew and continually cued him to become involved in the time management activity. This interaction seemed to increase John's resistance to verbalize his ideas during the group session.

In such interactions, the client and the group are doing the best they can. The therapist's actions are not therapeutic because they trigger a conflict for the client within the group (Yalom, 1985). The new practitioner can assist this situation by always asking, "What is going on here?" Drew's reflection on the situation in supervision helped him to verbalize his thoughts and feelings and paved the way for newly gained critical knowing (Irwin, 1995). Thus, Drew was able to adjust his behavior to empower John in increments grounded in John's capacity to participate in making decisions.

When a stalemate occurs in goal setting or inadequate participation is evident in the therapeutic process, the practitioner must ask, "What kind of resistance is operating in the client, the group, and the practitioner?" The practitioner must embrace resistance, which is evident in all professional relationships, and should never view resistance as something bad or wrong (Laquercia, 1990; Sandler et al., 1995). When Drew recognized John's resistance in supervision, Drew could accept his negative feelings about being a "bad" practitioner who cannot help his clients. Instead of continuing to intrude on John during the problem-solving group, Drew embraced John's resistance by not making any contact with him unless John requested contact. Eventually, John became tired of his own passivity and of being ignored by the group and the leader. He began to interact slowly with others. When Drew believed that John was ready to say what was on his mind, Drew adapted the group to incorporate role-playing of vignettes that required time management strategies for success in daily life activities. Drew's understanding of the transference, his awareness of his own negative reactions, his ability to embrace the resistance instead of opposing it, his patience, and his ability to adapt the activity to meet the needs of John and the group were all important aspects of creating a therapeutic environment.

Treatment of Destructive Resistance

Sometimes clients or groups fear the success that goal setting brings and find ways to destroy the effects or purposes of therapy. Such attempts to destroy the effects and purposes of therapy are called *destructive resistances* (Spotnitz, 1985), and they happen in subtle ways. A client may not show up for the goal setting session, may arrive late, may want to leave early, or may refuse to consider constructive goals. Another client may drop out of a group and sabotage the cohesiveness of the group, may arrive late, may monopolize the group, or may behave in a manner that drives others out of the group.

The practitioner's reactions to these destructive behaviors may form a counter-resistance. When feeling discouraged by these behaviors, the practitioner may collude with the client or group by canceling a group or individual session, arriving late, forgetting to bring supplies for the activity, daydreaming instead of listening to clients, talking too much, responding without empathy, or attacking the client or other group members. All of these subtle behaviors may occur and work against the collaborative process. Working collaboratively does not mean the group activity will always be a pleasant experience. Sometimes both the practitioner and the client may be stressed by the client's illness, disability, or emotional barriers to performance. In such cases, the practitioner has the responsibility to choose appropriate therapeutic activities. Some activities like drama games, journaling, and letter writing may allow clients to recognize their feelings. Other activities such as role-playing provide opportunities for clients to express emotions and deal with the many aspects and pressures of their personal situations (Dayton, 1994). Throughout this process, the practitioner must engage in a process of self-examination and reflection during supervision.

Practitioners often have opportunities to work with family members, caregivers, or significant others. Sometimes family members appreciate the practitioner's attention and are eager to engage in goal setting. At other times, family members, caregivers, or significant others may be stressed and expect the practitioner to do all the work. In some cases, the family members, caregivers, or significant others may want the practitioner to take care of them. Thus, the practitioner may have to cope with the multiple transferences of these persons. Likewise, practitioners must examine their own countertransferences.

Case Scenario 6

The mother of twins with developmental disabilities is responsible for coordinating therapy services and carrying out necessary interventions, is perhaps working, and is doing all of the other tasks of a new mother. With one child on a ventilator, she finds that medical procedures dominate her family life. As part of the intervention plan, the mother joins a group for mothers who have young children with disabilities. Although she attends regularly, the team is concerned with her apparent level of stress and underlying depression.

A mother in this circumstance may feel desperate about her children and all of their needs. She may want the practitioner to do something about the situation and to teach her what she needs to do. Her concern may focus on her child's needs and not on her own. While experiencing this stress, the mother may become demanding. During the group sessions, the practitioner may sense powerful feelings of hopelessness in the family members and want to withdraw from the case. Practitioners must identify these personal feelings and explore with group members realistic and achievable goals and objectives. Activities that address natural events in the home are often the most therapeutic and meaningful for these clients. Family members, caregivers, and significant others can engage in and plan for events in the home such as cooking and eating meals together, going shopping, or attending medical visits. During all of these activities, practitioners must attend to transferences and their own countertransferences.

Collaboration With the Team

Team members and the ways that they function vary depending on the service delivery model and the location of the intervention. Practitioners who work in home care may have little contact with a structured team, whereas in a hospital, school, or long-term care setting, a practitioner may be a member of a structured team with specific functions to perform. In all cases, each team member brings a particular perspective. Whether the occupational therapy practitioner is working with the team on the telephone or in a conference room, the same principles of transference, countertransference, and resistance are in effect. Practitioners meet the best interests of the clients and groups when a team functions in a mature, cooperative manner. Open communication among team members develops out of the willingness of each member to clarify feelings. When team member's interactions are oppositional, hopeless, or competitive, team members should spend time dealing with these issues. Teams that work cooperatively are important vehicles to create interventions that move the therapy forward for the clients.

Dynamics of Implementing Goals in the Group Process: Resistances

As an activity group forms, individual members initially look to the practitioner rather than each other for interaction. Progressive engagement between group members is a process that the occupational therapy practitioner facilitates through the activity selected to achieve the group goals. Group interaction among members is necessary to teach members how to help each other to meet their individual goals instead of relying on the practitioner.

Case Scenario 7

One activity group had a group goal of increasing empathy in social interaction between members. This group decided to use role-playing techniques to explore the range of possible responses. Each member had an individual goal that represented working through a particular obstacle in responding to others with empathy. One group member, who always felt left out, wanted to know how he would feel in the others' predicaments. Another member who frequently cried wanted to have more control over showing strong emotions.

These obstacles to achieving a client's individual goals are resistances to function in a particular way.

When the group presents a shared obstacle to achieving the group goal, that is a group resistance (Rosenthal, 1985). In this case, if the group began to giggle when a member presented a difficulty in achieving some aspect of performance, then the group would be resisting expressing difficult feelings in the member's presentation. If all group members arrived late to each session, then investigation of this resistance would likely reveal avoidance of negative feelings that the group could not express. Resistances are barriers to cooperative function that the person or group does not express in words.

Monopolizing

Sometimes groups do not deal with resistances, and this may affect the integrity of the group. Monopolizing is a destructive resistance found in groups because it denies others their treatment time (Rosenthal, 1994). When left unresolved, this resistance can have a deleterious effect on the group.

Case Scenario 8

In a highly functioning music group at a senior center with a group goal to achieve emotional wellness, a group member named Sam had the need to be the favorite of the leader. To gain the leader's attention, he would come early to speak with her, struggle with technique problems that would require her lengthy attention during the music activity, and talk to the group at any opportunity about his knowledge of composers. This group member's insistence on monopolizing the leader and the group created tension and disharmony among the group members. Group members communicated this with nonverbal facial expressions. Marcy, the occupational therapy leader of the group, was uncomfortable with her own feelings and the disinterest she was beginning to sense in the group. Ultimately, the group resistance in this case, unexpressed hostility toward a monopolizing group member, was enacted. The rest of the group began ignoring Sam and lost interest in the project, and the group leader withdrew emotionally.

The group triggered Marcy's counterresistance in a way that demonstrated that she was not comfortable with using her own feelings to help the group work cooperatively within the context of the activity. Marcy did not realize that she was angry with the group, and, because she worked in a community setting as a consultant occupational therapy practitioner, she had no supervisor with whom to discuss the dynamics of her group. Unwittingly, she tried a new musical activity that would curtail Sam's monopolizing. Marcy selected two other group members for a duet, thus leaving out the member who wanted attention. Although the two members selected were delighted, Sam experienced a feeling of rejection and dropped out of the group without any notice. With the exit of the rejected group member, the rest of the group felt abandoned and at the same time guilty for regaining their opportunity to interact freely. They no longer wanted to work together, and the group soon fell apart.

Exercise 1

Can you think of how you would have intervened in this circumstance?

The person and group resistances that occurred in this activity group were wonderful opportunities to explore the emotions that interfered with cooperative group function. When practitioners understand their own reactions in response to group members, they can intervene with appropriate activities that will free persons to express their thoughts and feelings in a way that will be maturational for themselves and the group. In this case, Marcy should have considered including some psychodrama activities, such as sculpting. Sculpting is a living picture of a family or group that involves the main character and other role-players (Dayton, 1994). This type of activity may have helped the group to learn about their own past roles in their families and in the present when confronted with a monopolizer.

Rivalry

Another powerful group resistance is rivalry (Rosenthal, 1985). Rivalry in groups can operate to reject new group members. Once a group has become cohesive and is working well on individual and group goals, a sense of boundary and bonding develops. The practitioner, however, is responsible for keeping the group alive with enough members. If members drop out, either because of illness, moving away, or anger, the practitioner must bring in new members (Yalom, 1985). The entrance of a new group member can trigger a multitude of feelings in the group, and the group may have a desire to eject him or her as soon as possible. The group's desire to "get rid of the new baby" is resistance when the group excludes the new member, tells the group member horrible stories about group members who have since left, attacks the new member, or demands that the new member reveal personal details in the first two meetings. Often, the group is angry at the leader for bringing in someone new and displaces the anger onto the new group member rather than risk jeopardizing the relationship with the leader. Adequate preparation of the group for the new member's entrance may temper this reaction.

Group members learn that the practitioner and each client can handle thoughts and feelings. When the practitioner handles this situation properly by embracing these resistances, the group members, depending on their level of understanding, will talk in some way about their fears of loss and desire for dominance in the face of a new member. Many group members will remember conflicts they experienced in their early family life. With the occupational therapy practitioner's help, members can appreciate this history and how it interferes with their own effectiveness in achieving their personal goals. A practitioner should carefully select an activity that highlights the group member's reactions to changes in the group. A historical time line activity can provide the opportunity for the group member to identify patterns of responses and adaptations to changes. A mural art project that involves modalities of collage (e.g., pattern, torn paper, cut paper, texture, and paint) can offer the group an opportunity for an emotional, sensory, and symbolic representation of their experiences with time for processing this aspect of their experience (Silberstein-Sorfer & Jones, 1982; Thomson, 1997).

Sabotage

Sabotage, or uncooperative behavior, is another form of resistance that interferes with goal achievement. Sabotage of the treatment goals can occur when the person or group believes a change is necessary, and they cannot find or are unable to communicate this need in an appropriate way. When the practitioner discovers the purpose of the sabotage, he or she has the opportunity to evaluate, in collaboration with clients, which goals to change.

Case Scenario 9

In working with school-age children in a private office, occupational therapy practitioners have the opportunity to set the time, frequency, and fee for sessions and to collaborate with the child and family members on goal setting. In one case, a parent unwittingly sabotaged the occupational therapy of her son, Lance, by bringing him to the sessions more than 20 min late each time. Tina, the occupational therapist, was in a difficult position because the child, Lance, who was working on increasing social competence skills, was upset that he was arriving late and was afraid to let his mother know that he wanted to be at the sessions on time. Tina, with the child's permission, invited the mother and his twin sister to the sessions. During the course of several sessions, the family members worked together on group art projects such as making masks and tissue paper collage lunch boxes with a group goal to have fun together and verbalize individual needs. Lance confidently began to tell his mother that he wanted to be on time and found being late stressful. As his mother listened, she explained that she was stressed and tired, and as a result, she found leaving early in the morning for the therapy sessions difficult. She herself needed new activities to balance the long hours of working in an office. Tina, by selecting a family events calendar, was able to engage the mother and her child in a discussion of what they could do together to resolve both of their issues.

Had the mother of this child behaved compliantly by getting to the sessions on time, the practitioner would not have explored a hidden problem that was affecting the entire family. Tina needed to address the resistance in a way that empowered Lance with his newly achieved assertiveness. This new skill likewise helped Lance's mother. Activity group process is an excellent medium for developing new skills and new ways of relating and empowering a sense of self. When occupational therapy practitioners conduct the activity group in a safe environment with low stimulation (i.e., the practitioner allows the process to unfold and responds to the communications of the members), they establish an optimum setting for goal achievement.

Transferring and Applying Goals to the Community

Clients in occupational therapy are eventually ready to leave individual therapy or the activity group. Sometimes clients leave the treatment setting prematurely because of external circumstances, curtailment of insurance coverage, or the closing of a program. Discharge from occupational therapy, whether an agreed-on termination or a premature termination, requires that clients transfer what they have learned to a new setting or a familiar setting in the community. These settings may be classrooms, job sites, homes, recreational centers, or institutions (e.g., long-term care facilities, prisons). These settings may be in a different state, county, or even a different country.

Activity–Goal Partners–Peer Collaboration

Peer collaboration by pairing one client with another is a method in which clients can support each other as they transition back to the community. With a link to a resource support person from a group, the client has the help of a peer who can troubleshoot or serve as a consultant in difficult situations. Peer support gives clients someone to whom they can relate regularly as they adjust to demands of their postdischarge communities. These relationships help to support group members for many years as they face new obstacles and challenges to the goals they set for themselves. Many self-help groups use this structure.

Case Scenario 10

A coed group of adolescents hospitalized for depression were members of an activity group to promote assertiveness in school, work, family relationships, and friendships. Each member had been working on individual goals such as speaking up, taking their appropriate share of time in the group, becoming aware of others' needs and offering assistance, controlling urges to withdraw, and resolving to engage in tasks. The group goal was to become a cooperative group in which members have their own needs met while helping others to meet their needs. Over time, the group became cohesive with members supporting each other. When discharge time arrived, the practitioner presented group members with the task of how they could support each other once back in the community. The group members wanted to maintain contact with each other and spent several sessions planning a support network. Their final plan included pairing members (activity goal partners) with each other around activities that occur in their communities. Each pair of activity goal partners has someone with whom they can go to a movie, have dinner or coffee, or just talk.

Group Linking Collaboration

Another method of easing the transition from an institutional group to a community setting is to establish a connection with the support systems within the community. In these situations, occupational therapy practitioners must know about available resources in the community. Additionally, they must establish relationships with practitioners and other service providers within communities. When group linking, practitioners work with the clients to prepare them for postdischarge services. During the transition, occupational therapy practitioners serve as consultants to the new group in the community and become an important link in the rehabilitation of the client.

Case Scenario 11

Mr. Allen, an elderly gentleman residing in a health care facility, was recovering from a mild stroke that left him with some weakness on the dominant side of his body. He was referred to an activity group in occupational therapy to enhance functional skills. After 3 months, Mr. Allen had learned to doff and don a shirt, tie his shoes, and handle all his grooming activities. He was uncertain about cooking and cleaning his apartment, and he was worried about being isolated in the community without any friends. Recently, many of his friends had died. In planning for his discharge, the occupational therapy practitioner and Mr. Allen went to visit his new residence in the community. As the practitioner evaluated the new living quarters, Mr. Allen expressed a need for a support network of activities in the community. The practitioner knew of several senior day programs that offered activity groups. With Mr. Allen's permission, she worked with the team to refer him to an activity group at a program for seniors in the new neighborhood. At discharge, she met with the occupational therapy practitioner at the new setting. Mr. Allen and both practitioners talked about the carryover of his goals to the new group. Although the new practitioner would make her own evaluation, Mr. Allen had the support he needed during this important transition to a new group in the community.

Ethics in the Goal Setting Process

The Occupational Therapy Code of Ethics (AOTA, 1994a) provides guidelines for ethical behavior that assists practitioners when dealing with the complexities that emerge when collaborating with clients and activity groups in the goal setting process. Embedded in all phases of the collaborative relationship are issues of beneficence, confidentiality, autonomy, competence, justice, and veracity (Bailey & Schwartzberg, 1995; Mosey, 1996). The interplay between ethical behavior and difficult feelings that erupts in practitioners, clients, and groups during the goal setting process requires practitioners to take professional responsibility for the therapeutic relationship and obtain supervision as necessary (New York State Board for Occupational Therapy, 1998).

Supervision: Competence, Confidentiality, and Feelings

Beginning practitioners, practitioners who are returning to the profession, and experienced practitioners who decide to work with a new population all benefit from a supervisory relationship. All practitioners must be competent in the areas in which they practice. Although a practitioner who is a beginner or working in a new area may have some insecure feelings, competence will develop over time with experience. Ongoing supervision is an essential way to ensure that practitioners meet the ethical demands of a therapeutic relationship. Supervision ensures that the competence of practitioners coincides with the progress of the therapy.

Case Scenario 12

Jane, an occupational therapy practitioner, had been leading an activity group for geriatric residents in a long-term care facility for several months. As a new practitioner, Jane had weekly supervision to discuss issues and interactions that came up in her group. During supervision, she related that she observed patterns of silence emerge in the group when one member, Mrs. Smith, stopped attending the group because of a serious illness. To complicate matters, Jane had information about Mrs. Smith's cardiac problems that Mrs. Smith had shared before her hospitalization. Mrs. Smith did not want anyone to know the nature of her illness and had asked Jane to keep the information confidential. Jane realized that, without Mrs. Smith in attendance, several group members were fragile and had difficulty tolerating painful feelings, and she did not discuss Mrs. Smith. Several weeks later, a group member mentioned that Mrs. Smith had been hospitalized and asked Jane, "What is wrong with Mrs. Smith? Tell us why she had to go to the hospital." Jane faced an ethical dilemma. She was ethically bound to honor the confidence of Mrs. Smith.

During supervision, Jane discussed that some group members had unexpressed feelings and fears about Mrs. Smith leaving the group. Jane observed that the group members never dealt with the Mrs. Smith as a group member. Jane and her supervisor questioned whether the members should help each other talk about illness, death, and dying or whether such a strategy would do harm? Although Jane realized that she must respect the group resistance, she became aware that she, as a therapist, had to assist clients in dealing with these issues. Faced with this conflict and not wanting to do any harm, Jane, with the guidance of her supervisor, began the next session of the group by asking members about information they already had about Mrs. Smith. After two sessions, the group members began to explore their own feelings about loss, and they talked about themselves, experiences they had in the hospital, and fears about death. During these sessions, Jane introduced a range of activities such as designing get well cards, listening to music, reminiscing and sharing stories, sharing photographs of family traditions, and finally making a welcome back collage to encourage Mrs. Smith to return to the group. Through supervision and guided by the principles to do no harm and to honor the person's right to confidentiality, Jane acted competently by paying attention to her own feelings. Supervision gave Jane support while she struggled through the ethical dilemma of how to maintain Mrs. Smith's confidentiality. Furthermore, Jane succeeded in her role as an occupational therapist in this situation by choosing activities that were meaningful and lifegiving to her activity group.

Practitioners must honor the privacy and confidentiality of their clients and activity groups. When clients and groups consider what they want to achieve, they may talk about sensitive issues and become empowered to make appropriate choices. Clients must know that practitioners are concerned for their well-being and will respect their right to confidentiality. Practitioners must not give into the pressures of persons who want personal information regarding their child, spouse, partner, or friend who is in therapy.

When working with clients who have a history of acting out violently or sexually, practitioners must acknowledge their fears to decide whether they can work with a particular client. Should a practitioner not feel physically safe with a client, the practitioner has the right to request that someone else work with the client. If this is not possible, then practitioners should structure the therapy group situation so that they neutralize any potential for aggressive or sexual acting-out behavior. Careful examination of a practitioner's reactions to difficult clients can prevent catastrophic incidents. Difficult clients can induce aggressive and sexual impulses in practitioners that cause the practitioner to act impulsively or unethically toward others. Here again, supervision offers practitioners opportunities to reflect on and analyze their areas of difficulty and to create alternative strategies for dealing with these issues. For example, a practitioner who fears a violent psychotic patient on a closed psychiatric unit in a state hospital could work in a space with low stimulation and with an aide always present. Feelings remain the practitioner's personal source of information necessary to understand the dynamics in a therapeutic situation. Reflection and supervision provide the means that practitioners use to reconstruct these feelings to help clients or activity groups meet their goals.

Summary

Activity group work can be stimulating, revealing, gratifying, turbulent, and curative. Just as with any other therapeutic intervention, activity group work can be challenging because it demands our intellectual and social cognitive skill and the emotional use of self. Activity group work is a complex modality because it involves adding the dimension of activities to group structure and interaction. We hope you come to enjoy using activities in groups therapeutically by observing your participants' growth as they and you support their rehabilitative efforts. ■

References

Allen, C. K., Earhart, C. A., & Blue, T. (1992). *Occupational therapy treatment goals for the physically and cognitively disabled.* Rockville, MD: American Occupational Therapy Association.

American Occupational Therapy Association. (1994a). Occupational therapy code of ethics. *American Journal of Occupational Therapy, 48,* 1037–1038.

American Occupational Therapy Association. (1994b). Uniform terminology for occupational therapy—Third edition. *American Journal of Occupational Therapy, 48,* 1047–1054.

Asher, I. E. (1996). *Occupational therapy assessment tools: An annotated index* (2nd ed.). Bethesda, MD: American Occupational Therapy Association.

Bailey, D. M., & Schwartzberg, S. L. (1995). *Ethical and legal dilemmas in occupational therapy.* Philadelphia: F. A. Davis.

Bair, J. (1998, December). Response to American Journal of Psychiatry article. *OT Week,* 10–11.

Barth, T. (1978). *Barth time construction.* New York: Health Related Consulting Services.

Bollas, C. (1987). *The shadow of the object: Psychoanalysis of the unthought known.* New York: Columbia University Press.

Bruce, M., & Borg, B. (1993). *Psychosocial occupational therapy: Frames of reference for intervention* (2nd ed.). Thorofare, NJ: Slack.

Christiansen, C., & Baum, C. (Eds.). (1997). *Occupational therapy: Enabling function and well-being.* Thorofare, NJ: Slack.

Cole, M. (1998). *Group dynamics in occupational therapy: The theoretical basis and practice application of group treatment* (2nd ed.). Thorofare, NJ: Slack.

Dayton, T. (1994). *The drama within: Psychodrama and experiential therapy.* Deerfield Field, FL: Health Communications.

Donohue, M. V. (1998). *The Group Level of Function Scale: Adult version.* Unpublished manuscript, New York University.

Donohue, M. V., Blount, M. L., & Swarbrick, P. (1996). *The Group Level of Function Scale: 18 months to 18 years old and adult version.* Unpublished manuscript, New York University.

Duncombe, L. W., & Howe, M. C. (1985). Group work in occupational therapy: A survey of practice. *American Journal of Occupational Therapy, 39,* 163–170.

Early, M. B. (1993). *Mental health concepts and techniques for the occupational therapy assistant* (2nd ed.). New York: Raven.

Freud, S. (1912). The dynamics of transference. *Standard Edition, 12,* 97–108.

Hemphill, B. (1988). *Mental health assessment in occupational therapy: An integrative approach to the evaluation process.* Thorofare, NJ: Slack.

Howe, M. C., & Schwartzberg, S. L. (1995). *A functional approach to group work in occupational therapy* (2nd ed.). Philadelphia: Lippincott.

Irwin, R. L. (1995). *A circle of empowerment: Women, education and leadership.* Buffalo, NY: State University of New York.

Johnson, D., & Johnson, F. (1991). *Joining together: Group theory and group skills* (4th ed.). Boston: Allyn & Bacon.

Kaplan, K. L. (1988). *Directive group therapy: Innovative mental health treatment.* Thorofare, NJ: Slack.

King, L. J. (1974). A sensory integrative approach to schizophrenia. *American Journal of Occupational Therapy, 28,* 259–536.

Kirman, W. J. (1982). Modern psychoanalysis of learning in the classroom. *Modern Psychoanalysis, 7,* 87–89.

Laquercia, T. (1990). Family involvement in the treatment of psychosis. *Modern Psychoanalysis, 7,* 7–28.

Locke, D. C. (1992). *Increasing multicultural understanding: A comprehensive model.* Newbury Park, CA: Sage.

Mosey, A. C. (1986). *Psychosocial components of occupational therapy.* New York: Raven Press.

Mosey, A. C. (1996). *Applied scientific inquiry in the health professions: An epistemological orientation* (2nd ed.). Bethesda, MD: American Occupational Therapy Association.

New York State Board for Occupational Therapy. (1998, August). Guidelines for supervision. *News From the Office of the State Board for Occupational Therapy,* 1–2.

Posthuma, B. W. (1996). *Small groups in counseling and therapy: Process and leadership* (2nd ed.). Needham Heights, MA: Allyn & Bacon.

Rosenthal, L. (1985). A modern analytic approach to group resistances. *Modern Psychoanalysis, 10,* 165–181.

Rosenthal, L. (1994). *Resolving resistance in group psychotherapy.* Northvale, NJ: Jason Aronson.

Ross, M. (1997). *Interactive group therapy: Mobilizing coping abilities with the five-stage group.* Bethesda, MD: American Occupational Therapy Association.

Sandler, J., Dare, C., & Holder, A. (1995). *The patient and the analyst: The basis of psychoanalytic process* (2nd ed.). Madison, CT: International Universities Press.

Silberstein-Sorfer, M., & Jones, M. (1982). *Doing art together: The remarkable parent–child workshop of the Metropolitan Museum of Art.* New York: Simon & Schuster.

Spotnitz, H. (1985). *Modern psychoanalysis of the schizophrenic patient: Theory of the technique* (2nd ed.). New York: Human Sciences Press.

Steward, E. C. (1972). *American cultural patterns.* La Grange Park, IL: Intercultural Network.

Thomson, M. (1997). *On art and therapy: An exploration.* London: Free Association Books.

Toglia, J. P. (1993). *Contextual Memory Test.* Tucson, AZ: Therapy Skill Builders.

Yalof, J. A. (1996). *Training and teaching the mental health professional.* Northvale, NJ: Jason Aronson.

Yalom, I. D. (1985). *The theory and practice of group psychotherapy* (3rd ed.). New York: Basic Books.

Zeitlin, S., Williamson, G. G., & Szczepanski, M. (1988). *Early coping inventory.* Bensenville, IL: Scholastic Testing Service.

9

The Ability/Disability Continuum and Activity Match

Lisa E. Cyzner, MS, OTR

The totality of the impact of serious physical impairment on conscious thought, as well as its firm implantation in the unconscious mind, gives disability a far stronger purchase on one's sense of who and what he is than do any social roles—even key ones such as age, occupation, and ethnicity. These can be manipulated, neutralized, and suspended, and in this way can become adjusted somewhat to each other. (Murphy, 1990, p. 105)

In his book, The Body Silent (Murphy, 1990), Robert Murphy, a retired professor from the Department of Anthropology at Columbia University in New York, described his experiences living with a chronic illness as the most challenging journey of his life. By invoking the metaphor of a journey, Murphy related how learning that he had a spinal cord tumor that eventually developed into quadriplegia affected every aspect of his life. If life is the journey, then the body is our vessel through which we experience life. The body is our physical, psychological, philosophical, and sociological connection to the world through which we strive to create meaningful lives.

As occupational therapy practitioners working with persons with disabilities, we must incorporate this multifaceted approach of considering physical, psychological, sociological, and philosophical perspectives into our evaluation and intervention with purposeful activities. In a sense, we can embrace Murphy's anthropological perspective as a way to individualize our approach. For each person, the journey is different. For some persons, the journey begins at birth; for others, the journey begins after a traumatic event. Family members, friends, and significant others of persons with disabilities are part of this journey as well. For many, the journey of living with a chronic illness is a lifelong process.

This chapter has two major sections. The first section explores each of the four life perspectives that we, as occupational therapy practitioners, should explore during both the evaluation and intervention processes for persons with disabilities. The latter half of this section includes a graphic representation of the four perspectives. The second section includes a framework with explanations about how we can help persons construct or reconstruct their lifestyles by using purposeful activities, with the belief that the process of reconstructing lifestyles for many is an evolving, ever changing process. The chapter additionally includes a worksheet developed from this framework to use in daily practice.

An Exploration and Integration of the Four Perspectives: Physical, Psychological, Philosophical, and Sociological

The World Health Organization Model

In an effort to provide a framework for health professionals who deliver services for persons with disabilities, the World Health Organization (WHO) published the *International Classification of Impairments, Disabilities, and Handicaps* (1980). Complete with definitions and information regarding the consequences of disease, the WHO publication presented a continuum (an illness trajectory) through which health professionals can communicate by using more uniform terminology than they had used in the past (Knussen & Cunningham, 1988; Rogers & Holm, 1994; Wood, 1980). This continuum is shown in Figure 1.

Impairment, disability, and handicap are all consequences of disease. Rogers and Holm (1994) cautioned that the WHO publication only defined these concepts in terms of dysfunction and did not include aspects of remediation or compensation; however, the definitions are useful and lay a groundwork through which we can begin to explore the physical, psychological, and sociological perspectives of disability. Furthermore, Coster and Haley (1992) noted that, although the WHO model is hierarchical in that each of the four components represents "increasingly, complex integrated activities" (p. 13), health professionals should not necessarily view this continuum as linear. Coster and Haley (1992) explained that, even though a person presents with problems indicative of a certain component or level of the WHO model, one cannot presume that the same person additionally has problems indicative of another component along the continuum. Coster and Haley provided the example of a child with a below-elbow amputation resulting from trauma (an impairment) who can perform all activities of daily living (ADL) independently with his prosthesis.

Disease ⇒ Impairment ⇒ Disability ⇒ Handicap

Figure 1. The WHO (1980) continuum.

Thus, according to the WHO system, although he has an impairment, this child is not *disabled* because he is able to perform all ADL independently. Therefore, what we as occupational therapy practitioners must ask is: What is the person able to do, and what is he or she not able to do? We must likewise consider what he or she chooses to do and what level of assistance may or may not be necessary.

Coster and Haley (1992) continued to explain that other models of disablement are conceptually clearer than the WHO model, such as the model proposed by Nagi (1965, 1991). Nagi, unlike the WHO model, linked impairment and disability through functional limitations. Functional limitations encompass a person's ability to perform tasks and to carry out obligations that are part of his or her roles or daily activities.

To discuss the WHO model and definitions in more detail, *impairment* is any type of loss or abnormality in physical or psychological functioning or anatomical structure. On the continuum, impairment is at the organ level and may be temporary or permanent. Examples of impairments include the loss of a limb or organ, as in the case Coster and Haley (1992) presented of the child with a below-elbow amputation. Impairments may include a temporary or permanent loss of mental functioning such as impairments of consciousness and wakefulness or impairments of autonomic response control mechanisms such as severe anxiety mechanisms (WHO, 1980). At the beginning of the continuum, both physical and psychological functioning are integrated. This holistic approach is a part of occupational therapy practice.

Disability is the consequence of impairment that affects a person's activity performance. Therefore, according to the WHO model, disability is at the person level of the continuum. Disabilities can result from any type of excesses or deficiencies of usual activity performance. As with an impairment, a disability may be temporary or permanent and may be a direct response to an impairment or a person's psychological response to a physical, sensory, or other type of impairment. Furthermore, a disability is any disruption in ADL such as problems with modulating one's behavior, communicating, carrying out self-care activities, moving through space (ambulating), determining body position, and dexterity. Disabilities may be situational or environmental (e.g., difficulty tolerating temperature changes) and may relate to particular skills or activity restrictions (WHO, 1980).

Many of these subcategories of disability in the WHO model are similar to those areas of human experience in which occupational therapy practitioners have expertise. These subcategories reflect elements of our domain of concern (Mosey, 1996). Note, however, that as we, as a profession, witness the reemphasis on and redirection toward occupation, we must consider the larger activity performance areas that a disability affects (Clark et al., 1997; Coster, 1998; Jackson, Carlson, Mandel, Zemke, & Clark, 1998; Wood, 1998).

Whether the performance of the activity relates to work, play, leisure, recreation, friendships, family interaction, or ADL, some members of the occupational therapy profession advocate that we should examine these areas first, along with considering context, rather than initially evaluating and subsequently basing treatment on problems related to the underlying components affecting the performance. This concept is better known as a "top–down" approach to evaluation (Coster, 1998; Trombly, 1993).

When using a top–down approach with a client, an occupational therapist initially tries to determine the person's ability to perform certain roles and the meaning that the person attaches to these roles. This information helps to determine which activities the person may want to address in occupational therapy sessions. Those roles and related activities in which a person engaged before becoming disabled or before beginning occupational therapy (as a result of a recent event or more chronic disability) become the focus of evaluation. If the occupational therapist determines that a difference exists between past, present, and future role performances, then the therapist implements treatment. The occupational therapist explores with the client those role performances and activities he or she wants to do and investigates why he or she is unable to do them. This aids in helping the client understand the need for treatment and what its focus will be (Trombly, 1993).

Finally, *handicap*, according to WHO (1980), encompasses the disadvantages that a person experiences as a result of an impairment or a disability. Handicap is a reflection of the person's interaction with and adaptation to his or her environment (WHO, 1980). This part of the continuum reflects yet another dimension of occupational therapy evaluation and intervention: the importance of context. Coster and Haley (1992) cautioned that some consider the term *handicap* to be demeaning in nature. We should be cognizant of the terminology we choose to use when describing clients' life situations and their ability to negotiate and to interact with their respective environments.

A Psychological Continuum: The Disability Process

Much of the psychological literature describing persons' reactions to disabilities and the processes they undergo deals with the areas of bereavement and loss and stress and coping (Carroll, 1961; Clegg, 1988; Knussen & Cunningham, 1988; Lazarus & Folkman, 1991; Parkes, 1979; Parkes & Weiss, 1983). Clegg (1988) defined *bereavement* as a state that follows an actual or perceived loss. She stated that bereavement includes changes in all dimensions of a person's life (physical, psychological, and behavioral) as a result of the loss. Persons may display their reactions to this actual or perceived loss through their own social, cognitive, physical, and emotional behaviors.

As described earlier, a disability results from a loss or deficit in activity performance. One particular continuum found in the literature specifically resulted from research related to bereavement (Parkes & Weiss, 1983). Some of the authors' research related to the bereavement process focused on participants who had acquired disabilities. Their continuum is presented in Figure 2.

Clegg (1988) described that, in life, we tend to live each day on a set of assumptions; a loss disrupts these assumptions (see "Philosophical Underpinnings: Self,

---

Intellectual recognition and explanation of loss ⇒ Emotional acceptance ⇒
Adoption of a new identity

Figure 2. The tasks of grieving (Parkes and Weiss, 1983).

Skills, and Ideas" in this chapter). Clegg explained that Parkes and Weiss viewed the grieving process as a person's letting go of one set of assumptions and adopting another set when dealing with such losses as a disability (Figure 2). Parkes and Weiss (1983) believed that a person must go through this grieving process before truly accepting the loss. They stated that a person facing a recent loss must try to make sense of what happened. The person must do this to begin to answer the omnipresent question "Why?"

Persons then move along the continuum toward emotional acceptance when they begin to feel less of a need to avoid reminders of the loss that may evoke other painful feelings and emotional responses including denial. Some persons who receive occupational therapy will never fully come to this level of emotional acceptance. For many, the process may be slow. Each person's experience and ways of dealing with loss are unique, and we must be vigilant and sensitive to a client's place along this continuum.

Finally, Parkes and Weiss (1983) described the adoption of a new identity as dichotomous, as "maintaining one identity while acting in another" (p. 159). In other words, if we believe that our identity reflects the set of assumptions or ideas that we have about ourselves, then these are the same ideas that affect our choices, our activity selections. This emphasis on choice, on engaging in meaningful activity, is central to the profession of occupational therapy. Whether using activities in evaluation or treatment to remediate or to compensate for a particular disability, the activities must be meaningful to the person. Choosing activities for treatment as part of helping a person reconstruct a lifestyle after a disability is specific to the person (American Occupational Therapy Association, 1993). An activity match is critical.

Philosophical Underpinnings: Self, Skills, and Ideas

From a philosophical perspective, the concept of figure–ground perception appears to have direct application in examining how a disability affects a person's physical and psychological well-being and essentially how a person learns to cope with the loss (Bateson, 1972, 1979; Idhe, 1991; Popper, 1985, 1994). Similar to the ideas of Parkes and Weiss (1983), the assumptions on which we operate and carry out our daily activities are part of our "ground," part of what we do not necessarily consciously think about during the course of a day. The ground is our background knowledge and is what we oftentimes take for granted. Even habits can become part of our background knowledge. When we have an event that brings about change, or "rupture," we see the figure (Idhe, 1991; Moglia, 1998). In other words, the figure must come out of the background for us to realize all that we do automatically. Thus, when a person becomes disabled, when he or she can no longer perform activities as before, the disability becomes part of the figure. A person may realize what he or she had taken for granted in the past. To try to go back to the ground is often a difficult journey.

Related both to the concept of figure–ground perception and to the idea that we, as human beings, tend to live by a certain set of assumptions is the idea that we tend to attach our ideas and skills (and essentially many of our daily activities) to ourselves (Figure 3). Essentially, we embody ideas. We adhere to the belief that our ideas and our skills define who we are. If we relinquish an idea or a skill, especially if we lose a skill and can no longer perform an activity the way in which we were accustomed, then a piece of who we are "dies" (Idhe, 1991; Moglia, 1998; Popper, 1985, 1994).

Until we are able to view those same ideas and skills outside of ourselves, we cannot begin to criticize our ideas and our skills needed to engage in activities. This fact is what makes the process so difficult: accepting that some of our ideas and skills are fallible, and often we must make mistakes to learn more about ourselves. Only then can we improve on our ideas and skills (Popper, 1984, 1995). This idea is analogous to a person accepting that he or she may not be able to perform an activity the way he or she used to or learning that he or she can still perform the same activity, but modifications may be necessary to carry it out independently. Assistance may be necessary for a person to continue to participate in an activity that was part of his or her daily life before becoming disabled. Furthermore, for persons living with chronic illness, if their symptoms progress, the level to which they may be able to perform certain activities will change. As the conditions change, so may the need for modifications or assistance.

This theme of embodiment of ideas and skills is apparent in the occupational therapy literature. This chapter uses only a few works as examples, yet others exist. For example, in her Eleanor Clark Slagle Lecture, Florence Clark (1993) presented her story about Prof. Penny Richardson from the University of Southern California. Clark

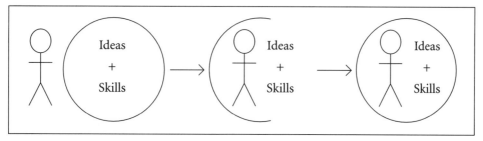

Figure 3. We as human beings tend to live by a certain set of assumptions and attach our ideas and skills.

poignantly told of the process that Prof. Richardson went through to rediscover herself, to realize how she had defined herself before surviving the traumatic event of an aneurysm, and what she would have to do to discover a new self. Clark described that, through the use of narrative, she was able to help Richardson through the process of recovery and "how rehabilitation can be experienced by the survivor as a rite of passage in which a person is moved to disability status and then abandoned" (Clark, 1993, p. 1067). Prof. Richardson made Clark aware "that occupations were important because they marked the new you versus the old you" (Clark, 1993, p. 1072). These statements not only echo the information presented in the tasks of grieving that Parkes and Weiss (1983) described, but also they echo the notion that our ideas and our skills—our occupations and the activities that constitutes them—define who we are.

Similar to Clark's (1993) work, Price-Lackey and Cashman (1996) presented information gained from life history interviews to describe how one person, Jenny (the second author of the work and a graduate student of library science and archeology), experienced and adapted to becoming disabled after a traumatic brain injury. The authors presented Jenny's use of daily activities that had meaning for her and a narrative construction to help her in the recovery process to regain a sense of identity. Like Robert Murphy, Jenny viewed her recovery process as a challenging journey. The following is an excerpt from Jenny's postscript to her head injury experience, which was included in the article.

> The process of healing and redefinition has also been a profound experience, providing new depth and richness to my life. The fact that my life has changed is no longer a source of grief to me, but something I embrace. I am writing again—not in the way I wrote before, but in a new way, and that feels like a gift. . . . I am at this point, working on a book about my experience and my journey. It is somehow fitting that I celebrated my 5-year anniversary of my accident on an archeological dig in Egypt. The joy this gave me makes it clear that I have found my new path, so I have committed to working on the excavation for at least the next five campaigns. Then I'll see what happens next. Life is, after all, an eternal process of being and becoming. (Price-Lackey & Cashman, 1996, p. 312)

Price-Lackey and Cashman (1996) suggested the following to occupational therapy practitioners.

- Practitioners must understand which daily activities their clients engaged in before becoming ill or disabled. This information is important because descriptions of patterns of activities (occupations) may inform practitioners about clients' self-identities, and this information is integral to the recovery process.

- Goal setting should be a collaborative effort between the occupational therapy practitioner and the client.

- In treatment, occupational therapy practitioners should consider both the doing aspects of occupations and the narrative meaning the client expresses regarding his or her daily occupations. By doing so, practitioners can truly begin to value the personal meaning that daily, purposeful activities bring to their clients' lives.

We need not only look to the literature to find examples of the embodiment of ideas and how persons attach their ideas to themselves as a way of forming and reforming their own identities. We can see this happening in our everyday practice, and we can see this happening in ourselves. Until we can understand this process in ourselves, we will have difficulty recognizing the effect of this process when helping others.

As occupational therapists, we must determine the type of learner our client is and which type of learning styles may affect his or her intervention and recovery process. A person's learning style may evolve as intervention progresses. Thus, creating an environment in which persons are comfortable learning and through which they can learn by trial and error, by making mistakes, and by creating their own knowledge as they begin to construct or reconstruct their lifestyles living with a disability is important. Perkinson (1984, 1993) described what he called an *educative environment* that may be helpful to practitioners. Although Perkinson mainly described the environment a teacher creates for his or her students, his ideas are applicable to occupational therapy practitioners in determining the type of treatment environment to arrange for their clients, whether children or adults. Perkinson (1993) suggested that we do the following when making decisions about the environment to help clients learn.

- Create an environment in which the persons feel free to "disclose their present knowledge" (Perkinson, 1993, p. 34).

- Create an environment that provides critical feedback regarding persons' present knowledge. (This feedback can come from various sources.)

- Create a supportive environment so that persons can accept criticism about their present knowledge and begin to eliminate errors.

Thus, simultaneously, we must question whether the clients we work with truly understand what we have asked them to do. Again, we must question ourselves and ask: "Because my client can perform a certain action while engaging in activity, does he or she really understand the nature of why I have asked him or her to perform this activity in a certain way (with the understanding that the person chose the activity)?" In other words, can we make the assumption that, if we setup behavioral objectives A, we will achieve outcome B (Perkinson, 1993)? Or, as Bridgman (1927, 1950) described, ideas lead to action; if one is able to act on an idea, then the idea appears to be true. We must be sure that, when a person is performing a certain activity, he or she should understand why and for what purpose. The person can then begin generalizing the knowledge learned from these experiences of performing activities during treatment to other activities in their daily lives. Again, an activity match among the activity itself, the underlying reasons for performing it, and the person is critical.

Sociological Perspective and Personal Transformation

Disability in many ways is a culture (Campbell & Oliver, 1996). In a sense, we can all think of at least one activity we do that the culture has defined for us, or even an activity that we may actually resist engaging in because the culture has deemed it unacceptable. When reflecting on the disability movement in Britain and disability movements in general, Campbell and Oliver (1996) described these movements as redefining "the problem of disability as the product of a disabling society rather than individual limitations or loss, despite the fact that the rest of society continues to see disabled people as chance victims of a tragic fate" (p. 105).

For a person who has become disabled, Campbell and Oliver (1996) explained that part of this redefining is a sociological process that includes redefining oneself and realizing that part of one's personal issues surrounding disability may, in fact, be political. These issues give rise to social movement. Therefore, when examining the change process that affects persons with disabilities, the change is twofold in that one examines the changes in oneself and how these changes affect society. The authors described this duality as transforming both a personal and social consciousness, as "promoting self-understanding as a platform for change" (Campbell & Oliver, 1996, p. 145). Certainly, we have evidence of this idea in American society with the passage of the American With Disabilities Act of 1990 (Pub. L. 101–336) and the reauthorization of the Individuals With Disabilities Education Act in 1997 (Pub. L. 101–476) (Bailey & Schwartzberg, 1995; Johnson, 1996; Metzler, 1997, 1998). Advocacy groups, often consisting of persons with disabilities and their family members, lobbied for the passage of these laws. This active participation in advocacy groups and other organizations often becomes a highly valued activity for persons with disabilities.

Furthermore, when deciding how to describe this change process to others, Campbell and Oliver (1996) resisted separating information and issues surrounding disability, including social theory, political history, action research, individual biography, and personal experience. Each of these areas related to disability influences the other, which is reflected in what appears to be yet another continuum regarding disability that examines changes that occur on both a personal and social level. Thus, two smaller continua are representative of the sociological perspective regarding disability and the change process associated with it. This chapter concentrates on a personal transformation continuum that eventually affects the social transformation process as well (see Figure 4).

Regarding personal transformation, Campbell and Oliver (1996) suggested that the following must occur. First, persons may deny that they have a problem. Their initial response may be to assimilate with the rest of society and view the disability as part of their identity. Campbell and Oliver (1996) then suggested that persons must be grateful and reasonable. In other words, persons with disabilities must somehow learn to balance accepting and being grateful to others who want to help them and simultaneously be reasonable and more conscious of what they should accept and even tolerate from society (e.g., knowing when to report discriminatory acts).

Denial ⇒ Be grateful and reasonable ⇒ Bearing witness ⇒
Understanding ourselves ⇒ Fighting back

Figure 4. A personal transformation continuum adapted from ideas presented by Campbell and Oliver (1996).

The next stage in the personal transformation process is that of bearing witness. This stage bridges the personal and societal transformations, including the act of sharing experiences with others (especially persons who have encountered similar problems), including societal issues. We can see how activities such as this may become vital for clients with whom we work to help them establish resources and to help them reestablish connections with their world. Frequently, others with similar disabilities teach clients the most, including information regarding which type of wheelchair lift to install in a van or which grocery store is the most easily accessible and accommodating to persons with disabilities.

Next along this continuum, persons with disabilities must learn to understand themselves and learn to differentiate what Campbell and Oliver (1996) believed is the difference between one's own personal problems and problems resulting from a disabling society. Finally, these authors suggested that persons can fight back, especially against the stereotypes in society. Fighting back involves rejecting what one believes is the dominant disabling culture, getting involved in "cultural production" (e.g., the arts) as a way to express what has happened to the person in his or her life, and engaging in political practice by becoming involved in political organizations and increasing empowerment. Speaking from personal experience, Campbell and Oliver (1996) described their journey, like many others, as difficult ones.

When reflecting on the four life perspectives that affect activity performance for persons with disabilities, we see that parallels exist between them. The perspectives overlap in the information presented regarding the change processes that take place in the person and the fact that these processes occur simultaneously. Changes occur within oneself and within one's environment. We can then view disability sociologically as a "gap between a person's capabilities and the demands of the environment" (Committee on a National Agenda for the Prevention of Disabilities, 1991, p. 1). Thus, to begin to examine how to help persons construct or reconstruct their lifestyles by using activities, we must consider information from all four of these perspectives. We can obtain this information in many ways, most often through clinical interviews with the person, his or her family members, significant others, and caregivers. What becomes an overriding theme for our activity reasoning process is that we must continually ask ourselves the question at the beginning of this chapter: What is the person able to do, and what is he or she not able to do regarding his or her activity performance? This is represented by *A* in Figure 5 (*B, C, D,* and *E* represent the physical, psychological, philosophical, and sociological perspectives, respectively). What we may consider includes but is certainly not limited to a person's resources, background knowledge, level of assistance needed, understanding what he or she is able to do, and level of motivation. As always, for each person, his or her experiences, feelings, and life situations will be unique.

A Framework: Helping Clients Construct and Reconstruct Their Lifestyles By Using Activities

According to the philosopher Karl Popper (1985, 1994), for human beings to learn, we must criticize our ideas and look for errors. Essentially, we often learn best through the process of trial and error and by making mistakes. Criticizing our own ideas or making guesses about other ways in which to solve problems is difficult when we are accustomed to addressing problems in a certain manner. Thus, Popper (1985,

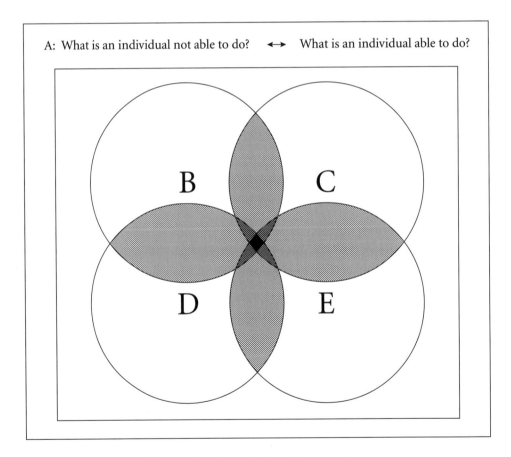

Figure 5. Integration of the continua from the four life perspectives.

1994) described one way in which we can learn more (and gain knowledge) about how to address our problems: accepting the idea that a true solution may never exist. Popper explained that, once we have identified a problem, we should make guesses about how we can address these problems and then criticize each of these guesses. By discovering problems, we advance knowledge. The metaphor of the staircase for Popper's ideas, as described by Greg Moglia (personal communication, June 1, 1998), allows us to go through a process of presentation or description of the problem, make a guess, criticize the guess, and make a better guess. This process continues and evolves with each level of the staircase. Thus, by ascending this knowledge staircase, as we are able to see our mistakes, take on deeper problems, and develop better guesses. No finite end exists, only the process to make better guesses (Moglia, 1997; Popper, 1985, 1994).

The occupational therapy reflective staircase illustrates this process (Figure 6). When we are near the top level of the staircase, we may reach the point at which we must reframe the problem. What we thought was the original problem either resolved or changed, or perhaps deeper problems existed within the original problem (Schön, 1983). An example of this is that, once initiating treatment, we begin to realize that a person's depression is affecting physical activity performance more than we had believed on initial evaluation. Thus, we may need to address the depression before continuing treatment or concurrently with treatment, or we may need the help of other professionals who may be able to assist the person in addressing this problem.

As occupational therapy practitioners working with persons with disabilities, this process appears similar to our clinical reasoning process. When thinking about how to use activities to help persons with disabilities construct or reconstruct their lifestyles, the incorporation of this staircase and essentially the process of analysis (of the problem) and synthesis (making guesses to arrive at possible ways to address the problem) appear applicable and useful.

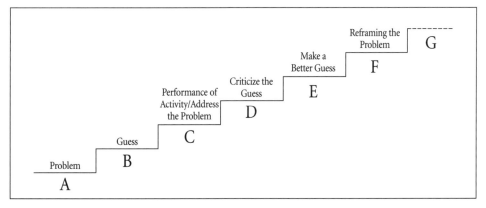

Figure 6. The occupational therapy reflective staircase: adapting and integrating the ideas of Moglia (1997, 1998), Popper (1985, 1994), and Schön (1983) for practice.

Using the Staircase in Clinical Practice: The Process

Problem

As part of the evaluation process, we may ask several questions regarding the person's current and past level of activity performance. Essentially, the information we, as occupational therapists, are seeking both through interview and observation of activity performance is: What is the person able or not able to do? More specifically, what does the person identify as a problem related to activity performance that is interfering with his or her ability to function as independently as possible (on the basis of the activity that he or she has chosen)? What does the caregiver identify as a problem related to activity performance? What purpose does the activity serve? For example, is the activity part of the person's daily routine, is it a leisure activity, or is it an activity that aids the caregiver in assisting the person? For each person, the focus will be different. Having a clear description and understanding what the problem is before proceeding with the rest of the process is important.

Case Scenarios

Consider the following two brief case scenarios. Embedded within them are problems we may choose to address as part of helping these persons construct and or reconstruct their lifestyles with activities. More than likely, we would need more information to develop a complete intervention plan. However, these scenarios may begin to stimulate your thinking.

After reading the case scenarios, ask yourself: What is one potential problem related to activity performance that occupational therapy could address? What other information could an occupational therapist need? Then describe the problem in your own words. (See the worksheet in the Appendix of this chapter for more guidance.)

Case Scenario 1

Mr. Johnson is a man 28 years of age who recently developed paraplegia after a motor vehicle crash. Before his accident, he was a manager of a local business supply store. His physiatrist referred him to inpatient occupational therapy now that he is stabilized; thus, he can safely participate in a rehabilitation program. During an interview, Mr. Johnson relates that he lives alone and plans on returning to his apartment on discharge. His nearest relatives are 400 miles away. On weekends, close friends and family members have been visiting him in the hospital. His initial requests during the occupational therapy evaluation are that he wants to be able to dress himself and to bathe himself. At this time, he is completely reliant on others to carry out these daily living tasks for him. Furthermore, later in the interview, Mr. Johnson describes that he was a member of a men's sports league before his crash and that he has enjoyed competitive sports since childhood.

Case Scenario 2

Karen is a girl 5 years of age who attends public school in a regular education classroom. On initial evaluation, you determine that she is sensory defensive. (Sensory defensiveness is a defensive reaction to sensations that most persons do not consider noxious [Wilbarger & Wilbarger, 1991, 1997].) Her prekindergarten teacher initially referred her to you, the school occupational therapist. Her teacher reported that Karen refuses to participate in most of the daily activities in which the children engage such as arts and crafts and snack preparation and that she becomes upset (e.g., crying, running around the room attempting to find a place to hide) when she sees that she may have to touch any type of "messy" materials such as glue or cookie dough. In addition, she is quite fearful of playing on any moving playground equipment, which results in her playing alone during recess. She has difficulty making friends. Her mother relates to you that Karen is unable to do many self-care activities independently, such as buttoning her shirt. You additionally notice that Karen has a weak grasp when drawing with crayons, and Karen herself tells you that, when she grows up, she wants to be an artist.

Guess

To begin to make a guess about how to address these problems, your initial question at this point in the process is: What is constraining activity performance? Similar to using a top–down approach, after determining the meaning attached to a person's activities and roles, we must explore with the person (or the caregiver) the possibilities regarding why he or she is unable to carry out certain activities. This process helps to form the focus on treatment (Trombly, 1993). We can use several guesses or strategies concerning how to address the problem related to activity performance. For example, we may choose to modify the activity itself, provide adaptive equipment, modify the environment, or provide physical assistance to help someone perform an activity that he or she has identified.

Exercise 1

Considering the two case studies, think about what some of your possible guesses would be to address these problems. Again, remember that no one correct guess exists and that several ways may exist to address the problem. In addition, when comparing the two scenarios, other issues may affect your thinking such as Mr. Johnson appearing concerned with reconstructing certain activities that were part of his lifestyle before the crash. For a child like Karen, however, she has never constructed certain lifestyle activities because of her sensory defensiveness. For example, because she has avoided touching many objects, the musculature in her hands may not be fully developed, which would affect her fine motor performance and choice of fine motor activities.

Performance of the Activity (Address the Problem)

We must observe clients performing the activity to determine whether the guess we made regarding the problem was appropriate. Thus, we can reflect on the performance to move to the next step of criticizing our guess.

Criticize the Guess

This step in the process is crucial in helping the person construct or reconstruct his or her lifestyle with activities because this is the point along the staircase in which he or she may see "the figure" (as described earlier in this chapter) of what he or she is still not able to do as a result of the disability.

Furthermore, if the person made errors during the performance of the activity, allow the person to see the error (Popper, 1994) to help him or her gain knowledge from the performance. As occupational therapy practitioners, we can gain valuable knowledge by looking at our guess, attempting to determine why it was appropriate or not, and why it worked or did not work in addressing the problem.

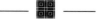

Exercise 2

Think about how you would provide feedback regarding errors or mistakes for both Mr. Johnson and Karen during their activity performances. For example, if Mr. Johnson attempted to use adaptive equipment during a dressing activity and used it in such a way that he seemed to be expending too much energy, how would you make him aware of this? How could you use the activity as an element of change in helping him to incorporate energy conservation techniques into his lifestyle? For Karen, if she continues to use a weak or incorrect grasp with her pencil or crayons, how will you make her aware of this? Because she is sensitive to touch, will you physically cue her to place her fingers differently on the shaft of the pencil, or will you devise other cueing systems such as modeling the grasp so that she can visually monitor the change necessary for more successful activity performance?

Make a Better Guess

Making a better guess involves several issues. Perhaps the activity you selected was appropriate for an initial treatment activity (i.e., the activity was within the person's capabilities with or without modifications), but the conditions (e.g., amount of time needed for performance of the activity in its entirety) or the context in which the person performed the activity may need changing or modification as well. Maybe a different but related activity would better match the person's or caregiver's current needs. Only through making these better guesses can we move persons along the staircase so that they can continue to construct or reconstruct their lifestyles.

Reframe the Problem

This process is continuous and evolves over time. However, when guesses still do not seem to be effective, we may need to reflect on all that we have done and reframe the problem (Schön, 1983). The original problem we chose to address may in fact not be the one we needed to address first to bring about change. As professionals, we must ask ourselves questions and reflect on the following ideas.

■ Is the person only physically unable to perform the activity (or elements of a larger activity), or are other life perspectives affecting performance?

■ Considering the question above, we could then ask ourselves: Are there underlying reasons why he or she cannot perform the activity (e.g., level of motivation, difficulty reaching an emotional level of acceptance of his or her disability, or difficulty separating ideas from self to learn).

■ Perhaps the underlying problem is in the environment or the objects used in the activity and not in the person's physical or psychological capabilities.

■ Perhaps the person can perform one element of the activity, so the problem now becomes the next element, which is making the activity more complex.

Summary

Together, we have taken the journey through learning how we must consider the four life perspectives and how these perspectives can affect persons with disabilities and the activity choices they make in their lives. The occupational therapy reflective staircase, which involves the process of problem, guess, performance of activity, criticizing the guess, making a better guess, and reframing the problem, can help guide us as we learn to help persons construct or reconstruct their lifestyles with activities.

> We can bestow a meaning upon our lives through our work, through our active conduct, through our whole way of life, and through the attitude we adopt towards our friends and our fellow men and towards the world. . . . In this way the quest for the meaning of life turns into an ethical question—the question "What tasks can I set myself in order to make my life meaningful?" (Popper, 1994, p. 138–139) ■

Appendix
Constructing and Reconstructing Lifestyles With Activities:
The Occupational Therapy Reflective Staircase Worksheet

Name:

Age:

Brief activity history:

Concerns, needs, wants, or priorities of the person that could guide evaluation and treatment related to activity performance:

Concerns, needs, wants, or priorities of the caregivers and significant others involved that could guide evaluation and treatment related to activity performance:

Additional notes (e.g., medical precautions, disposition plans, contexts in which the person performs the activities, other factors that may affect activity performance):

Problem (related to the activity chosen with the person):

Guess:

Performance of the activity to address the problem:

Criticize the guess:

Make a better guess:

Reframe the problem if necessary:

References

American Occupational Therapy Association. (1993). Position Paper: Purposeful activity. *American Journal of Occupational Therapy, 51,* 864–866.

Bailey, D. M., & Schwartzberg, S. L. (1995). Section 504 and Americans With Disabilities Act. In *Ethical and legal dilemmas in occupational therapy* (pp. 31–54). Philadelphia: F. A. Davis.

Bateson, G. (1972). *Steps to an ecology of mind.* San Francisco: Chandler.

Bateson, G. (1979). *Mind and nature: A necessary unity.* New York: Dutton.

Bridgman, P. W. (1927). *The logic of modern physics.* New York: Macmillan.

Bridgman, P. W. (1950). *Reflections of a physicist.* New York: Philosophical Library.

Campbell, J., & Oliver, M. (1996). *Disability politics: Understanding our past, changing our future.* London: Routledge.

Carroll, T. J. (1961). *Blindness: What it is, what it does, and how to live with it.* Boston: Little, Brown.

Clark, F. (1993). Occupation embedded in a real life: Interweaving occupational science and occupational therapy, 1993 Eleanor Clark Slagle lecture. *American Journal of Occupational Therapy, 47,* 1067–1078.

Clark, F., Azen, S. P., Zemke, R., Jackson, J., Carlson, M., Mandel, D., Hay, J., Josephson, K., Cherry, B., Hessel, C., Palmer, J., & Lipson, L. (1997). Occupational therapy for independent-living older adults: A randomized controlled study. *JAMA, 278,* 1321–1326.

Clegg, F. (1988). Bereavement. In S. Fisher & J. Reason (Eds.), *Handbook of life stress, cognition, and health* (pp. 61–78). Chichester, UK: Wiley.

Committee on a National Agenda for the Prevention of Disabilities. (1991). Executive summary. In A. M. Pope & A. R. Tarlov (Eds.), *Disability in America* (pp. 1–31). Washington, DC: National Academy Press.

Coster, W. (1998). Occupation-centered assessment of children. *American Journal of Occupational Therapy, 52,* 337–344.

Coster, W. J., & Haley, S. M. (1992). Conceptualization and measurement of disablement in infants and young children. *Infants and Young Children, 4,* 11–22.

ldhe, D. (1991). *Instrumental realism: The interface between philosophy of science and philosophy of technology.* Bloomington, IN: Indiana University Press.

Jackson, J., Carlson, M., Mandel, D., Zemke, R., & Clark, F. (1998). Occupation in lifestyle redesign: The Well Elderly Study occupational therapy program. *American Journal of Occupational Therapy, 52,* 326–336.

Johnson, J. (1996). School-based occupational therapy. In J. Case-Smith, A. S. Allen, & P. N. Pratt (Eds.), *Occupational therapy for children* (3rd ed., pp. 693–716). St. Louis: Mosby.

Knussen, C., & Cunningham, C. C. (1988). Stress, disability, and handicap. In S. Fisher & J. Reason (Eds.), *Handbook of life stress, cognition, and health* (pp. 335–350). Chichester, UK: Wiley.

Lazarus, R. S., & Folkman, S. (1991). The concept of coping. In A. Monat & R. S. Lazarus (Eds.), *Stress and coping: An anthology* (3rd ed., pp. 189–206). New York: Columbia University Press.

Metzler, C. (1997, July). A better idea. *OT Week, 11,* 14–15.

Metzler, C. (1998, February). Key issues in idea. *OT Week, 12,* 10.

Moglia, G. (1997, September). *Philosophy of scientific inquiry.* Lecture notes from New York University.

Moglia, G. (1998, April). *Science and the professions.* Lecture notes from New York University.

Mosey, A. C. (1996). *Applied scientific inquiry in the health professions: An epistemological orientation* (2nd ed.). Bethesda, MD: American Occupational Therapy Association.

Murphy, R. F. (1990). *The body silent.* New York: Norton.

Nagi, S. Z. (1965). Some conceptual issues in disability and rehabilitation. In M. B. Sussman (Ed.), *Sociology and rehabilitation* (pp. 104–113). Washington, DC: American Sociological Association.

Nagi, S. Z. (1991). Disability concepts revisited: Implications for prevention. In A. M. Pope, & A. R. Tarlov (Eds.), *Disability in America* (pp. 309–327). Washington, DC: National Academy Press.

Parkes, C. M. (1979). *Bereavement: Studies of grief in adult life.* New York: New International Universities Press.

Parkes, C. M., & Weiss, R. S. (1983). The recovery process. In C. M. Parkes & R. S. Weiss (Eds.), *Recovery from bereavement* (pp. 155–168). New York: Basic Books.

Perkinson, H. J. (1984). *Learning from our mistakes: A reinterpretation of twentieth century educational theory.* Westport, CT: Greenwood Press.

Perkinson, H. J. (1993). *Teachers without goals, students without purposes.* New York: McGrawHill.

Popper, K. R. (1985). In D. Miller (Ed.), *Popper selections.* Princeton, NJ: Princeton University Press.

Popper, K. R. (1994). The growth of scientific knowledge. *In search of a better world: Lectures and essays from thirty years* (L. J. Bennett, Trans.) (pp. 171–180). London: Routledge.

Price-Lackey, P., & Cashman, J. (1996). Jenny's story: Reinventing oneself through occupation and narrative configuration. *American Journal of Occupational Therapy, 50,* 306–314.

Rogers, J. C., & Holm, M. B. (1994). Nationally Speaking: Accepting the challenge of outcome research: Examining the effectiveness of occupational therapy practice. *American Journal of Occupational Therapy, 48,* 871–876.

Schön, D. A. (1983). *The reflective practitioner: How professionals think in action.* New York: Basic Books.

Trombly, C. (1993). The Issue Is—Anticipating the future: Assessment of occupational function. *American Journal of Occupational Therapy, 47,* 253–257.

Wilbarger, P., & Wilbarger, J. L. (1991). *Sensory defensiveness in children aged 2-12: An intervention guide for parents and other caretakers.* Santa Barbara, CA: Avanti Educational Programs.

Wilbarger, P., & Wilbarger, J. L. (1997). *Sensory defensiveness and related social/emotional and neurological problems* [Course syllabus]. Oak Park Heights, MN: Professional Development Programs.

Wood, P. H. N. (1980). Appreciating the consequences of disease: The international classification of impairments, disabilities, and handicaps. *WHO Chronicle, 34,* 376–380.

Wood, W. (1998). Nationally Speaking—It is jump time for occupational therapy. *American Journal of Occupational Therapy, 52,* 403–411.

World Health Organization. (1980). *International classification of impairments, disabilities, and handicaps.* Geneva: Author.

10

Using Activities as Challenges To Facilitate Development of Functional Skills

Joyce Shapero Sabari, PhD, OTR, BCN

Previous chapters of this text have discussed how we use activities in occupational therapy as an end goal. Occupational therapists determine which performance areas that are meaningful to a person are now difficult to perform. Interventions include development of compensatory strategies, selection and modification of available assistive devices, design and fabrication of unique assistive devices, and focused practice of relevant tasks.

Critical interventions exist to enable clients to improve performance in selected activities. If underlying impairments remain unchanged, however, these improvements will not likely generalize to performance of other occupations. When occupational therapy evaluation determines that a person demonstrates the potential to improve underlying impairments (or performance components), the person deserves the opportunity to work toward restoration of foundational motor, cognitive, or interactive skills.

Think about the goals you would set for yourself or a loved one if faced with limitations in activity performance. Suppose your friend is unable to perform instrumental activities of daily living because traumatic brain injury has affected his organizational and problem-solving skills. If he exhibits the potential to improve these underlying cognitive skills, would an occupational therapy program consisting only of specific task practice be sufficient? What if your younger sister demonstrates impairments in hand coordination that limit her ability to learn handwriting skills? You would want the occupational therapy intervention to offer her the opportunity to improve her underlying limitations in addition to specific handwriting practice or to offer her adapted writing utensils. Suppose your grandfather has survived a stroke with intact cognition. He demonstrates some movement throughout his paretic left arm but is unable to use the arm for task performance. Would you be satisfied with an occupational therapy program that is limited to teaching one-handed self-care techniques?

Chapter 9 discussed the World Health Organization model of pathology, impairment, disability, and societal limitation. Figure 1 illustrates an occupational therapy practitioner's implementation of activity-based intervention to

■   maximize each person's potential to improve impairments,

■   minimize disabilities by enabling each person to perform relevant daily life tasks, and

■   reduce handicaps and societal limitations by facilitating task performance and role achievement (Figures 1 and 2).

Improvements at the impairment level are critical to the occupational therapy process because they enable persons to perform an infinite number of tasks in various situations. Such improvements empower persons to create and discover unanticipated occupations and roles.

This chapter explores the use of "occupation as means" (Trombly, 1995) or "enabling activities" (Pedretti, 1996) in which occupational therapy practitioners design activities to provide structured challenges to improve skills in specific areas of impairment. Occupational therapy practitioners use activities in three major ways to enable clients to improve performance components.

1.   Practitioners present an activity to provide the interest level that enables persons to exert more effort, complete more repetitions of a desired behavior, or sustain performance for a longer duration.

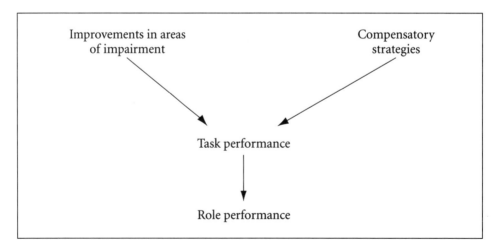

Figure 1. Occupational therapy practitioners implement activity-based intervention. *Note.* From *Stroke Rehabilitation: A Function Based Approach*, by G. Gillen and A. Burkhardt, 1997, St. Louis, MO: Mosby. Copyright 1997 by Mosby. Reprinted with permission.

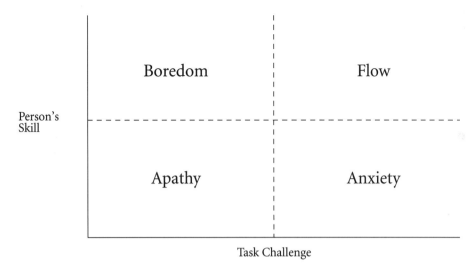

Figure 2. This figure illustrates that a state of flow depends on the person's sense that balance exists between a task's challenge and his or her own current skill level. *Note.* From "Introduction to Part IV," by M. Csikszentmihalyi and I. S. Csikszentmihalyi, in *Optimal Experience: Psychological Studies of Flow in Consciousness*, M. Csikszentmihalyi and I. S. Csikszentmihalyi, Eds., 1988, New York: Cambridge University Press. Copyright 1988 by Cambridge University Press. Reprinted with permission.

2. Practitioners manipulate selected activity and environmental conditions to present graded challenges to specific skills.

3. Practitioners select activities that will provide "problems" that challenge the client to develop effective cognitive or motor strategies that he or she can generalize to an unlimited variety of future situations.

Although categories overlap somewhat, occupational therapy students must understand when each of these types of occupation as means may be most appropriate and which concepts are most relevant to apply when using occupation as means in each of these three ways.

Using Activities To Elicit Greater Effort, Repetition, or Duration Than Traditional Exercise

Historically, the earliest use of activities in occupational therapy may have been as a medium to facilitate improvement in underlying performance components (Taylor, 1929). Research findings (Bloch, Smith, & Nelson, 1989; Kircher, 1984; Steinbeck, 1986) have indicated that healthy adults exert greater cardiovascular and muscular effort (as evidenced by a more rapid heart rate and increased electromyographic activity in selected muscles) when performing activities that they perceive to be fun (e.g., jumping rope) compared with exercises with similar motor components that they do not perceive to be fun (e.g., jumping in place). Using activities as interventions for this purpose is relevant when treatment goals are to improve cardiopulmonary endurance and specific muscle endurance.

Performance of interesting activities additionally promotes greater repetition and prolonged duration of physical output than does performance of routine exercise programs (DeKuiper, Nelson, & White, 1993; Hsieh, Nelson, Smith, & Peterson, 1996; Lang, Nelson, & Bush, 1992; Miller & Nelson, 1987; Nelson et al., 1996; Riccio, Nelson, & Bush, 1990; Steinbeck, 1986; Yoder, Nelson, & Smith, 1989). This concept is well understood in current popular culture as evidenced by the use of dance routines and embedded games during aerobic exercise and muscle toning sessions at community fitness centers. When muscle endurance or joint flexibility are treatment goals, the person should produce more repetitions for a longer duration of actions that demand optimal levels of muscle output or soft-tissue elongation (Downey & Darling, 1994). When seeking to decrease distal limb edema, repetitive isotonic contractions of muscles in the targeted body segment are a recognized complement to medical and positioning interventions (Burkhardt, 1998; Trombly, 1995).

Research findings provide evidence that persons with disabilities exhibit greater range of motion (ROM) (i.e., perform closer to their maximal potential) when engaged in interesting activities compared with performing activities under conventional exercise conditions. In one study, Van der Weel, van der Meer, and Lee (1991) encouraged children with cerebral palsy who exhibited right hemiparesis to perform actively the forearm movements of pronation and supination. While performing within the experimental condition, the researchers instructed the children to use a drumstick to bang on drums that were positioned to require full forearm ROM. During the control condition, the researchers instructed the same children to move the drumstick back and forth as far as they could in the frontal plane. Movement ROM was notably greater when banging the drums than during the abstract exercise condition.

Sietsema, Nelson, Mulder, Mervau-Scheidel, and White (1993) had similar findings in their study of forward reach in adults with hemiparesis resulting from traumatic brain injury. The researchers used neurodevelopmental treatment strategies to prepare subjects for forward reach from the sitting position. In the exercise condition, participants reached out their hands as far as they could in a rote manner. In the activity condition, they reached forward to control "Simon," a popular computer-controlled game that challenges players to repeat its sequences of flashing lights and sounds by pressing colored panels. Data collected through computerized motion analysis revealed that subjects displayed notably greater mobility when engaged in the activity compared with when they attempted to reach forward in a purely exercise context.

In pediatrics intervention, the use of playful, inviting sensory integration equipment serves in part to pique children's interest in and sustain their performance of activities that provide vestibular, tactile, or proprioceptive stimuli that they might otherwise avoid. The introduction of imaginative play may serve to engage the child still further and thus encourage longer duration of involvement and expenditure of greater effort during treatment sessions.

What makes an activity engaging enough that it will entice a person to continue its performance while repetitively performing a prescribed exercise or practicing a new skill? The answer depends on each person. Complex myriad factors affect a person's interest in specific activities, including the person's cultural background, age, and previous experiences. Csikszentmihalyi and Csikszentmihalyi (1988) coined the term *flow* to describe the extremely positive state in which a person is so involved in an activity that nothing else seems to matter. *Flow activities* are those sequences of action that make achieving this optimal experience state easy. During flow activities, participants reach a state of focused attention, they believe that the activity's outcomes are under their own control, and the process becomes as enjoyable as reaching the activity goal.

Understanding the characteristics of flow activities is useful to occupational therapy practitioners when designing activities that will motivate persons to participate in therapeutic interventions. Figure 2 illustrates that a state of flow depends on the person's sense that a balance exists between a task's challenge and his or her own current skill level. Apathy will ensue when the person perceives both the skill and the task challenge to be low. When a person views his or her skill as far exceeding the task challenge, boredom results. When task challenges exceed the person's skill, the person is likely to experience anxiety. Only when a task challenge is well balanced with a person's skill can a sense of flow occur (Figure 2). Csikszentmihalyi and Csikszentmihalyi (1988) gave two additional criteria for flow activities.

1. The goals of the activity must be clear to the participant.

2. The activity itself provides a continuous source of unambiguous feedback about how well the person is doing.

In our attempt to create activities that will serve as ways to entice persons to perform repetitive practice of specific movements or skills, occupational therapy practitioners may be tempted to present tasks that are so contrived that they hold little meaning for our clients (Fisher, 1998). If an occupational therapy activity does little to facilitate a flow experience, then choosing activity over exercise as an intervention has no advantage.

The occupational therapy practitioner has the responsibility to learn as much as possible about each client's previous skills, interests, and activity background. This information, combined with knowledge about the person's current strengths and limitations, is critical to setting feasible treatment goals. Although this information may be helpful when selecting therapeutic activities, flow activities do not necessarily need to relate to a person's previous repertoire of activity interests. "It does not matter whether one originally wanted to do the activity, whether one expected to enjoy it, or not. Even a frustrating job may suddenly become exciting if one hits upon the right balance" (Csikszentmihalyi & Csikszentmihalyi, 1988, p. 32). For many adults, an enabling activity need not have been a favorite previous pastime. In fact, sometimes a well-meaning occupational therapy practitioner is disappointed to learn that selection of favorite tasks as therapeutic intervention serves to frustrate rather than bring pleasure to the client. The man who worked as an electrician may become disheartened to see that simple wiring tasks are now excessively challenging. The avid puzzle solver may be dismayed to be practicing crossword puzzles designed for children. Instead, the match between the intrinsic interest level of an activity and the person's understanding of why practice is the key in determining how successful an activity will be in eliciting pleasure during sustained performance. As in all other aspects of occupational therapy, active involvement in the total therapeutic process enhances a client's motivation to participate.

Occupational therapy practitioners must consider a few critical words of caution when using activities to elicit repetitive performance of prescribed movement sequences. First, the person should perform repetitive movements only from a position of optimal alignment. The therapist has the responsibility to avoid activities that are ergonomically unsound and to provide appropriate therapeutic positioning and handling that will enhance the person's performance and comfort. Second, the therapist should not introduce therapeutic activities unless the person demonstrates adequate prerequisite skills. For example, introducing a task that requires repetitive active reaching has no therapeutic value unless the person exhibits the necessary joint play and muscle distensibility to allow adequate passive ROM at all of the joints of the shoulder complex. Finally, therapists must remember that repetition must occur naturally within the activity performance. Setting up a checkerboard affords the opportunity for repetitive practice of reach, grasp, and release. The activity component, however, is maintained only if this initial placement of game pieces is followed by an actual game of checkers (with a family member, a volunteer, or another client). In an effort to foster even more repetition, a therapist may want to ask a client to remove the checkers and begin the task again. Although this contrivance may be effective once or twice, it quickly reduces what may have begun as an interesting activity to a rote exercise that is unlikely to maintain the person's interest over time.

Case Scenario 1

Jack is a man 19 years of age who sustained a spinal cord injury resulting from a fracture of the sixth cervical vertebra 4 weeks ago in a motor vehicle crash. At this time, he demonstrates good strength bilaterally in the deltoid, rotator cuff, pectoralis major, biceps, pronator teres, and extensor carpi radialis longus and brevis. One current goal is to develop skill functionally by using a tenodesis grasp pattern. This grasp requires repetitive practice in picking up lightweight objects by coordinating active wrist extension with the resultant passive tenodesis flexion of his fingers. By wearing an orthosis that maintains his thumb, index, and middle fingers in optimal alignment, Jack develops new skills by playing the solitary board game "Think and Jump." He finds pleasure in trying to surpass his record of jumping over and removing pieces from the playing board. For each game of "Think and Jump," he completes, including setting up the game board, Jack practices tenodesis grasp and release up to 74 times.

Using Activities To Provide Graded Challenges

Repetition alone will not promote improvements in all performance components. When client goals are to enhance muscle strength, ROM, balance, or coordination, practice sessions must provide opportunities for incremental increases in appropriate demands. The key to using activities effectively to provide graded challenges is the therapist's identification of a specific, relevant continuum on which the therapist will introduce gradations. For example, if the client's goal is to improve active hip and pelvic mobility when sitting, placement of activity objects in relation to the client will represent a relevant continuum. Because the weight or the size of activity objects will essentially be irrelevant to the specific performance component of active hip motion, the therapist will not manipulate these factors when making incremental changes to the activity demands. Gentile's (1972, 1987) term *regulatory conditions* refers to environmental features that directly influence a person's choice of strategies for performing a selected task. Occupational therapy practitioners, when designing activities to present graded challenges, determine which features in the environment and the selected task are "regulatory" to the performance components in question (Sabari, 1991). Figure 3 illustrates the various regulatory conditions that therapists can manipulate to influence the performance requirements for engaging in therapeutic tasks.

Goal objects and tools are items that a person must act on or manipulate within the course of task performance. The therapist can adapt them according to size, shape, weight, and texture (Hinojosa, Sabari, & Pedretti, 1993; Trombly, 1995). In addition, the position of goal objects and tools in relation to the participant will greatly influence which movements and balance adjustments are necessary for task performance. Goal objects may vary between being static (e.g., a jar of paint next to an easel) or being in motion (e.g., a ball during a game of catch or the action figures in a computer game). When goal objects are moving, their trajectories may be either predictable or unpredictable. Each of these variations places different demands on the participant's requirements to use perceptual-motor skills.

Rules guide performance of hobbies, crafts, games, and sports. Creative adaptations in rules can tailor an activity to allow for grading along dimensions as varied as taking turns, cognitive complexity, social interaction, use of imagination, and specific motor skills. The therapist can grade supporting structures to provide incremental challenges to balance and dynamic motor performance. Whether a supporting structure is a chair, a bolster, a floor surface on which the client stands, or

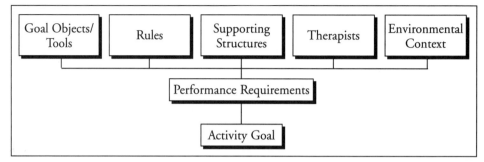

Figure 3. Regulatory conditions that the therapist can grade in therapeutic activities.

a piece of suspended play equipment, the occupational therapy practitioner can create variations in shape, weight, texture, base of support, and degree of external support. In addition, the therapist can grade supporting structures along a continuum beginning with stationary support to increasingly unstable or dynamic surfaces.

The therapist may consider himself or herself as a regulatory condition that influences the client's performance requirements. Therapists can vary the ways in which they provide instructions and feedback and the ways in which they provide physical handling to support or assist a client in task performance. The therapist grades down such assistance in an incremental fashion to provide clients with opportunities to develop increasing ability in the performance components in question.

Finally, the environmental context introduces various additional regulatory conditions. Competitive noises or visual distractions place higher demands on attention skills, and the therapist can grade these distractions through adaptations to the setting of the therapeutic intervention. Physical obstacles, even when they are not central to the actual activity, can pose graded cognitive, perceptual, and motor challenges. Table 1 offers examples of selected performance components and corresponding "regulatory features" that would be appropriate to adjust when the intervention presents relevant, graded challenges.

The following case scenario provides an example of how one occupational therapy practitioner uses activity grading within a group setting to assist clients in achieving specific goals related to trusting others and developing a repertoire of wellness behaviors.

Case Scenario 2

Cynthia is coordinating a relaxation group for six members who attend an outpatient community mental health day program. All clients have severe and persistent mental illness. This group is part of a larger wellness program in which

Table 1
Regulatory Features of Tasks That Correspond With Grading To Challenge Specific Performance Components

Performance Components	Intervention Strategies
Figure–ground perception	Complexity of the visual background, similarity between the visual background and the key foreground object (provided in real-life hide-and-seek games or paper-and-pencil puzzles)
Active ROM: Shoulder flexion	Height of object placement
Active ROM: Finger flexion	Size of handles to grasp
Strength of specific muscles	Placement of objects in relation to gravity (gravity eliminated to lightweight objects to be moved against gravity) to increased weight (resistance) against gravity, length of lever arm (short resistance arm to progressively longer resistance arm)
Praxis	Complexity of a novel motor task
Fine motor coordination and dexterity	Size and shape of tool (gross to fine grasp); size, texture, and shape of objects to be manipulated; increased demands on speed of performance; increased demands on manipulation of objects
Standing balance	Size and stability of base of support (progress from larger, most stable base to smaller base, less stable base), amount of weight shift required in all planes of motion (achieved through placement of goal objects in relation to the person)
Attention span	Increased time necessary to complete a task
Social interaction	The interactive nature of tasks, which may progress from parallel task performance alongside another person, to activities requiring dyadic interaction, to activities requiring increasing amounts of sharing views and feelings with one or more persons

Note. ROM = range of motion.

participants learn to manage their psychiatric symptoms and develop healthier lifestyles. Group members have difficulty committing themselves to new styles of behavior and exposing their vulnerabilities to others. Cynthia will grade the group's activities along a continuum of increasing trust within a group framework and will use the clients' strengths and interests in maintaining good health.

At the first session, participants must take off their coats, hang them on wall hooks that are clearly visible in the same room, and sit in a circle on wooden chairs. Initial activities include practicing deep breathing strategies and performing active stretching of neck muscles. At subsequent sessions, participants remove their shoes and then progress to facial exercises with their eyeglasses off. Cynthia encourages group members to appreciate the humor in their facial expressions when frowning, grinning, and pouting to enhance their level of trust. Gradually, Cynthia adds larger body movements to the group repertoire. Eventually, Cynthia demonstrates relaxation activities while supine on a floor mat and encourages group members to try these at home. One ultimate goal of this grading process is for participants to reach a comfort level in which they are able to sufficiently trust the group to engage in a full repertoire of relaxation exercises that are popular and healthful in the larger society.

Note. From Suzanne White, MA, OTR, Senior Occupational Therapist, St. Luke's Hospital, Start II Psychosocial Rehabilitation, New York.

———

Similar precautions to those used with activities that promote repetitive, sustained performance are necessary when occupational therapy practitioners present activities as a series of graded challenges. The therapist must ensure that, in any activity requiring movement, the person is performing from a position of optimal body alignment. Particularly when altering a support surface or introducing objects that have been strategically placed at increasingly more challenging locations to grade the task, the therapist has the responsibility to pay close attention to the person's general body posture and to maintain appropriate alignment at specific body segments. If not, what the therapist planned as a therapeutic intervention may promote inefficient and potentially harmful motor strategies.

Before selecting a treatment sequence on the basis of graded activity performance, the therapist must determine whether the person demonstrates the potential to benefit from this type of intervention. Simply providing increasingly difficult challenges to a performance component will not necessarily result in functional improvements. Occupational therapy practitioners must collaborate with other team members to determine what combination of medical, orthotic, physical, or educational measures should precede or accompany graded activity performance.

Occupational therapy practitioners should strive to avoid two common mistakes when using activity grading as a therapeutic intervention. First, activity grading becomes counterproductive when the client perceives it to be an unfair "tease." In this situation, a well-meaning but overzealous therapist continually upgrades the challenge of therapeutic tasks so that the client never achieves the satisfaction of performing activities more easily. For example, after struggling to achieve improved reach in the context of making a macramé rug, the client deserves an opportunity to work with the materials positioned within reasonable access. The therapist, however, in an attempt to challenge the person's improving abilities, continually repositions the wall-mounted rug so that it is always just out of comfortable reach. Blanche (1997) warned therapists who use toys as lures to motivate young children to reach or ambulate that the practice becomes misguided if the therapist continually moves the toy further and further away as the child approaches in an attempt to upgrade the child's efforts.

A second problem occurs when a client participates in an occupational therapy program designed to promote improvements in multiple performance components. For example, a child may be working to improve cognitive and gross mobility skills. Grading treatment activities so that cognitive and gross mobility challenges are simultaneously increased is a mistake. Rather, the therapist should account for the likelihood that increased demands to one performance component may negatively affect the child's demonstrated skills in other performance components. Consider how you would function if someone challenged you to your ultimate limits in trying to perform a triple-axle ice-skating jump. Would that be the best moment for you to grapple with a difficult mathematics problem? Similarly, a person who demonstrates dual problems with balance and fine hand coordination may have recently become able to sit unsupported in a standard chair. When confronted with a challenging task in which she must manipulate objects with both hands, however, her ability to function at her highest level in maintaining sitting balance may be temporarily diminished. In another example, a young woman who has survived a traumatic brain injury may demonstrate problems related to socially appropriate behavior, cognitive processing, and motor control. When the treatment emphasizes upgrading demands for social interaction, the intellectual and motor challenges of a group activity must be kept as simple as possible. The skillful occupational therapy practitioner knows how to alter a task's regulatory conditions so that, when grading up on one dimension, demands to other performance components remain at manageable levels. In many cases, the therapist will structure the activity so that competing demands are temporarily graded down.

Using Activities To Promote the Development of Effective Strategies

For many persons who require occupational therapy, the process of overcoming impairments is a process of learning. Teaching and learning as part of an occupational therapy intervention are necessary for clients of all ages whose goals are to improve postural control, motor control, cognitive abilities, interpersonal skills, and coping mechanisms. Neither activity repetition nor activity grading may be sufficient interventions when the therapeutic goal is to assist clients in learning and generalizing effective strategies for their performance of daily tasks.

Strategies are organized plans or sets of rules that guide action in various situations (Sabari, 1998). Each of us has developed various strategies that serve as foundational guidelines for our effective participation in daily activities. We have learned many of these strategies so well that they seem to be automatic. Without them, however, the challenges of performing occupations would be overwhelming.

Motor strategies include the vast repertoire of kinematic and kinetic linkages that underlie the performance of skilled, efficient movement. For example, when reaching forward to turn on a computer, the strategy of anteriorly tilting the pelvis ensures sufficient mobility of the trunk and scapula. The strategy of abducting and upwardly rotating the scapula enhances the smooth mobility of the arm's trajectory (Norkin & Levangie, 1992). Specific hand shaping (Jeannerod, 1990) and visual guidance (Shumway-Cook & Woollacott, 1995; Wing & Frazer, 1983) strategies enable the index finger to reach the start button with minimal effort. Other motor strategies include automatic plans of action that enable us to maintain our balance throughout infinite varieties of environmental support and challenges to our centers of mass. In addition, we routinely implement strategies that will ensure our "postural readiness" (Abreu, 1998) to perform desired tasks. Think back to the task of turning on the computer. What strategies can you implement for establishing a base of support and alignment of body segments that ultimately make accomplishing your goal easier and more efficient?

Cognitive strategies include the multiple and varied tactics we use to facilitate processing, storing, retrieving, and manipulating information. What cognitive strategies have you found to be useful in negotiating the academic demands of being a college (or graduate) student? Sitting close to a lecturer and jotting down questions to ask after class may be effective strategies that enable you to process information in a large, noninteractive class setting. Reorganizing and rewording class notes on a regular basis may aid in storing course information. Categorizing and drawing your own visual models may be helpful in storing, retrieving, and manipulating information. Cognitive strategies influence our performance of all activities, whether they are simple or complex. Grocery shopping is more efficient if one uses the strategies of taking a kitchen inventory, generating a shopping list, organizing the list according to the supermarket layout, and assembling appropriate discount coupons. When basic self-care tasks are challenging to persons because of brain injury or developmental disabilities, selection and use of appropriate cognitive strategies allow persons to achieve independence and autonomy.

Interpersonal strategies assist in our social interactions with other persons. During child and adolescent development, and every time we join a new group, we learn the normative practices of social engagement within a given context. Interpersonal strategies are necessary for forming and maintaining friendships, for expressing our opinions in various situations, for enlisting the assistance of strangers or family members, and for conducting routine transactions within our communities. Many persons requiring occupational therapy intervention can benefit from the opportunity to develop more effective interpersonal strategies.

Coping strategies allow persons to adapt constructively to stress (Giles & Neistadt, 1998). Persons experience stress when we perceive that events or factors in our environment exceed our current resources. Effective coping strategies are critical in preventing negative physiological, cognitive, and emotional sequela to stressful situations. A framework that Williamson, Szczepanski, and Zeitlin (1993) developed postulates that a sequence of interactions between a person and the environment elicits coping strategies in a four-step interrelated process. During the first step, the person determines the meaning of a stressful event or situation. A useful strategy at this step is to review logically the factors that the person perceives to be stressful and to analyze the demands of the situation in relation to one's own resources. During this process of "primary appraisal," the person determines whether and to what degree the perceived stressor is indeed harmful or challenging. The strategy of distancing oneself temporarily from the stressful situation may facilitate this appraisal process. The tactic of "cognitive restructuring" (Giles & Neistadt, 1998) may assist the person in identifying cognitive distortions that may lead to inappropriate interpretations of stress.

The second step is to develop an action plan. Effective strategies at this phase include the practice of taking stock of all available options and enlisting appropriate assistance from others. The choice of an action plan that accurately capitalizes on one's own resources and accounts for one's limitations is critical to the effectiveness of the coping process.

Implementing a coping effort on the basis of the action plan is the next step to cope effectively with a stressor. This coping effort produces an outcome that will elicit feedback from the environment. The fourth step, evaluating effectiveness of the coping effort, depends on the person's ability to evaluate cues from the social and physical environment effectively in relation to his or her own actions. A strategy of identifying and taking pleasure from small achievements is helpful in deriving feelings of success in situations that the person may otherwise perceive as overwhelming.

Therapists should view strategies as frameworks rather than as recipes. Strategies provide us with foundational skills to adapt to the ever changing demands of the occupations in which we engage and the infinite variations of multiple environments. Although one correct strategy does not exist, some strategies may have a negative effect on a person's future success or well-being. The occupational therapy practitioner has the responsibility to guide clients toward developing strategies that are likely to have long-term positive implications.

Persons develop strategies through a process of encountering problems, implementing solutions, and monitoring the effects of our solutions. "In child development, an experienced adult guides the child through problem-solving activities and structures the child's learning environment by selecting, focusing, and organizing incoming stimuli" (Toglia, 1998, p. 12). "Through transactions in the environment, children try out, practice, and integrate coping strategies into their behavioral repertoire" (Williamson et al., 1993, p. 396).

Strategy development continues throughout our lives. New jobs, new relation-ships, and new hobbies present us with new sets of problems to solve. Changes in our physical status, concomitant with normal aging, disease, or disability, create the need for altered strategies when performing familiar tasks.

Sometimes we are lucky enough to receive advice or instruction to guide us in the formation of new strategies. We enhance our success in tennis if we learn early on some basic rules about postural set and kinematic linkages and offensive and defen-sive tactics. We will promote facility at the computer keyboard if we practice touch-typing techniques. Ergonomic strategies for positioning workstation materials will have a positive effect on our long-term visual and musculoskeletal health. A coworker's advice about how to interact with a particular administrator will guide us in developing effective on-the-job strategies.

How do occupational therapy practitioners use activities to assist clients in developing useful strategies? Therapists structure tasks within a safe environment that provides clients with opportunities to try out different solutions to actual problems. The practitioner selects problems in accordance with the performance component goals for each person. For Trina, a preschool child with a balance dysfunction, the problem may be to determine how she can stay upright while pushing a doll carriage. Instead of providing solutions, the therapist offers suggestions to Trina through phys-ical handling and artful structuring of the play situation (Pierce, 1997). For Scott, a young adult with schizophrenia, a set of problems arises within the context of work-ing as a salesperson in the hospital-run thrift shop. Potential problems may include the challenge of interacting appropriately with customers or the challenge of main-taining interest in the work when business is slow. The therapist's role is to assist Scott in reflecting on the effectiveness of the solutions he has chosen and to help him deter-mine strategies that may guide his future performance in this and other work expe-riences. The ultimate goal in this type of activity intervention is that the client will develop strategies that he or she can generalize to a wide variety of occupations and environments.

Case Scenario 3

Tommy is a boy 4 years of age who has been referred to occupational therapy because his excessive activity level, impulsiveness, and motor incoordination are affecting his ability to function successfully in his preschool classroom. The occupational therapist has determined that Tommy has difficulty identifying environmental cues that are important to successful activity outcomes. Therefore, one occupational therapy goal is to help him to develop strategies to improve his ability to match his motor acts to the requirements of the task.

Because Tommy demonstrates great interest in the "clown" bean bag toss board, the occupational therapist presents a problem. She informs Tommy that the clown has not eaten today and is hungry. She places a bucket of bean bags that are chocolate flavored (chocolate is the clown's favorite food) at a distance that is challenging but still possible for Tommy to be able to throw the food through the clown's mouth. The therapist asks Tommy, "What shall we do?" By asking Tommy to tell her what he intends to do before he does it, the occupational therapist ensures that Tommy focuses on the relevant characteristics of distance, size, and position of the clown's mouth and the size and weight of the bean bags. His interest level in the activity will help him learn to screen out extraneous environmental stimuli. After Tommy throws the "food," he must tell the occupational therapist what happened. To help him learn to evaluate his own performance, the occupational therapist gives feedback such as "you threw the food too hard" or "look at the mouth when you throw." The occupational therapist can help Tommy to learn to modify his strategies as necessary by encouraging him to "try another way" or asking him "What can you do differently?"

The occupational therapist creates a safe environment with a playful atmosphere in which Tommy is comfortable in experimenting and making mistakes. In this way, Tommy will learn to engage in the following strategies.

- Focus on characteristics that are relevant to the task

- Evaluate his own behavior and actions regarding outcome and performance

- Implement changes in his behavior and actions on the basis of the evaluation

In addition, the occupational therapist has collaborated with Tommy's teacher to develop ways of encouraging Tommy to use these strategies during classroom activities.

Note. From Margaret Kaplan, MA, OTR, Clinical Assistant Professor, Occupational Therapy Program, State University of New York, Health Science Center at Brooklyn.

Self-awareness and self-monitoring skills are critical prerequisites to a person's ability to generate and apply appropriate strategies. *Metacognition* (Katz & Hartman-Maier, 1998) is the knowledge and regulation of personal cognitive processes and capacities and includes an awareness of personal strengths and limitations and the abilities to evaluate task difficulty, plan ahead, choose appropriate strategies, and shift strategies in response to environmental cues.

Toglia's (1991, 1998) dynamic interactional model for persons with cognitive impairments after brain injury emphasizes the importance of metacognition. In this treatment approach, occupational therapy intervention begins by helping clients developing insight about personal strengths and deficits through a program that challenges them to estimate task difficulty, predict outcomes, and evaluate personal performance. The occupational therapy practitioner then presents tasks to selected challenges and guides the client in selecting appropriate strategies for meeting these challenges. Self-review of one's own performance and guided planning for tackling the challenges of future tasks are key factors in the therapeutic process.

Persons who need to develop improved interpersonal or coping strategies likewise benefit from therapeutic attention to metacognitive processes. The occupational therapy practitioner plays an important role in guiding the client's self-reflection on relevant components of task performance.

Self-awareness is valuable to persons with impairments in motor or postural control who want to learn effective strategies for movement and task performance. Just as evaluation of one's cognitive or interpersonal strengths and weaknesses is critical to developing strategies in these areas, the child with cerebral palsy and the woman who has experienced a stroke must accurately evaluate when their body segments are optimally aligned or when they are posturally ready to perform particular activities. The occupational therapy practitioner provides effective feedback about kinematic aspects of performance and graded physical guidance to assist these persons in developing effective self-monitoring of their movement strategies (Sabari, 1998).

The use of activities to stimulate strategy development requires extensive knowledge and creativity. Whether the practitioner directs the intervention toward developing motor, cognitive, interpersonal, or coping strategies, he or she must be an expert in that area of function. A thorough knowledge base, skill in analyzing performance, and the ability to anticipate how environmental and task demands are likely to affect function are necessary for effective intervention.

Activity challenges must take place in a safe environment that allows for mistakes, self-reflection, and dynamic interaction with the practitioner. Although providing this type of activity intervention in a naturalistic environment may be valuable, the practitioner must consider that public spaces may be embarrassing places for persons to develop basic strategies. For example, a supermarket or public library may not be an appropriate place to try new motor or cognitive strategies. Occupational therapy interventions should avoid contributing to making our clients feel like objects of pity in social or community situations. Rather, the practitioner can simulate challenges in the client's home or in a therapy setting that may be emotionally and physically safer to begin the process of strategy development. Once the person has sufficiently mastered the necessary strategies, then the practitioner can provide opportunities to practice in real-world environments.

Summary

The use of activities as interventions to promote the development of performance components, skills, or strategies is an important component of occupational therapy. On the basis of a client's goals, the practitioner determines whether the activity program will focus on

- eliciting repetition or longer duration of a desired behavior,

- presenting graded challenges to specific skills, or

- providing problems that challenge the person to develop appropriate strategies.

Regardless of the treatment setting, client background, or type of activity intervention, the activity must meet several criteria. First, the person must be ready to participate in the selected activity. The therapist must evaluate prerequisite skills for performance and initiate interventions to reduce physical, cognitive, or emotional factors that may constrain performance. Such constraints to performance can render an activity intervention useless or even harmful to a client. Second, the practitioner must synthesize the activity for each person. This is necessary to ensure that the activity will both be useful in developing skills that are specifically relevant for that person and will meet the third criteria and that the activity must provide some level of inherent interest to the person. In addition, the person must understand the dual purpose of the activity. The occupational therapy process confuses many clients. When the therapist designs an occupational therapy intervention to promote improvements in underlying performance components, clients must be able to differentiate the underlying therapeutic purposes from the activity itself. Finally, occupational therapy intervention to improve performance components is never isolated from the projected effect on a person's ability to perform meaningful tasks. The ultimate goal is always to facilitate performance of activities and roles that are meaningful to the person in the context of his or her own life. ■

References

Abreu, B. (1998). The quadraphonic approach: Holistic rehabilitation for brain injury. In N. Katz (Ed.), *Cognition and occupation in rehabilitation: Cognitive models for intervention in occupational therapy* (pp. 51–98). Bethesda, MD: American Occupational Therapy Association.

Blanche, E. I. (1997). Doing with—Not doing to: Play and the child with cerebral palsy. In L. D. Parham & L. S. Fazio (Eds.), *Play in occupational therapy for children* (pp. 202–218). St. Louis: Mosby.

Bloch, M. W., Smith, D. A., & Nelson, D. L. (1989). Heart rate, activity, duration, and affect in added-purpose versus single-purpose jumping activities. *American Journal of Occupational Therapy, 43,* 25–30.

Burkhardt, A. (1998). Edema control. In G. Gillen & A. Burkhardt (Eds.), *Stroke rehabilitation: A function-based approach* (pp. 152–160). St. Louis: Mosby.

Csikszentmihalyi, M., & Csikszentmihalyi, I. S. (Eds.). (1988). *Optimal experience: Psychological studies of flow in consciousness.* New York: Cambridge University Press.

DeKuiper, W. P., Nelson, D. L., & White, B. E. (1993). Materials-based occupation versus rote exercise: A replication and extension. *Occupational Therapy Journal of Research, 13,* 183–197.

Downey, J., & Darling, R. (Eds.). (1994). *Physiological basis of rehabilitation medicine* (2nd ed.). Boston: Butterworth-Heinemann.

Fisher, A. G. (1998). Uniting practice and theory in an occupational framework. *American Journal of Occupational Therapy, 52,* 509–519.

Gentile, A. M. (1972). A working model of skill acquisition with application to teaching. *Quest, 17,* 3–23.

Gentile, A. M. (1987). Skill acquisition: Action, movement, and neuromotor processes. In J. H. Carr, R. B. Shepherd, J. Gordon, A. M. Gentile, & J. N. Held (Eds.), *Movement science: Foundations for physical therapy in rehabilitation* (pp. 93–154). Rockville, MD: Aspen Publishers.

Giles, G. M., & Neistadt, M. E. (1998). Treatment for psychosocial components: Stress management. In M. E. Neistadt, & E. B. Crepeau (Eds.), *Willard & Spackman's occupational therapy* (9th ed., pp. 458–470). Philadelphia: Lippincott.

Hinojosa, J., Sabari, J., & Pedretti, L. (1993). Position Paper: Purposeful activity. *American Journal of Occupational Therapy, 47,* 1081–1082.

Hsieh, C. L., Nelson, D. L., Smith, D. A., & Peterson, C. Q. (1996). A comparison of performance in added-purpose occupations and rote exercise for dynamic standing balance in persons with hemiplegia. *American Journal of Occupational Therapy, 50,* 10–16.

Jeannerod, M. (1990). *The neural and behavioral organization of goal-directed movements.* Oxford, UK: Clarendon Press.

Katz, N., & Hartman-Maier, A. (1998). Metacognition: The relationships of awareness and executive functions to occupational performance. In N. Katz (Ed.), *Cognition and occupation in rehabilitation: Cognitive models for intervention in occupational therapy* (pp. 323–342). Bethesda, MD: American Occupational Therapy Association.

Kircher, M. A. (1984). Motivation as a factor of perceived exertion in purposeful versus non-purposeful activity. *American Journal of Occupational Therapy, 38,* 165–170.

Lang, E. M., Nelson, D. L., & Bush, M. A. (1992). Comparison of performance in materials-based occupation, imagery-based occupation, and rote exercise in nursing home residents. *American Journal of Occupational Therapy, 46,* 607–611.

Miller, L., & Nelson, D. L. (1987). Dual-purpose activity versus single-purpose activity in terms of duration of task, exertion level, and affect. *Occupational Therapy in Mental Health, 1,* 55–67.

Nelson, D. L., Konosky, K., Fleharty, K., Webb, R., Newer, K., Hazboun, V. P., Fontane, C., & Licht, B. C. (1996). The effects of an occupationally embedded exercise on bilaterally assisted supination in persons with hemiplegia. *Journal of Occupational Therapy, 50,* 639–646.

Norkin, C. C., & Levangie, P. K. (1992). *Joint structure and function: A comprehensive analysis* (2nd ed.). Philadelphia: F. A. Davis.

Pedretti, L. W. (Ed.). (1996). Occupational therapy practice skills for physical dysfunction (4th ed.). St. Louis: Mosby.

Pierce, D. (1997). The power of object play for infants and toddlers at risk for developmental delays. In L. D. Parham & L. S. Fazio (Eds.), *Play in occupational therapy for children* (pp. 86–111). St. Louis: Mosby.

Riccio, C. M., Nelson, D. L., & Bush, M. A. (1990). Adding purpose to the repetitive exercise of elderly women through imagery. *American Journal Occupational Therapy, 44,* 714–719.

Sabari, J. (1991). Motor learning concepts applied to activity-based intervention with adults with hemiplegia. *American Journal of Occupational Therapy, 45,* 523–530.

Sabari, J. (1998). Application of learning and environmental strategies to activity based treatment. In G. Gillen and A. Burkhardt (Eds.), *Stroke rehabilitation: A function-based approach* (pp. 31–46). St. Louis: Mosby.

Shumway-Cook, A., & Woollacott, M. (1995). *Motor control: Theory and practical applications.* Baltimore: Williams & Wilkins.

Sietsema, J. M., Nelson, D. L., Mulder, R. M., Mervau-Scheidel, D., & White, B. E. (1993). The use of a game to promote arm reach in persons with traumatic brain injury. *American Journal of Occupational Therapy, 47,* 19–24.

Steinbeck, T. M. (1986). Purposeful activity and performance. *American Journal of Occupational Therapy, 40,* 529–534.

Taylor, M. (1929). Occupational therapy in industrial inquiries. *Occupational Therapy and Rehabilitation, 8,* 335–338.

Toglia, J. (1991). Generalization of treatment: A multicontext approach to cognitive perceptual impairment in adults with brain injury. *American Journal of Occupational Therapy, 45,* 505–515.

Toglia, J. (1998). A dynamic interactional model to cognitive rehabilitation. In N. Katz (Ed.), *Cognition and occupation in rehabilitation: Cognitive models for intervention in occupational therapy* (pp. 5–50). Bethesda, MD: American Occupational Therapy Association.

Trombly, C. A. (1995). Purposeful activity. In C. A. Trombly (Ed.), *Occupational therapy in physical dysfunction* (4th ed., pp. 237–253). Baltimore: Williams & Wilkins.

Van der Weel, F. R., van der Meer, A. L. H., & Lee D. N. (1991). Effect of task on movement control in cerebral palsy: Implications for assessment and therapy. *Developmental Medicine and Child Neurology, 33,* 419–426.

Williamson, G. G., Szczepanski, M., & Zeitlin, S. (1993). Coping frame of reference. In P. Kramer & J. Hinojosa (Eds.), *Frames of reference for pediatric occupational therapy* (pp. 395–436). Baltimore: Williams & Wilkins.

Wing, A. M., & Frazer, C. (1983). The contribution of the thumb to reaching movements. *Quarterly Journal of Experimental Psychology, 35A,* 297–309.

Yoder, R. M., Nelson, D. L., & Smith, D. A. (1989). Added-purpose versus rote exercise in female nursing home residents. *American Journal of Occupational Therapy, 43,* 581–586.

11

Moving From Simulation to Real Life

Anita Perr, MA, OT, ATP
Paulette F. Bell, MA, OT

The focus of this chapter is the importance of activities as a part of the last steps in the habilitation or rehabilitation process, or the transition to real life. Although many textbooks concentrate on occupational therapy and its use of purposeful activities in controlled environments, such as occupational therapy clinics or laboratories and a client's room or home, this chapter addresses the value of client-centered activities as part of the end goal of occupational therapy—a client's return to real life. Real life involves a client's participation in activities outside a controlled therapeutic environment and often requires that a client engage in activities that he or she commonly performed in specific contexts and settings before his or her illness or injury. Real life for a client with disabilities often also requires that he or she engage in new activities and perform a task in new ways. These new activities may be necessary to address changes in the client's functional abilities, home responsibilities, interest in learning new hobbies, or employment.

The occupational therapy practitioner can assume a critical role in the integration of a client into his or her natural environments. By using the therapeutic value of active engagement in activities, occupational therapy practitioners work in collaboration with the client, caregivers, significant others, and other professionals to match the client's engagement in an activity with therapeutic goals. The process by which a client reintegrates into his or her environment involves a transition along a continuum from performance of contrived activities in a clinical or controlled environment (e.g., stacking blocks), to performance of simulated activities in clinical environments (e.g., role-playing a job interview with other clients), to performance of simulated activities in real environments (e.g., pretending to brush one's teeth at the bathroom sink), to real activities in simulated environments (e.g., shaving at the sink in the occupational therapy clinic), to performance of real activities in real environments (e.g., taking a bus to school, making a meal at home). Figure 1 illustrates this process in a flowchart. Simulation is a central concept in this transition and is discussed in this chapter.

Real Life as the Goal of Occupational Therapy Intervention

The ability to function in real life is the ultimate goal for clients receiving occupational therapy. Through a collaborative process, each client and occupational therapy practitioner identify and develop client-centered goals, which means that the occupational therapist develops goals with the client and his or her significant others to meet the client's needs and address the issues relevant to the particular environments in which the client will live and engage in activities.

Closely aligned with this concept of real life is the idea that real-life functioning assumes that the client is able to perform activities independently. Occupational therapy practitioners are often concerned with the client's independence and his or her ability to complete tasks alone. This goal, however, is only relevant if it is acceptable and appropriate for the client. The therapist and client should consider the client's culture, support systems, and values when defining independence goals. Independence is important because many persons associate independence with the ability to perform or complete specific tasks, activities, or occupations. Occupational therapy practitioners define the concept of independence from the client's perspective, in other words, the ability of the client to direct his or her life. Therapists do not view independence on the basis of the performance of the various tasks; rather, inde-

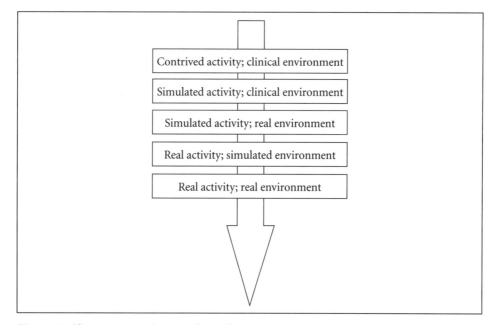

Figure 1. Client reintegration into his or her environment.

pendence is the ability to execute the tasks in a manner that is acceptable to the client. Thus, independence for one client may be quite different from independence for another client. For example, a client who has never cooked and can afford to eat out may not want to prepare food but would be independent in his or her ability to acquire food or to be fed. Another person who needs or wants to prepare food would need to be able to complete various tasks to be independent in food preparation. This view of independence becomes complex when one begins to adapt an activity or use assistive devices. Society often judges persons with disabilities by a different standard than it judges persons without disabilities and views persons with disabilities as limited in independence because of the use of an adaptation or assistive device. For example, a client may need to write a list to remember what to do during the day. He or she would be independent related to organization of daily routines. A person with a disability is often independent with assistance, which means that he or she needs to write a daily list of reminders.

When independence is a goal, occupational therapy practitioners may use environmental modifications, assistive technology, or other compensatory strategies to facilitate the client's performance or engagement in an activity. For example, one goal for a person who is paralyzed after a cervical spinal cord injury may be to navigate the environment by using a manual or powered wheelchair. In this case, independence requires the use of a wheelchair (or assistive technology). Ultimately, from an occupational therapy practitioner's view, the client would be independent in mobility once the client fully integrates the wheelchair into his or her real-life routine and can move around independently in various environments. The use of a compensatory strategy then does not negate a person's independence; rather, such strategies are simply the means by which the person is independent.

Some clients may not be capable of or desire full independence. For a client who does not believe that he or she is capable of full independence in a particular activity, the occupational therapist must first evaluate the client to identify the obstacles. Do cognitive, psychological, or physical impairments limit independence? Is partial independence feasible? The practitioner may intervene by downgrading or simplifying the activity to match the client's level of function and thus encourage the client's participation. In addition, the occupational therapy practitioner may adapt the activity, manipulate the environment, or teach the client to use assistive devices and compensatory techniques to facilitate task performance. The practitioner may train the client in instructing others to meet the client's needs.

In the following example, the occupational therapist and the client determine the client's potential for partial independence and select activities leading to this goal. Although the client wants to dress independently, the client is unable to do so fully because of paralysis in the right-dominant upper extremity, decreased dexterity in the nondominant left hand, and difficulty sequencing the dressing activity.

The practitioner's initial intervention may include a simulated activity in the clinic (e.g., having the client manipulate various clothing fasteners on a dressing board to improve dexterity in the left hand). Next, the client may learn compensatory one-handed dressing techniques with the use of assistive devices, such as a button hook and elastic shoelaces, during dressing at the bedside. In addition, the practitioner may provide a contrived or simulated activity in the clinic to improve the client's ability to sequence dressing. The client may then progress to applying sequencing strategies to dressing during the morning routine. After the client has maximized the ability to dress, he or she still may only be partially independent in this area. The client may then need to problem solve when and how to ask for assistance appropriately.

A client who does not want to perform all aspects of his or her daily activities personally may still exert control over his or her routine by determining which activities to delegate to others. The practitioner's intervention may include activities that help the client to improve the clarity and the manner in which the client gives instructions to caregivers. The practitioner and client may role-play situations to optimize client–caregiver interactions. Activities that begin as simulations (e.g., role-playing) in the controlled environment transition into real life as the client directs the caregiver at home.

The goal of many clients is to become as independent as possible. Let us examine a client who was paralyzed after a spinal cord injury for an example of real-life activities that require assistance. This example illustrates how the client defines independence.

Case Scenario 1

During the rehabilitation process, the client, Daphne, participates in a seating and wheeled mobility evaluation and eventually receives a powered wheelchair and seating system that enable her to negotiate smooth and uneven terrain both indoors and outdoors. She is able to transfer independently to and from her wheelchair. Daphne cannot perform one task. She has not been able to position her wheelchair for charging and to connect her wheelchair to the battery charger in the evening or to unplug the charger and position the wheelchair for her transfer in the morning. Daphne lives with a roommate who is able to assist her with these activities. Daphne considers herself an independent person and hopes that she will be able to devise a method to charge her wheelchair herself. But for now, she is satisfied with her roommate assisting so that she can spend her time on other tasks. For now, this is an aspect of her life in which she uses assistance. Daphne's independence hinges on her ability to instruct others in the appropriate care or assistance that she requires.

This case scenario makes three crucial points. First, Daphne is actively engaged in performing some tasks and in delegating others to her roommate. Second, Daphne's delegation does not diminish her sense of independence because she retains control over which tasks she delegates. Third, Daphne continues to strive for even greater independence for the future. Although Daphne requires help in managing the maintenance of her wheelchair, she is independent in managing her routine in this area. Daphne is not, however, independent in performing the task of wheelchair maintenance.

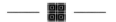

Exercise 1

Consider life as a student away from home and answer the following questions.

- The context in which you perform activities has changed; the human environment no longer includes your parents. How do you define your new level of independence?
- Does this independence differ from the independence you had living at home with your family members? If so, in what ways?
- Consider your level of freedom. Who controls or directs your activities?
- Consider the different ways in which persons with disabilities may experience independence?

You may consider yourself independent because you have the freedom and the responsibility to make your own decisions, prioritize your activities, and accept the consequences of your decisions. In the same manner, a person with a disability may experience independence by personal performance, by making the decision to delegate a time-consuming or difficult task, and by directing others to meet his or her needs.

Dependent or Independent?

Independence is a simple word, yet the more one explores it, the more complex it becomes. Try answering the following series of questions. Be open-minded, and take time to think about your answers.

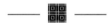

Exercise 2

Independent meal preparation 1: Answer the following questions on the basis of your experience.

- What is independent meal preparation?
- Does independent meal preparation require cooking? Using a microwave oven? Using the stove top or range? Following a recipe? Does preparation of a cold meal count?
- Does independent meal preparation include getting packages from cabinets and the refrigerator and opening them, or is the client still independent in meal preparation if someone else cooks and puts together the meals and the client merely puts the meal on the table?

- Does independent meal preparation require independently obtaining the food? Does it require shopping? Making a shopping list? Carrying food home?

- Is the task still independent meal preparation if your client orders a meal from a restaurant or from a local delivery service? Does money management matter? Can a personal assistant leave money? Can the client run a tab that someone else pays?

Now answer the above questions for a person who has a disability. Select one of the following: a woman who has had a stroke resulting in left hemiparesis, a young man with depression, or a young woman with cerebral palsy resulting in spastic diplegia.

Do your answers differ? Why would we hold a person with a disability to a different standard than we do for ourselves? Does this mean that planning for your client to order food in or having someone else prepare meals so that you do not have to do kitchen activities during therapy is acceptable? Absolutely not. You must know your client, his or her family members and support system, and his or her needs and then plan treatment accordingly.

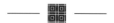

Exercise 3

Independent meal preparation 2: Answer the following questions on the basis of your experience.

- What is independent home management? Does this mean your client must be able to mow a lawn?

- What if he or she lives in an apartment and has no lawn? What if he or she does have a lawn?

The client's neighbor may have a lawn care service, or a child in the neighborhood may do the work. If this is acceptable for the neighbor, is it acceptable for your client? What if no one else in the neighborhood has this service? You can ask similar questions for every activity. Why is it acceptable for persons without disabilities to hire a maid, but we find it so important for our clients to be able to make a bed or iron a shirt?

Alternative techniques and compensatory strategies may allow independent performance of skills. For example, persons commonly use a checklist or "to-do" list if their memory is impaired because of a brain injury or other neurological insult. Persons with maladaptive behaviors may be taught strategies such as counting to 10 before responding in anger. The provision and use of adaptive equipment and assistive technology includes the process of recommending and providing assistive technology. This process is complex, and the unpredictability of real life makes it even more so.

What is important actually depends on the client and his or her own situation. As occupational therapy practitioners, we should not force our values on our clients. Our role is to help our clients meet their needs as they define them, so if the ability to manage household help is what is important to the client, then *that* is what is important.

Habilitation and Rehabilitation: A Collection of Transitions and Activity Simulations

As mentioned previously, the process of moving to independence involves numerous transitions, and therapists can facilitate these transitions by using various simulations (i.e., performance of contrived activities in a clinical environment and simulated activities in a real environment) (see Figure 1). When discussing habilitation and rehabilitation, we are concerned with independence and real life. Many changes occur during the transition to real life. Most persons like to organize events in some sort of order. Thinking of the process of habilitation or rehabilitation as a series of transitions that occur in some order may be helpful. The chronology of these transitions generally progresses a person from dependence (or difficulty and inability in performing life skills) to independence (or the ability to perform life skills without assistance). Each step along the way involves a transition, and at the completion of each transition, the person is closer to the end goal of independence. At each transition, the client actively participates in selecting and performing activities that promote the acquisition of skills toward a goal.

The process of habilitation or rehabilitation does not often occur in an orderly, predetermined way. Some persons start the process with total dependence and may require contrived activities in the clinic or another externally structured environment to master initial subskills. Contrived activities can be meaningful to the client if he or she understands their place in the overall treatment plan. The client should understand that these activities are temporary and transitional in nature and provide an opportunity for him or her to learn skills that he or she will later integrate into performance of the real-life task.

Case Scenario 2

Consider the case of Dana, who has severe anxiety attacks whenever he takes the elevator to his job on the 15th floor of a high-rise office building. Dana's goal is to become independent in taking the elevator by himself. Presently, however, he becomes physically ill when simply contemplating the idea. Because of his dependence in this activity, the occupational therapist has decided to initiate intervention by engaging Dana in simple, nonthreatening activities that involve the elevator. Dana and his therapist discuss the activities, and, with Dana's input, they make slight modifications. They decide on the following: Dana will watch the elevator doors open and close, watch persons get on and off, push the button to summon the elevator, and quickly walk on and off the stationary elevator.

During these activities, the therapist encourages Dana to discuss his level of comfort or discomfort, and the therapist in turn provides support and encouragement. Although contrived, these activities are meaningful to Dana and actively engage him.

Other persons start somewhere further along the continuum and focus on learning or relearning actual skills in a simulated environment. Still others start at different points in different performance areas. For example, one client may be dependent in one area (e.g., dressing) and be further along the continuum in another area (e.g., work activities, computer use). In this example, the difference may be because the person has relatively intact fine motor coordination for computer use but has impaired balance and gross motor performance for dressing while sitting on the edge of the bed.

The process or movement through the stages varies among clients and even between the expectations and the actual process for an individual client. No one can say exactly how long a person will stay in any stage of the process or whether he or she will move forward and backward several times during the progression. Some persons never make the journey all the way to the end. They achieve some level of independence, but they may not achieve total independence or perhaps not the level of independence that they or their family members expected. In addition, a client may choose to receive assistance for a gross motor task that is tiring and time consuming to save his or her energy for another task in which independent performance is a higher priority.

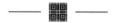

Exercise 4

John is a bright 6-year-old boy who, after months of therapy, is now able to maintain good dynamic balance in long sitting. John's goal is to learn to put on his socks and shoes by himself. Where along the continuum would you begin your occupational therapy intervention and why? Which of these activities would you select?

- Teach John the concepts of "on" and "off" as he places and removes large plastic rings on a pole as he sits on the clinic floor?

- Teach him how to put the socks and shoes on the Raggedy Andy doll?

- Teach him how to position himself so that he can put the socks on his own feet?

- How would you grade the activity you chose?

Occupational therapy intervention should continue by teaching John how to position himself and how to move to put on his socks and shoes. He is a bright boy and has already mastered the concepts of "on" and "off." Now that his dynamic balance in long sitting is good, he can build on this ability by performing the actual task. Dressing the doll would be an unnecessary detour toward his goal.

Instead of a neat, predictable timetable, the process of habilitation or rehabilitation winds sometimes forward, sometimes backward, and sometimes in a circular pattern. Occupational therapy practitioners set goals and expectations in conjunction with their clients on the basis of a wealth of information, including the occupational therapy practitioner's previous experiences, the client's current level of functioning, the context of activity performance, and the occupational therapy practitioner's knowledge of the pathology involved. The therapist adjusts treatment sessions and revises goals when necessary in response to the winding trail of progress.

Most persons would prefer that the process be more predictable, but this is not possible because of the unpredictable nature of habilitation and rehabilitation. People are not machines, and influences such as personality, physical health, and environment affect their ability to participate in therapy programs and to perform activities. This unpredictable nature is sometimes unsettling for occupational therapy students, and clients and family members may have difficulty accepting this as well. Clients and family members often view the repetition of previously learned skills as a step backward. Occupational therapy practitioners must reassure clients, family members, and others that the process is complex and somewhat unpredictable and that repetition or movement to a previous step does not signify failure. As occupational therapy practitioners gain more experience, their expectations may match the actual outcome more closely, but the expected procedure will always require some modification. Clinicians and clients must accept this fact and adjust the program and expectations to meet the clients' current needs and abilities. Occupational therapy will otherwise be less meaningful and less effective.

Although the exact process is unpredictable, some trends are evident in the timing and order of the transitions and stages (see Figure 2). At each level of transition, simulation of real-life activity plays a role in the occupational therapy program. The first transition is one that occurs when someone detects a problem, dysfunction, or condition. At that instant, the client changes (or transitions) from being a person without a disability to a person with a disability.

After a traumatic injury or illness, the client has a period of medical recovery. During this period, the primary focus for the client is survival. Initiating occupational therapy may be possible at this point. As a result of the client's condition, occupational therapists often limit sessions to activities that do not closely resemble real life. For example, the therapist may ask the client to grasp objects of various shapes and sizes, place and release these objects in various planes, and perform certain movement patterns while sitting or lying in bed. These activities, although contrived, are crucial to promote joint range of motion and muscle flexibility throughout the upper extremities. The client may not associate these actions with the accomplishment of an activity (such as self-feeding) that he or she will perform in the future. At this stage, the client performs contrived activities in a clinical environment (see Figure 1).

As the person becomes more medically stable, he or she may be better able to participate in therapy. During this stage of transition, learning various skills is the focus of occupational therapy. The therapist may teach the skills individually, and the skills may or may not be related to each other and are sometimes referred to

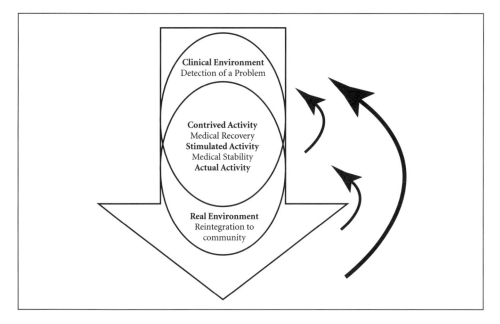

Figure 2. Stages of progression through habilitation or rehabilitation.

as *subskills.* After the client masters the subskills to some degree, the therapist combines the skills in various groupings to simulate various real-life activities. In this case, the client performs simulated activities in a clinical environment (see Figure 1).

As therapy progresses, activities more closely resemble real life. Simulation of activities varies greatly, and we address this topic in greater detail later in this chapter. Initially, a client's treatment session may seem quite different from the expected, eventual activity performance. The client sometimes has difficulty identifying the usefulness of a given task in relation to his or her own needs. The client may perform individual skills out of sequence or in awkward ways. The client may overlook some steps or skills altogether at this point. The treatment sessions may seem to be some abstract representation of real life. This can be frustrating for the client and for others involved in the client's progression. For this reason, the occupational therapy practitioner must reassure the client and family members that the simulations reflect real-life situations and that the actual activities will be brought into the clinical environment. The simulation is crucial to treatment, and the simulations become increasingly more realistic. At the end of this phase, the client performs simulations in real environments to prepare for real activity performance in the real environment. As discussed previously, therapists may skip steps along this continuum or revisit them until the client achieves maximal performance of the activity in the real environment. The following example demonstrates that the client may learn individual skills out of sequence and then later integrate them into a real-life activity.

Case Scenario 3

In an outpatient mental health clinic, a client has learned, at different times, strategies to control impulsive behavior, to foster taking turns and basic money management skills, and to be appropriately assertive. The client eagerly participated in the activities to learn these skills and was able to master them individually. Next, the client and the occupational therapist planned a trip to the local supermarket to shop for the upcoming holiday party. In this situation, the client has the opportunity to integrate learned skills into a successful shopping experience.

Simulation

According to *Webster's Ninth New Collegiate Dictionary* (1986), to simulate is

> to assume the outward qualities or appearance of, often with the intent to deceive . . . imitative representation of the functioning of one system or process by means of the functioning of another . . . enables an operator to reproduce or represent under test conditions phenomena likely to occur in actual performance. (p. 1099)

Thinking about human performance in terms of using simulation to develop expertise is not unique to habilitation or rehabilitation. Each of us can remember numerous times when we have practiced each component of a skill before putting them together to practice the entire skill in a protected environment before performing the skill in the real environment. Learning a balance beam routine is one example of this process. A gymnast may begin by practicing each jump and flip on a mat. He or she may practice walking a straight line marked on a floor. For the gymnast, these are subskills. These subskills only distantly resemble the final routine. Once the client masters the individual skills, he or she then combines the skills. The routine is still not exactly like the form it has in real life, and this is simulation. For example, the gymnast may perform the routine more slowly or on a low or wide beam. Finally, the gymnast performs the routine in its appropriate context, and the gymnast completes the simulation phase of mastery. For the gymnast, real-life performance of the routine occurs during a competition or exhibition. At any time, however, the gymnast may return to simulation to refine the individual skills.

Simulation is commonplace in other human endeavors, such as in engineering; product design, development, and testing; and marketing. These efforts have shown that mechanical simulations or mock-ups, computer-driven simulations, virtual reality, and interactive simulations can provide an accurate representation of the real world. We can analyze product testing, efficiency, and worker and consumer behaviors via simulations. In marketing, the value of testing a concept and then building and testing a prototype is that one can measure the viability of ideas long before the product is actually manufactured, thus saving valuable time, effort, and money (Eastlack, 1968). We cannot overstate the value of rigorous testing simulations to determine the durability, effectiveness, and viability of these and similar products. In the following paragraphs, we discuss a few examples of industry-based simulation.

The Visionary Shopper from Canada Market Research is a computer-driven simulation that uses a virtual reality store to study the purchasing behavior of shoppers (Marney, 1997). Consumers sit at a computer monitor and simulate their purchasing preferences. Consumers can "lift and move" product packages to inspect and read packaging material from different angles. Market researchers are able to determine whether the package design has emotional appeal and provides useful information to encourage purchase.

The *SIMUL8* is a computer software visual simulation package designed for use in general engineering (Visual Thinking International, 1998). This simulation software allows time tracking of particular products and assigns fixed and variable costs to simulated activities. The package tracks use of resources, inventory storage, and costs incurred by stocking products and allows engineers to explore plant improvements and make recommendations for changes in a timely and cost-effective way.

Physical interactive simulation is a dynamic technique that goes beyond computer simulation or visual interactive simulation to provide a highly accurate representation of the real world (Winarchick & Caldwell, 1997). Through physical interactive simulation, one can simulate and evaluate human performance on an actual three-dimensional physical model. Delphi Chassis Systems and Sinclair Community College, both of Dayton, Ohio, worked together to establish a workplace prototype laboratory in which analysis of modeling an entire process before pilot production has saved Delphi Chassis Systems millions of dollars. Users of physical interactive simulation are able to interact with models before determining their work-site setups to maximize productivity and to save time and money in development. The models are easy to construct, rearrange, and modify to provide various analyses, including motion economy and ergonomics (Winarchick & Caldwell, 1997).

The Fatigue Phenomenon

Product durability has long been a crucial issue not only for the designer and manufacturer of the product (e.g., the automobile, the airplane), but also for the end user. Automobile manufacturers have produced test programs that simulate road profiles, weather conditions, and the most aggressive maneuvers to ensure that a product meets a desirable target for durability (Weal, Liefooghe, & Dressler, 1997). Impact tests determine the fatigue strength or crash worthiness of automobiles. Computer-aided engineering models test the durability of automobiles and validate design assumptions. Laboratory simulations are efficient and flexible ways of determining the durability of products from design through manufacturing.

Simulation plays a major role in the aeronautics industry. One example is the development of airplane engines. Initially, designers make gross drawings to design specifications. Next follow computer-aided simulations of the designs and a critical design review. Solid mock-up airplane engine parts are then made according to the specifications of the critical design review team. These parts are assembled in test-cell engines under simulated conditions of aircraft usage. A constant flow of information exchanges between the designers and those testing the products in simulation (S. Rausch, personal communication, October 15, 1998).

Virtual reality is the ultimate simulation. Through environmental immersion, a person believes that he or she is in an alternative reality. Forms of input of virtual reality include visual, auditory, and tactile. Headsets cover the eyes and ears and allow only input from computer-generated information and thus prevent outside stimuli from affecting the person. In addition, the sense of touch, through the field of haptics, is involved whereby a person acquires the ability to "feel" his or her environment, which increases the intensity of virtual reality (G. Bell, personal communication, October 2, l998). The PHANToM is one example of a haptic device that may have applications in occupational therapy (MIT Artificial Intelligence Laboratory, 1998). This computer input device allows the user to feel virtual objects. The device exerts an external force on the user's fingertips to provide information about the shape and texture of solid virtual objects. With the PHANToM, a user can control a virtual pencil or paintbrush to draw or paint by using movements that are free and unimpeded in virtual space.

Occupational therapists currently use virtual reality alongside more traditional interventions. According to Cunningham (1998), virtual reality provided multisensory input and feedback to clients with stroke who were working to improve their perception, cognition, gross and fine motor coordination, praxis, posture, and safety awareness. Cunningham further stated that, "the [virtual reality] modality allows therapists to work in several problem areas at one time" (p. 19).

Simulation in Occupational Therapy

Occupational therapy practitioners use various tools to help clients achieve their highest level of independence; simulation is one of these important tools. Simulation is an effective tool in various occupational therapy settings, including acute care, rehabilitation, long-term care, home care, and outpatient settings, and is an appropriate tool to use with persons who have various cognitive, emotional, physical, and psychological conditions. Simulation is useful regardless of age, ethnic or cultural background, and gender. In almost every scenario, simulation can be a tool to develop independence.

In psychotherapy, role-playing is an education tool in which therapists provide persons with situations in which they can act out imaginary situations. This acting out or participating in an imaginary experience can lead to self-understanding and to improved skills and behaviors. Role-playing provides the participants with simulated examples of how others act in specific situations and how they themselves may act (Corsini, 1966). Role-playing involves the repetition of situations in a therapeutic environment, which allows practice while encouraging exploration and spontaneity. Role-playing in which the participants understand that they are participating in an imaginary situation is commonly part of the simulation process in occupational therapy.

Occupational therapy practitioners plan treatment by designing activities that simulate real life. Practitioners identify activities to simulate on the basis of client evaluation data. After determining which activities to simulate, the practitioner selects and creates an opportunity to engage in the activities in the occupational therapy clinic, the classroom, the home, or a community setting. While the client is engaged in the activities, the occupational therapy practitioner uses cues and assistance to allow the client to work with only the challenge that is useful and that he or she can tolerate to ensure a positive learning experience. These treatments often involve imagination, and the practitioner asks the client to imagine the circumstances and the context in which the client will perform occupations.

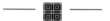

Exercise 5

You are working with a 14-year-old boy who recently underwent right below-elbow amputation as a result of a traumatic injury. This boy was previously right-hand dominant. As a result of the occupational therapy evaluation, you outline goals with input from both the child and his parents. One long-term goal is for the boy to perform activities of daily living (ADL) and schoolwork by using the right upper extremity (which has been fitted with a mechanical prosthesis) as an assist. Another goal is to retrain the boy to use his left upper extremity as dominant. Describe one activity that you could use to meet the goal of changing dominance. After you have described the activity, answer the following questions.

- How have you set up the treatment environment to replicate the real-life setting in which the activity will take place?

- What are the differences between your simulated environment and the real-life environment?

- How does the activity itself differ from real life in your simulation?

- How can you change the demands of the activity and the structure of the environment to meet the changing needs of the client as his skills improve?

In the previous activity, we asked you to use simulation to target completion of one task that is important to your client. You created the environment in which your client played the role of task performer, and you provided the structure that was necessary to match the client's abilities and was sufficiently challenging and important to motivate the client to work hard.

Simulation involves the use of some elements of real life and allows the client to explore real-life performance in a protected environment. Because the occupational therapy practitioner can control some aspects of the simulation, he or she can design it to meet the client's needs and abilities at any given time. For example, early in the process, the occupational therapy practitioner may plan the activity so that successful performance is likely. Later, the client can accept more of the responsibility for success. The following is a series of treatment sessions that illustrate this point.

Case Scenario 4

Brenda is an occupational therapist who works in a community-based center. Her clients are primarily persons who live on the street and do not work. Brenda works in a program with social workers, psychologists, and vocational rehabilitation counselors. One goal of the program is to improve the work habits and skills of the clients. Her group meets for 3 months. The group starts by talking about what they would like to do in the future and what steps are necessary in reaching that goal. After a short period, attendance and participation in the group activities becomes the "work" of its members.

This case scenario of Brenda's community-based program provides a clear example of when a simulation is paramount to the activities. During the group meetings, members discuss work behaviors like grooming, timeliness, punctuality, and other responsibilities. During some sections, Brenda encourages group members to role-play specific situations.

The group members then begin to work in the center's gift shop to develop their work skills further. Group members, who are at this point group employees, punch time clocks and meet with their supervisor on a daily basis. In addition to working in the gift shop, the members continue to meet in their discussion group. During the discussion group, they learn skills to use when interviewing, how to write a résumé, and how to complete a job application. Group members play the roles of the interviewer and the interviewee to practice job interviews. At this point, the group members can apply for specific jobs in the center's shop. For example, some persons are interested in working in the stock room, others are interested in working as a cashier, and others are interested in management.

The clients and the group leaders then work together to answer newspaper advertisements and to work with job placement services. Clients go to their interviews sometimes with a job coach or assistant and begin their jobs with the help of a job coach, which is the highest level of simulation. The situation is not quite real life because the job coach influences performance and success by assisting, supervising, and encouraging the client. The job coach continues to work with the client for the required amount of time and then removes himself or herself. At this point, the client is in real life as it relates to working. The client may contact the group leaders anytime, and the group leaders often ask graduates of the group to return to talk to new members about the process and the result.

The ways that occupational therapy practitioners use simulations as part of their interventions is similar in all areas of practice. The process begins with a comprehensive evaluation, development of specific goals, determination of which performance components need improvement, and finally which performance skills would benefit from a simulated situation. Of course, the client's motivation, willingness, and preferences are key factors to consider before engaging him or her in a simulated activity. For some clients, simulations are motivating and fun. For other clients, simulations may have seemingly no value, and clients may perceive the simulations to be like child's play. Simulations are often the key to engaging young children in a meaningful learning activity.

Case Scenario 5

Belle, a woman 75 years of age who has had a cerebrovascular accident, needs to improve her toileting skills. Initially, Belle participated in tasks and exercises focused on individual steps in the activity. The occupational therapy program included the following: activities in sitting to improve balance and the ability to shift weight, activities in sitting that encourage weight bearing through the upper and lower extremities, activities requiring a forward weight shift and unweighting of the buttocks, fine motor activities and bimanual tasks in preparation for lower-extremity garment management, activities in standing to improve balance, and activities to improve compensation for a visual field cut.

This is the point during early recovery when treatment appears to be the least representative of real life. The simulation is rather abstract. After mastery or partial mastery of the individual components of an activity, the client compiles and performs the components in a protected environment. The treatment environment is a safe place to practice each component and many combinations or collections of components. This environment allows clients to make mistakes and to learn from them, to explore alternatives, and to develop strategies for improved performance. Initially, the practitioner sets up the environment to protect the person from distractions and to encourage successful completion of the task.

At this next stage of intervention for Belle, the occupational therapist uses one or more treatment sessions to bring Belle to a private bathroom where she can practice transfers to and from the commode. During these sessions, the therapist does not address other components of the activity, such as lower-extremity garment management and hygiene after toileting. At some point, the client will perform these simulated activities in a real trial. Belle, initially with assistance and later with supervision, toilets in the private bathroom. Belle may practice by herself any task that is difficult for her.

Other occupational therapy sessions focus only on lower-extremity garment management. For example, during part of one treatment session, Belle worked on buttoning and unbuttoning buttons and zipping and unzipping zippers on a dressing board. The therapist designed the activity to begin with large buttons and loose buttonholes and move on to smaller buttons and tighter buttonholes. Another treatment session began with large zippers on slippery tracks and moved on to smaller zippers with more resistant tracks. Once Belle mastered the tasks on the dressing board, the next step was to lay a pair of pants smoothly in her lap. The therapist assisted by holding the clothing taut, exposing the zipper, or holding the buttonhole steady. As Belle gained the ability to perform this task, the therapist provided less assistance. the next step in this sequence was to have

Belle practice the tasks of buttoning and unbuttoning and zipping and unzipping on her own pants. After she mastered this step, the therapist and Belle worked on removing and replacing the lower-extremity garments in preparation for toileting.

Other interventions focused on the activities of toilet paper management and hygiene. These interventions followed the same procedure of practice and mastery. The therapist used other activities to address areas in which Belle had difficulty. For example, the therapist used paper-and-pencil tasks, bed making, and computer games to increase her awareness of the visual field cut.

As you can see from this example, practitioners address each component of an activity individually. The client practices and masters the tasks and components of each activity and then groups them together until he or she has addressed the entire occupation (in this case, toileting) sufficiently.

When Belle is able, she completes each activity by herself. This may, however, only be when conditions are optimal, such as when she is already in her wheelchair and is wearing sturdy shoes with nonslip soles. In the evenings, when Belle is fatigued, she may continue to require assistance from her husband to perform this task safely. When planning treatment with Belle, the long-term goal is to toilet independently regardless of the time of day, the type of clothing she is wearing, or even the layout of the bathroom. When she is able to achieve this goal, Belle will be independent in performing this task in real life. Her occupational therapy sessions will no longer address this task.

Occupational therapy practitioners frequently use simulation as a key aspect of the intervention plan. The following are a few examples of the way practitioners use simulation to ensure that activities are purposeful in occupational therapy. Work-centered rehabilitation often uses simulation. Work samples such as *Valpar Work Samples* (Valpar Corporation, 1974) and the Baltimore Therapeutic Equipment Work Simulator™ replicate various job skills (see Figure 3). Work samples or work simulations can be evaluation tools to determine a client's abilities and to measure the progress a client makes toward returning to work. Not only are work samples useful for evaluation, but also components of some work samples can be treatment tools. By using these simulation tools, practitioners can target specific work skills in an objective, measurable, and repeatable way.

In one Valpar activity, the user must piece together three small metal objects and place them in moving holes on a round track. The rate of movement is adjustable so that the holes move faster as the person's fine motor coordination and speed increase. The practitioner may adjust the time allotted for this activity to meet or challenge the user's endurance. The therapist counts the number of sets of objects placed in the holes while the person works. The practitioner and client can track progress in several ways: by noting the client's ability as the speed quickens, by noting the amount of time that the client participates in the activity, and by noting the number of sets that the client completes in a fixed or consistent amount of time. This Valpar activity, which simulates the manipulation of small objects and in turn simulates repetitious assembly-line work, is useful for several reasons, such as preparing an assembly-line worker for his or her return to work, improving a person's fine motor and bimanual coordination, increasing endurance for fine motor tasks, or even increasing tolerance for repetitious work. This tool may be appropriate for persons with various disabling conditions, including traumatic hand injury, medical conditions like diabetes that involve associated sensory impairments, visual impairments in which the purpose of occupational therapy is to improve tactile compensatory strategies, and mental illness that affects a person's concentration and attention span.

Another work-centered simulation involves adults in work rehabilitation who simulate jobs as part of a program (Ellexson, 1989). In a work-hardening program, activities simulate those work skills on which the client must concentrate. Inpatient or outpatient groups may take contracts from other companies to complete work. For example, a group of adults with developmental disabilities may work in a program that has a contract to package plastic knives, forks, and spoons. This job includes counting the utensils, placing them in bags, sealing the bags, labeling the bags, and

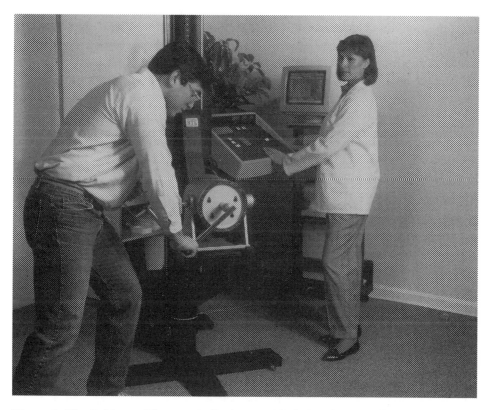

Figure 3. The Baltimore Therapeutic Equipment Work Simulator Model WS20 with the Quest computer system can simulate work activities in a clinical setting. Note. Reprinted with permission from Valpar International Corporation.

placing the bags in boxes. This activity demonstrates how simulation allows an occupational therapy practitioner to organize the environment, break down tasks into components, and offer clients purposeful activity as a treatment tool.

Occupational therapy clinics have long included specially built treatment areas that provide clients with treatment in a setting that simulates real life. Examples of this are specific areas in the occupational therapy department such as a kitchen, a bathroom, and a bedroom or living area in which clients practice certain basic ADL skills and instrumental ADL (IADL) tasks. These treatment locations are useful when the client has improved to the point at which a setting that is more realistic than the occupational therapy clinic or laboratory encourages further progress. A training apartment, for example, may be useful after the client has completed wheelchair transfers in a hospital room and meal preparation in the occupational therapy kitchen area. A client's family members may join him or her in the training apartment so that they can practice the skills of caregiving before discharge. The training apartment offers a transition between the contrived and simulated activities in the clinic and performing activities in real life (in this case, at home).

Occupational therapy practitioners working with children and adolescents often use simulation as part of their interventions. Children develop and explore their environment through the use of their imaginations. Children with disabilities may not be able to use their imaginations or be able to explore their environment as they would without their disabilities. The role of the occupational therapy practitioner is, in part, to create the environment for children to use their imaginations to develop new skills or to become secure or confident with their abilities. Children use play to explore and learn about their environment and to receive the sensory stimulation that they need for development. A child with a disability may be unable to participate in play sufficiently to meet his or her other needs.

Case Scenario 6

Ricardo is a 5-year-old boy 5 in kindergarten. He has a learning disability and attention deficit hyperactivity disorder. He attends regular classes and has occupational, physical, and speech therapy three times weekly. Ricardo switches hand dominance for different activities; he throws a ball with his left hand, but he writes and uses scissors with his right hand. The occupational therapist observed the following problems during writing activities in the classroom: impaired fine motor coordination of both hands, associated reactions in the left hand and arm, squeezing the pencil too hard, pressing too hard on the paper, and difficulty releasing the pencil when finished and repositioning it when writing.

The occupational therapist, Isadore (Izzy), decided that Ricardo needs a fun way to learn to regulate pressure and to learn to grasp and release the pencil appropriately. Izzy decided to play "Blockhead" with Ricardo. "Blockhead" is a game in which the players take turns balancing oddly shaped wood blocks on top of one another until one person causes the tower to topple. The person who causes the tower to topple is the "blockhead." Because Ricardo does not have the attention span, motor skills, or perceptual skills to play "Blockhead," Izzy, by using the rules of that game, created a game with Styrofoam™ and paper. These materials require Ricardo to regulate his grip pressure and to use larger gross motor skills. Izzy required Ricardo to play the game while assuming different positions with both hands. Sometimes Ricardo played while seated at a table and other times while standing. Sometimes Ricardo played while lying in a prone position and resting on his forearms when upper-extremity weight bearing was necessary. Izzy talked with Ricardo's mother, and she reported that she bought "Blockhead" and that he enjoys playing at home with her and his older brother.

After playing a simulated "Blockhead" game, Ricardo learned the appropriate rules and developed an attention span adequate to play the real game. Izzy noted that Ricardo's writing skills likewise improved.

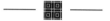

Exercise 6

Think about the above case scenario and answer the following questions.

- What real-life activity does this therapeutic intervention address?
- How did the occupational therapist use simulation to simulate the real-life activity?
- What modifications did the therapist make to the environment and the demands of the activity?
- How do the therapist and the family members provide assistance to make the activity possible?

Exercise 7

At this time, take a few minutes to think about more activities that could serve the same purpose for Ricardo.

- If you were the occupational therapy practitioner, what would you do? How would you set up the environment?
- How would you alter the assistance given to meet the changing needs of the child?
- How would you help the parents and siblings to do this?

Jacobs (1991) discussed the importance of introducing various activities that simulate adult roles in the transition to the adult worker. She discussed the use of exploratory play and role-playing activities even in children as young as preschool age. During these role-playing activities, children can explore the physical properties associated with various careers. Children are also able to try out different social skills and behaviors necessary for leadership and team work. Throughout school, these skills address and develop work behaviors. Behaviors such as punctuality and preparedness are necessary early in a child's schooling, and mastering these skills prepares a child for behaviors that will be necessary later in life at work. Older children may participate in programs in which they develop a mock business and provide some service or product to others.

In the recent past, several rehabilitation departments across North America have begun to use sophisticated, visually appealing, functional simulations of various environments called Easy Street Environments[SM] (Habitat, Inc., 1998). These custom environments include more than 30 areas of activity, such as a park, restaurant, bank, supermarket, department store, office, theater, and automobile. Easy Street Environments provide convenient, safe, low-risk, weather-free treatment spaces in which occupational therapy practitioners can effectively treat clients in all age groups who have a wide range of disabilities. The practitioner and client may address discharge readiness, community reentry, client and family member training, evaluation of possible home adaptations, and assistance necessary in the community with Easy Street Environments.

Easy Street Environments are at a level similar to the training apartment discussed earlier. These environments fill the gap between the occupational therapy clinic or laboratory and real life. After a client demonstrates the ability to perform contrived and simulated activities in an occupational therapy clinic or laboratory but is not yet ready for community reentry, the client can perform activities in the Easy Street Environments. Practitioners who have used these simulated environments claim that their clients' confidence in performing IADL has increased and that the practitioners can use their time more efficiently (Habitat, Inc., 1998). The more realistic the simulation is in the controlled setting, as in Easy Street Environments, the easier or smoother the clients' transition may be when performing these activities in real life.

Occupational therapy practitioners must not make the mistake of thinking that an excellent simulation supersedes real-life training and application. Simulation, by definition, is not real life. Although the amount of time and the intensity of simulation in occupational therapy may influence the ease of transition to real life, success in simulation does not ensure success in real life.

Simulation is useful in outpatient settings and can provide an even smoother transition to real life. Clients can work on a certain skill during their therapy sessions and practice the skill at home or in another real-life setting. This homework is actually an advanced form of simulation because, although still somewhat contrived, the homework is useful in maximizing a person's ability to perform an activity. When clients try techniques at home, they can bring questions back to therapy, and the occupational therapy practitioner can devise simulated activities to use during treatment that target those specific problems. Each time a client masters a skill in the clinic, he or she can perform the skill at home or in the real-life location as a check. As the client performs activities satisfactorily at home, the goals for treatment change. The practitioner can document progress and indicate whether occupational therapy should continue after satisfactory task performance in real life.

Real Life

In all of the previous examples, simulations prepare clients for real life. Transition to real life is the final step in the process we describe in this chapter. The occupational therapy practitioner can foster the transition to real life by keeping the focus on real life foremost in treatment throughout the habilitation or rehabilitation process. The ultimate goal of occupational therapy is for the client to be successful in his or her occupations. Real life is the usual environment in which any given activity takes place. Real-life environments include the home, workplace, school, places of leisure enjoyment, and private and public transportation. The occupational therapy intervention to prepare a client for real life is limited in scope. Predicting all of the environments in which a client may interact is impossible for the practitioner. Addressing many of the more likely environments in simulation is possible to ease the transition to real life. In occupational therapy, the client learns problem-solving skills and strategies that will enable him or her to generalize information to various real-life environments. Remember that simulations do not guarantee success in real life. Planning for the unexpected is essential and yet somehow is not entirely possible.

During therapy, an occupational therapy practitioner must address foundational performance components that are necessary to engage in performance areas essential for real life. Addressing the psychosocial requirements of an activity is important, including the acceptability of the methods and equipment, embarrassment or pride associated with performance, and support of family members, friends, and others. Real-life task performance includes using all of the appropriate performance components to engage in an occupation. Real life includes performing activities in the conventional manner, performing activities with alternative techniques and compensatory strategies, and performing activities with assistive technology.

When addressing the real world, occupational therapy practitioners often prescribe and provide adaptive equipment and assistive technology devices. Occupational therapy practitioners may focus on simulations with and without devices and ensure that the client can competently use the device to complete activities in the clinic environment. Everything changes at home, and the occupational therapy practitioner must address home issues. In Phillips and Zhao's (1993) study of technology abandonment, they described patterns of abandonment of devices recommended or provided to clients in a physical rehabilitation setting. Four factors were important in abandoning technology:

1. Lack of consideration of user opinion

2. Easy device procurement

3. Poor device performance

4. Change in user needs or priorities

The occupational therapy practitioner's role is to address those indicators. By ensuring that the device performs as it should, both in the protected therapeutic environment and in real life, the occupational therapy practitioner can help to provide the best possible solution to clients who require assistive technology. The client's home and other real-life environments should be the focus of treatment, and one should avoid assumptions such as, "If it works in the hospital room, it will work the same at home." In a related study, Bell and Hinojosa (1996) interviewed three participants regarding the effect of assistive devices on their ability to perform their daily routines. They concluded that successful use of these devices in the clinic setting did not necessarily transition to successful use of these devices at home. Follow-up at home, in home training, or during performance is crucial to using assistive devices or compensatory techniques successfully in the real-life, postdischarge setting.

The context in which the client performs any activity influences the realism of the simulation. For example, pretending to lift a heavy object in the proper way in an occupational therapy clinic is different from lifting an object of a similar weight on a busy factory floor. In the latter situation, the context includes noise, the space available, the presence of a supervisor and coworkers, and many distractions. These factors make real-life activity performance much more complex than simulated activity. Again, successful performance in a clinic does not necessarily guarantee success in real life.

Summary

As an occupational therapy practitioner becomes more experienced, evaluating the long-term goals of clients becomes easier. In turn, planning and organizing simulated activities to address these needs becomes easier. The visualization of the outcome of occupational therapy may not always be accurate because of the unpredictable nature of human beings, the unpredictability of the setting, and the other demands that influence performance. We believe that as a practitioner gains more experience and builds a repertoire of goal-setting and treatment skills, his or her predictions will be more accurate or will be accurate more often. The practitioner can outline some trends in performance and move from contrived to real activities in various environments that range from clinical or simulated to real. The ultimate goal is independent activity performance in a real environment, and occupational therapy practitioners use simulation in this effort. As in other industries, simulation in occupational therapy allows clients to test and practice techniques in a safe, controlled environment. Practitioners can address problems, gain insights, and explore solutions before real-life performance. Some occupational therapy practitioners believe that the ultimate setting for providing occupational therapy intervention is at the client's work site or in the client's home or community. In these cases, simulations are already in the real life-setting, which ensures the transition to more optimal real-life performance. ■

References

Bell, P., & Hinojosa, J. (1996). Perception of the impact of assistive devices on daily life of three individuals with quadriplegia. *Assistive Technology, 7,* 87–94.

Corsini, R. J. (1966). *Roleplaying in psychotherapy: A manual.* Chicago: Aldine.

Cunningham, D. (1998, April 27). In Alabama, OT is a virtual reality. *Advance for Occupational Therapists, 14,* 19.

Eastlack, J. O. (1968). New products for the seventies. In J. O. Eastlack & J. Tinker (Eds.), *New product development* (pp. 142–148). Chicago: American Marketing Association.

Ellexson, M. T. (1989). Work hardening. In S. Hertfelder & C. Gwin (Eds.), *Work in progress: Occupational therapy in work programs* (pp. 67–126). Bethesda, MD: American Occupational Therapy Association.

Habitat, Inc. (1998). *Easy street environments* [Brochure]. Tempe, AZ: Author.

Jacobs, K. (1991). *Occupational therapy: Work-related programs and assessments.* Boston: Little, Brown.

Marney, J. (1997). Design testing goes digital. *Marketing, 102,* 10.

MIT Artificial Intelligence Laboratory. (1998). *Haptics* [On-line]. (Available: www.ai.mit.edu/projects/handarm-haptics.html).

Phillips, B., & Zhao, H. (1993). Predictors of assistive technology abandonment. *Assistive Technology, 5,* 36–45.

Valpar Corporation. (1974). *Valpar work samples.* (Available: Valpar Corporation, 3801 East 34th Street, Suite 105, Tucson, AZ 85713)

Visual Thinking International. (1998). *SIMUL8* [On-line]. (Available: www.VTIL.com/simul8.htm)

Weal, P., Liefooghe, C., & Dressler, K. (1997). Product durability engineering: Improving the process. *Sound and Vibration, 31,* 68–79.

Webster's Ninth New Collegiate Dictionary. (1986). Springfield, MA: Merriam-Webster.

Winarchick, C., & Caldwell, R. (1997). Physical interactive simulation: A hands-on approach to facilities improvements. *IIE Solutions, 29,* 34–36.

12

Range of Human Activity: Leisure

Laurette J. Olson, MA, OTR, BCP, Elizabeth A. Roarty-O'Herron, MS, OTR

Leisure is . . . freedom from the necessity of labor.
Aristotle

Leisure is what we do in our spare time and may involve particular activities or a state of mind. Some persons define leisure as involvement in any activity that is not work. Others believe that within work are parts of the activity that a person may define as leisure. In this chapter, leisure encompasses meaningful activities that we choose to participate in during our discretionary time, but leisure is greater than the list of activities in which we engage in our spare time. Leisure happens when we engage in an activity that reflects our own true nature (Pieper, 1963). Leisure is a state of mind in which we are available and receptive to the experience of our physical, mental, and social selves. In leisure, we are free to participate or not without consequence, and the goals of the activity and the direction the activity takes come from ourselves. Leisure activities have no external judge of success or failure; only the participant decides whether his or her skill level of participation is adequate for personal enjoyment. Some leisure activities may require new learning, or we may use skills that we have already acquired. The former provide a challenge and intellectual stimulation. The latter may be purely for relaxation such as reading a novel, knitting, or gardening (Figure 1).

Leisure embodies a broad range of activities, including activities that provide entertainment, relaxation, fun and stimulation, or self-development. These activities may be active or passive. Watching television or listening to music are examples of passive activities, whereas traveling or playing a sport are examples of active activities. During leisure time, persons read, play sports, explore nature, dance, paint, tell jokes, solve puzzles, help others, engage in religious social activities, watch television, travel,

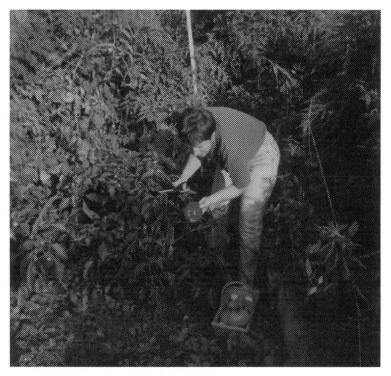

Figure 1. Gardening is an activity that relaxes some adults.

care for pets, drink, gamble, or daydream. Some leisure activities may resemble adult work, a child's school, or self-care activities. A businessperson may use leisure time to write a novel or to refinish old furniture, a high school student may explore astronomy, a retired teacher may volunteer a few days a week at a nursing home, and a homemaker may design and make clothing in his or her free time.

For adults, leisure requires that we discover our true nature and interests. Leisure involves becoming invested in an activity so that no other concern or goal matters for a time (Csikszentmihalyi, 1992). Leisure provides opportunities to seek out activities that we intrinsically find interesting. To have a satisfying leisure life, we must put as much energy into developing a leisure life as we put into work.

Although we frequently associate leisure with adolescence and adulthood, children's play is leisure. Leisure play occurs when children participate in an activity for no other reason than because the activity is interesting to them. During play, children have no overriding desire to please an adult and express their true nature in their interactions. Although children may develop motor, cognitive, or social skills in the process, these skills are not the primary goals for the children. Once children begin to experience the pleasure of mastery of the activity (e.g., jumping rope consecutively, swimming or diving into a pool), nothing else matters for a time, and other concerns or desires fade to the back of the children's minds.

—— ▦ ——

Exercise 1

Describe your active and passive leisure activities. What activities do you do for relaxation, fun and stimulation, entertainment, and personal development?

——————————

Needs Met Through Leisure

Why do persons seek out leisure? Why is leisure important throughout the life span? In modern, complex societies, a major amount of social control has been necessary for humans to maintain order and function every day. As members of society, people need to fulfill certain roles and put aside their own desires and impulses for immediate gratification. Sometimes people must contain their emotions so that work can proceed harmoniously. In these complex societies, leisure provides opportunities for people to put their commitments aside and to experience freedom in activities that satisfy their interests. Furthermore, participation in leisure activities provides opportunities for people to express their desires and their true range of emotions. This expression of emotions occurs with the approval of other persons (Neulinger, 1981). For example, an adolescent can write painfully honest poetry about loss and longing and receive praise from others for the beauty and depth of emotion of his or her writing. If the adolescent had shared these feelings at a part-time job, he or she may make his or her coworkers nervous, and coworkers may view the child as a troubled youth. Another example is the behavior characteristic of a football game, where fans cheer and jeer loudly while simultaneously sharing an intense camaraderie. This level of emotion in daily life would seem inappropriate or deviant.

Throughout our lives, the activities that have helped us develop, maintain, or strengthen relationships with others are often leisure activities. We plan and share special activities or events with family members or friends to bring pleasure and relaxation to all participants. When activities have the desired results, we associate the positive experience with the persons with whom we have interacted. This association strengthens these relationships, and we will most likely seek out these persons when we seek companionship in future activities. We may come to rely on these persons when we need assistance in our daily lives, and we will most likely be willing to help them as necessary. We will be more likely to tolerate and resolve disagreements and frustrations with others when they occur within a relationship that has a history of many pleasurable interactions (Figure 2). We most often sustain friendships throughout the life span through shared positive experiences that we associate with leisure.

Literature often emphasizes the relaxing nature of leisure (Kraus, 1994; Neulinger, 1981). Leisure provides us with opportunities to rejuvenate ourselves from the drudgery and stresses of everyday life. For some of us, leisure is an antidote to work, an opportunity to rest. Some of us seek relief by withdrawing from interactions and reading the newspaper or tending to our gardens. Others revive themselves

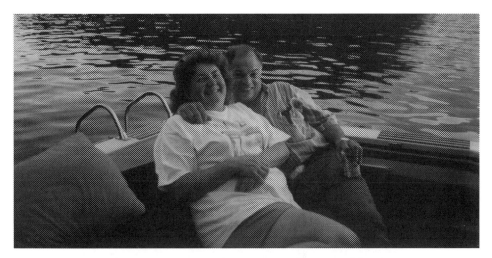

Figure 2. Enjoying leisure activities together can strengthen marital bonds.

through having special meals or drinks with others to create a relaxed mood for conversation and interaction.

Leisure provides opportunities to learn more about ourselves, to explore our interests, and to develop skills in activities that bring us pleasure. In our free time, we engage in activities that are interesting to us without concern about the activities' usefulness to others (Neulinger, 1981). We may learn to dance, kayak, paint, or play an instrument for no other reason than the pleasure that it brings us. Building our proficiency in an activity supports our internal sense of mastery and physical sense of control. Traveling may increase our awareness of other cultures, expand our understanding of ourselves and others, and foster an appreciation of activities from other cultures. For example, after a trip through the Middle East, a person may become more interested and invested in religion (Figure 3).

Engaging in leisure activities has the power to influence our mood and our view of possibilities for everyday living. Success in a leisure activity can be an antidote to a negative experience in another part of our lives. Successful leisure interests and experiences can lead one to have a renewed belief in his or her capacity to be effective in all parts of life. Furthermore, leisure activities or experiences can be a springboard for making changes in other parts of our lives. Some persons who are depressed or feel alienated from others benefit from taking up a new interest (leisure activity) to challenge themselves physically and mentally. Gulick (1998) reported the physical challenge that participating in a leisure activity can have for teenagers with spinal cord injuries who have taken up scuba diving, and Manuele (1998) reported such a challenge for adults with disabilities who learned to ride horses.

Learning new leisure activities within a structured group can lessen anxiety for learning and promote camaraderie and friendship that fosters enthusiasm for living and affirmation of the self. Developing the discipline one needs to master a new

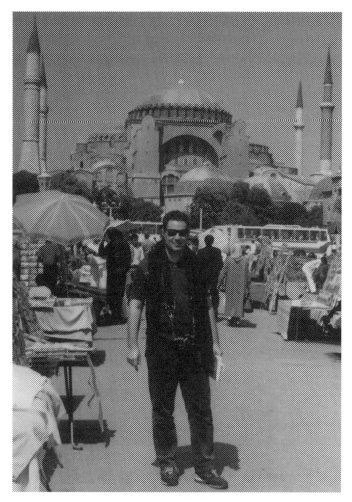

Figure 3. Traveling provides an opportunity to expand one's understanding of the range of human culture.

activity is often easier when one participates in a group of like-minded and equally skilled persons. The initial work of mastering a skill or preparing for participation can seem less daunting when we experience the camaraderie of others. Focusing our attention and completing an activity is easier when everyone is at the same skill level. When we are "in the same boat," we can share small triumphs and easily give support to each other when we stumble or make mistakes. Joining in with others and working harmoniously fosters engagement and continued interest in a challenging activity. In the United States, many nonprofit clubs, as well as profit-making companies, offer structured group activities. These groups afford various options for us to discover and explore new leisure activities either alone or with others. Joining in with others and working harmoniously fosters engagement and continued interest in a challenging activity.

Independent mastery of a leisure activity gives us pleasure. When we become overly compliant with external demands and lose our individuality among the needs and desires of others, our individuality disappears, and life becomes meaningless. During solitary time, we may learn to play a musical instrument, write, read, or perform a range of other activities for our own individual pleasure idiosyncratically. In an individual leisure activity, our activity pace is more likely unhurried, and our imaginative and creative abilities can flourish in the presence of only the self. Through this process, we get to know ourselves more deeply and gain an awareness of what moves us beyond the persons whom we love (Figure 4). Storr (1988) discussed two opposing human drives: the drive toward closeness to other human beings and the drive toward independence and self-sufficiency. Although love and friendship are important parts of what makes life worthwhile, solitude has great value. When we learn to make good use of solitude, we have the opportunity to focus on our own desires and interests separate from the needs and desires of others.

Persons seek leisure for emotional stimulation. Elias and Dunning (1986) stated that "Unless an organism is intermittently flushed and stirred by some exciting experience with the help of strong feelings, overall routinization and restraint . . . are apt to engender a dryness of emotions, a feeling of monotony" (p. 73). We can potentially experience a full range of human emotion that we avoid in everyday life in leisure activities. Many children love to frighten or be frightened on Halloween, and adults pay high ticket prices to become engrossed in the pain and suffering of characters in a play. Sloan (1979) reported studies suggesting that the heartbeat and stress level of fans at sporting events can be similar to that of the athletes participating in the sport. Tension and stress increase, but these feelings are different from and are pleasurable compared with tension and stress in everyday life. Aristotle's views that music and

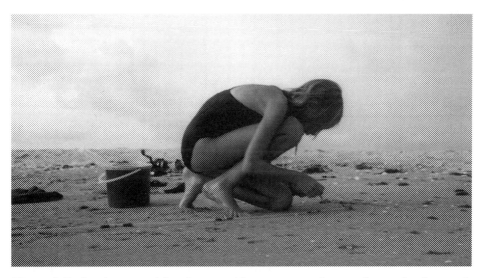

Figure 4. Performing an activity alone provides an opportunity to reflect and collect one's thoughts.

tragedy have a cathartic effect and move persons' souls the way sports relieve physical tension and energize the body is one that leisure theorists still assert today (Neulinger, 1981).

Leisure, as a social area for loosening nonleisure restraints, is evident in all societies and cultures. At a sporting event, a crowd may loudly express aggressive intentions toward an opposing team that would not be acceptable in a work environment. Roughness and aggression in game play, within the confines of the rules, facilitate enjoyment of watching or playing a game. Aggression ensures the participant and the fan of a high degree of competitiveness and human drama (Zillman, Sapolsky, & Bryant, 1979). Adolescents can express their sexuality more openly in social dance than they can in other environments. In some cultures, the expression of emotion is more acceptable than in others. A difference likewise exists in the openness with which persons of different ages show their tension and excitement through bodily movement. Older adults are generally more restrained compared with teenagers.

Spectator sports can provide fans with a strong emotional bond to a team. Persons can feel a sense of belonging to a larger, meaningful group. When the team wins, fans "bask in reflected glory" (Sloan, 1979, p. 235). Although fans cannot attain a sense of achievement as team players, they can experience a sense of triumph through cheering on their favorite teams. Spectator sports facilitate social interaction with other fans while watching the game or after the event. A shared love of sports can be the basis for days of enjoyable and stimulating conversations among some persons. Without the common focus on sporting events, these persons may have little to say to each other.

Leisure activities can provide an outlet or an adaptive way to ease the frustration of daily life. Through joke telling or sharing humorous vignettes about everyday experiences, children and adults alike can share and laugh about the absurdity of some life events that otherwise may produce intense anger or pain. Adults may tell jokes or stories about incompetent bosses or thoughtless spouses; children tell jokes about teachers and parents. Thinking about the absurdity of the antagonist removes the sting of the interaction.

For many of us, pets are an important part of our leisure time. Pets meet our needs for closeness and love that human interaction in our everyday life may not meet. A relationship with a cat or a dog is fraught with fewer complications than relationships with other persons. A pet owner can lavish attention on a pet in ways that he or she may not feel comfortable in showing other persons. An animal depends on its owner for sustenance. The pet's life centers around its owner. The pet is always present and provides a routine for its owner, companionship, unconditional acceptance, and, potentially, affection.

We can fulfill the need to be altruistic through leisure in ways that most work occupations do not meet. Many persons use some of their leisure time to help others and, in doing so, feed their own spirits. Altruistic acts often result in the participant feeling invigorated, effective, and in control.

Factors Affecting Leisure Participation

Persons of all ages participate in leisure activities for personal enjoyment and fulfillment of needs. Throughout life, participation in leisure activities is a critical safeguard for our mental health. When the external world of school, work, or everyday living does not offer us affirmation and a sense of mastery, we retreat into leisure to fend off depression and engender optimism in our self and our abilities, and we can use these leisure activities as a springboard for redirecting our life in a more satisfying and productive way.

The focus of leisure may be different at various points in our lives. In childhood, engaging parents or other children for fun and stimulation is a primary objective. Children need to engage others to receive sufficient nurturing, support, and stimulation for healthy development toward adulthood. Children need physical activity for skill development and physical well-being. Leisure is often a means through which children challenge their physical skills and, without conscious effort, develop the coordination and strength necessary for most human occupations.

Adolescents and young adults may focus on activities that are physically exciting and that offer the opportunity to meet new persons. Finding a significant other, a satisfying adult life separate from the family of origin, may be an outcome of leisure pursuits. Dating relationships that develop into marital ones in Western societies typically grow from sharing many positive leisure experiences before marriage. During young adulthood, participation in selected leisure activities may provide a career direction for later life. Adolescents and children often discover lifelong leisure or work interests through their leisure pursuits. A passion for exploring the outdoors may lead to a career as a naturalist or to participating in hiking and outdoor activities throughout the children's lives.

In adulthood, leisure activities provide a means to reconnect emotionally to spouses, children, and other adults; have a respite from work; and reaffirm or find a sense of self that may have been lost in everyday routines and responsibilities. In old age, leisure activities may be a means of making connections to others and defining a sense of identity, purpose, and personal meaning to life.

Personal Traits

Our temperament, our inborn style through which we approach and respond to the environment, influences our leisure pursuits. Our temperament affects our activity level, our approach and withdrawal tendencies in new situations, our adaptability to change, our sensory threshold, the quality and intensity of our mood states, our persistence, and our attention span (Chess & Thomas, 1984). When a person has a low activity level, he or she may seek out more sedentary leisure activities. When a person has a high activity level and a high sensory threshold, he or she may seek out high-intensity pursuits such as skydiving or hunting.

Likewise, our personality directs the activities in which we choose to participate and the extent to which we participate in them. If we are extroverted, then we tend to take advantage of many social opportunities and enjoy various group activities. If we are introverted, we may spend more time in solitary pursuits or activities requiring the participation of only a few persons.

Another personal trait that may influence our leisure activity selection is our physical stamina and skills. Some of us are suited physically to more strenuous physical activities such as skiing, swimming, or tennis. For those of us with less coordination, skill, stamina, and participation in these activities may seem like work.

Finally, our cognitive skill level or interests may determine in which leisure activities we are comfortable participating. Persons with highly abstract cognitive abilities may choose to play chess, do crossword puzzles, or play word games. Persons with different cognitive skills may find these same activities boring, confusing, or too demanding. Persons with less cognitive skill may find that participation in these activities seems like work.

Cultural Factors

Our family values and culture greatly affect our leisure participation. When our culture values productivity and usefulness to our family members and our community, leisure activities may revolve around activities related to organized religion or participation in doing practical crafts or hobbies that produce functional products. In some families that believe in the centrality of the family, leisure pursuits may center around family activities. In these situations, one's free time and creative talents focus on celebrating events or spending free time with family members. In other families that believe in one's self-fulfillment as a person, each member of the family may direct his or her time and energy exploring individual interests, which may lead to family members spending more time in solitary activity or in activities with like-minded persons outside of the family.

Cultural beliefs and values affect how our gender or age may determine our leisure activities. Some cultures delineate appropriate activities by age, gender, or marital status. Some cultures have specific rules about how and when men and women may participate in selected activities. For example, some cultural groups expect married women to spend their leisure time with family members and not in the community at large.

Personal Choice Considerations

How we use time outside of leisure may affect how we view and use leisure time. Some persons view their choice of activities relative to what they do in their career or vocation. Neulinger (1981) postulated that persons choose leisure activities that are the direct opposite of their daily work routine. Some examples are a person who works at a desk or a computer may spend free time in physically strenuous sport activities (e.g., ride a bike, hike); a mother who spends most of her time attending to family needs may seek out solitary activities where she can lose herself in an activity such as jogging, painting, or dancing; or a person who spends a lot of time in solitary work may actively seek group activities within a family or social network. Some persons seek leisure activities that are related to their chosen career or vocation. Some examples are a person who attends conferences and socializes with members of his or her profession, a high school English teacher who reads books and attends poetry readings, or a young carpenter who builds a boat in his free time.

Environmental Considerations

Our personal access to leisure environments, materials, and equipment strongly influences how we spend our free time and which activities we explore to meet our needs. If we live in a rural environment, we are likely to have the opportunity to explore and develop skills in many outdoor activities. In a city environment, we have a greater opportunity to participate as a spectator in a range of sporting and creative arts events. When we have economic resources, we can buy any materials or equipment that we need to participate in an activity of interest. Thus, personal resources have a major influence on which leisure activities we pursue.

Exercise 2

Think about your leisure pursuits. What factors influence your choice of these leisure activities?

Barriers to Participation in Leisure Activities

Developing healthy leisure pursuits is challenging and threatening. For some of us, work and other responsibilities seem to require every waking hour. We view leisure activities as frivolous. For some of us, leisure is threatening, frustrating, or a burden. We may be more comfortable having a consistent routine with required activities than having an expanse of time that we must fill with our own planned activities. Leisure concerns break away from our daily routine. Leisure requires us to challenge ourselves to participate in activities beyond those included in our daily routine. We have the right not to participate in leisure activities and to be passive in our free time. This lack of participation, however, is isolating and may lead to alienation and depression.

In the United States, we have many opportunities to be passive in our leisure time. A major American passive leisure activity is watching television. Television fills time. Television sometimes entertains us, relaxes us, and can be a learning tool.

Television, however, rarely helps us to understand ourselves more deeply, stretch the range of our intellect or emotions, or engage with others. Although watching television and participating in other passive activities can help us use our leisure time in a way that makes us feel better than we would if we had nothing to do, watching television can lead us away from learning to truly experience our leisure time.

When exploring alternative leisure activities, we must recognize that a major amount of corporate profit in Western society is related to mass consumption of leisure equipment and experiences. Corporations barrage us with advertising about the "perfect" use of leisure time that may interfere with searches for personal definitions of ideal leisure. Relentless advertising attempts to convince us that we want what they are offering. Some of us then begin to value only those leisure activities that are heavily advertised. The "right" pair of running shoes or sports equipment, belonging to the "right" gym, or going on the "right" vacations may become tied to our social status, which may result in our working more hours to afford leisure versus enjoying leisure. We may participate in few leisure activities or primarily passive ones because we believe that participation in active leisure activities requires a great deal of money.

Stereotypes of others can be an important barrier for leisure participation, especially for school-aged children, adolescents, and older adults. A group of children may decide that a particular child is "dumb" and therefore exclude that child from playground activities or from child-initiated clubs. Adolescents identify themselves and each other with groups who share certain observable behaviors (Brown, 1990). Typical identities in a high school may include "jocks," "brains," or "druggies." Certain groups have more socioeconomic status than others. An adolescent who is associated with an unpopular or negative group may experience rejection and discomfort in trying to participate in some leisure activities that are associated more with another group. A healthy elderly person may feel less included in some community activities that are typically associated with younger adults. The person may need to prove his or her competence before experiencing acceptance in some leisure group activities.

Other barriers to access to leisure activities are our personal character, racial background, religious practices, sexual orientation, community resources, and certain negative habits or behaviors. Some persons have personal character issues that interfere with the ability to engage in leisure activities with others. These persons may lack the internal resources (i.e., coping skills) or social skills to explore interests or to connect with others through personally meaningful and productive activity. For others, race, religious practices, or sexual orientation may limit the opportunities to join some leisure clubs or groups. If communities do not have facilities for creative arts or organized sports, then these leisure activities may not be available to persons in those communities. For elderly persons, a lack of transportation may severely limit their ability to participate. Finally, some barriers to participate result from a person's negative habits or behaviors such as abuse of drugs or alcohol. Participation in gangs, petty crime, or violence may become means of relaxation, excitement, and connecting with others.

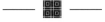

Exercise 3

Think about leisure pursuits that strongly interest you but in which you do not participate. What are the barriers to your participation?

Leisure Experiences Throughout the Life Span

Infancy Through Early Childhood

Leisure for children includes solitary activities and activities with caregivers or peers. Children's first leisure experiences are play. Play is child-initiated activity that adults have not structured to teach specific skills. The child engages in the activity because he or she wants to and because it is fun. The child is free to participate or to negotiate the activity with an adult or other children. A parent may approach an infant with a busy box, and the infant may bang on it for a few minutes but then crawl away and pick up a pot to bang. The infant is in control of the activity. Thus, this infant may look toward the parent when he or she wants the parent to join or may move away when he or she wants to play alone. An older child may build with Legos™ or solve a puzzle because he or she finds the activity interesting versus participating because a parent or teacher assigned the activity.

Erikson (1963) said that children's play "is not the equivalent of adult play . . . it is not recreation. The playing adult steps sidewards into another reality, the playing child advances to new stages of mastery" (p. 222). Children's play concerns exploration and discovery in all spheres of human existence. Children's play continuously evolves, and what was once interesting is now boring. Children develop new skills and use them in novel ways during play. Although improved functioning is not the purpose of play, through play, children become more competent in all areas of human functioning. They develop a capacity to cope with their environment, develop ego strength, and foster an investment in life (Cotton, 1984).

Playfulness is an important aspect of children's play. Playfulness exists when a child is intrinsically motivated, internally controlled, and able to suspend reality (Bundy, 1997). Intrinsic motivation means that the child participates in particular activities because of the innate rewards that the child experiences in the activity. The child does not participate in play activities because he or she is expecting a reward or praise. The child becomes involved to have fun. *Internal control* refers to the child having primary control over what occurs in the activity. When a child suspends reality, the child uses objects in new ways to discover new uses for everyday things, or the child participates in make-believe (i.e., imaginary play or games). A child frames an activity by giving cues to others regarding how they should act toward him or her. A child, for example, may cue a playmate to play house and state that he or she is going to be the parent. A child who wants to play superheroes and be the "bad guy" may frame the activity so that his or her peers must fight or run away. This cueing allows the child to experience life from the perspective of another.

Play begins in infancy when an infant learns to attend to the faces of caregivers. Caregivers smile and make soft sounds at infants and wait for infants to respond in kind. Over time, infants are ready to play peekaboo or to imitate the facial expressions and sounds that caregivers make. Infants begin to initiate the play, and the child and caregivers receive pleasure from the interaction. This mutual interaction evolves to social play when the child makes a different face or a sound. Through parent–child play experiences in infancy and early childhood, children develop the coping skills necessary for more complex play. According to Murphy and Moriarity (1976), the most important variable in the development of coping skills in young children is their mothers' leisure experience with them, in other words, their mother's enjoyment of their play (Figure 5).

Past successes and pleasures with the supportive guidance of caregivers give young children confidence that they will successfully participate in the activity and have fun. As children grow and enter middle childhood, some leisure activities become recreational ones. These activities have playful elements to them, but they are structured activities that occur as part of a team sport or within a club. Children who enter these activities have begun to accept rules as necessary for group activity. Without defined rules and some accepted order to activities, little pleasurable activity occurs. Children become interested in learning to draw or construct by following a set plan and learning new games and sports.

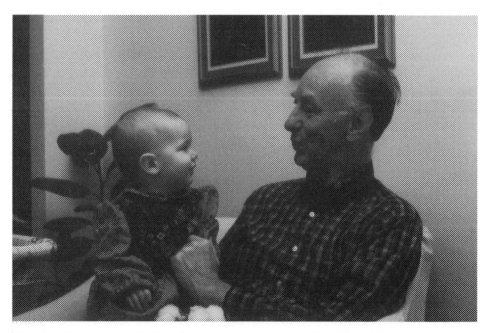

Figure 5. Caregivers and infants find mutual pleasure in social play.

Leisure for children begins to involve more complex games and group activities. Children master games of chance first, followed by games involving strategies. In games of chance, children learn first to modulate their intense excitement related to the process of being in the lead or losing a game and accept the outcome as "just a game" versus as a statement about their competence. The children learn to follow the rules and to inhibit negative emotions that may lead them to quit a game prematurely or to become aggressive when a game does not end in their favor. Depending on children's temperaments and innate skills, initially learning games may be challenging to children and to their caregivers. Children may be slow to learn or to acclimate to rules. Younger children often change the rules and cheat to win until losing becomes less threatening to them. Once children understand games and begin to accept rules, their animation, physical tension, and excitement in a simple game such as "Old Maid" can bring almost as much enjoyment to caregivers as it does to children.

Playing and interacting with other children is an important part of the leisure experiences of children from preschool age onward. Children share similar levels of physical activity, exuberance, and open emotional expression, which makes them more attractive to each other than adults are to them. Children share their interests with peers, and their enthusiasm for certain activities increases or decreases depending on the reactions of important peers to those activities. Children will more likely take chances and participate in new activities when other children are participating in those activities. Through leisure play experiences, children learn the joys of friendship and camaraderie and learn to negotiate and compromise in the interest of maintaining peer relationships (Figure 6).

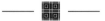

Exercise 4

Think about a child you know well. What activities does that child participate in that you would consider play or leisure? Why? What underlying skills does the child have that support the child's participation? What needs do you think the activities meet for the child? What effect, if any, do you think that the child's participation will have on his or her overall development?

Adolescence

Peer groups and peer culture are a central focus of adolescent leisure in the United States (Brown, 1990). Peer friendships serve as a primary source of activity, influence, and support for most adolescents. Adolescents report enjoying activities with friends more than they do with family members because they feel most understood by friends, and they can be most fully themselves in the company of friends (Savin-Williams & Berndt, 1990) (Figure 7). Adolescents tend to view themselves and their peers as fitting into particular groups. Where they fit within the adolescent culture of

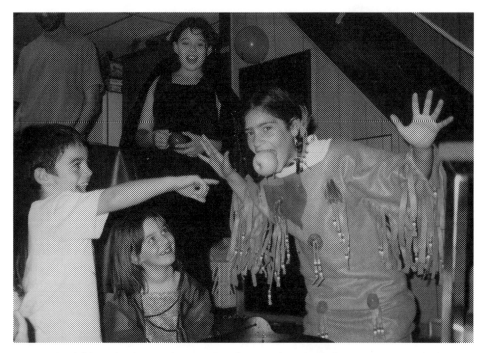

Figure 6. Children develop an appreciation of camaraderie through group games and activities.

their school and community increases or decreases group leisure opportunities. For example, a football player may receive invitations to many parties, whereas the president of the chess club may not. Although being a part of a high-status crowd may increase the number of group activities in which an adolescent participates, social status may not enhance the adolescent's experience of leisure. Less popular teens may actively pursue individual or small group activities for which they have a passion and may have deep and satisfying friendships.

American adolescents spend up to 40% of their time in leisure pursuits (Csikszentmihalyi & Larson, 1984). Adolescent moods are the most positive and activity level is the highest when adolescents are engaged in leisure activities versus work or school activities (Fine, Mortimer, & Roberts, 1990). How adolescents use such a large block of leisure time is important to their psychosocial development. Kleiber, Larson, and Csikszentmihalyi (1986) conceptualized adolescent leisure as consisting of two types: relaxed leisure and transitional leisure. Relaxed leisure includes activities that are pleasurable but are not challenging, such as listening to music, watching television, or hanging out with friends at a local mall or park. Transitional leisure activities prepare an adolescent for the serious aspects of the adult world. These activities promote concentration and challenge and may include extracurricular school activities, individual hobbies such as playing a musical instrument, or developing high-level painting or dancing skills. This type of activity participation correlates with adult occupational prestige.

When adolescents participate solely in relaxed leisure activities, they are more likely to be less focused and at risk for developing behavior problems that negatively

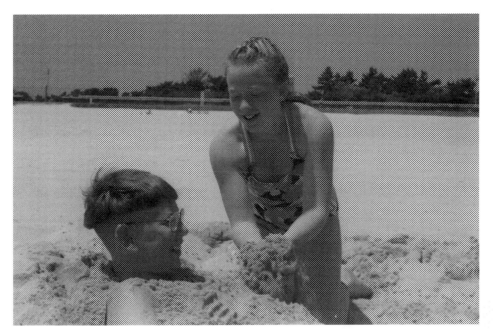

Figure 7. Interest in opposite-sex friendships increases in early adolescence.

affect their development. Without activities to channel their energies positively, they may be more likely to seek out adventure through drinking, drug experimentation, or early sexual activity. In contrast, adolescents who discover their particular talents and develop habits to cultivate their talents invest a major amount of time in related activities and develop comfort and the ability to use solitude effectively. As a result, these adolescents have a stronger grasp of their developing self-identity, and peers are less likely to negatively influence them. These teens tend to be more open to new experiences and exhibit higher levels of concentration than others. Of additional interest, many of these adolescents spend more time with their parents in leisure activities. Parental engagement provides adolescents with a sense of support and consistency, encourages their intensity and self-direction, and enhances their attentional capacities for finding and mastering challenges (Csikszentmihalyi, Rathunde, & Whalen, 1993).

Transitional leisure pursuits can be a sanctuary for adolescents. These activities most often occur in a safe and familiar setting that nurtures self-expression and exploration. These activities may involve visiting the science laboratory or an art room of a favorite teacher after school or participating in a club or extracurricular class. Wilson (as cited in John-Steiner, 1985) studied the experiences of a group of high school students in art class. The art room in a public high school was a retreat from the demands of the school environment. Within the room, these adolescents were able to "transcend the limitations of the structure, to engage in acts which are creative or ludic or subversive and to participate in a kind of communitas" (Wilson, as cited in John-Steiner, 1985, p. 94). Sports are important activities in the socialization of adolescents. Sports are strong foci of adolescent interest. Through sports, adolescents increase their exposure to peers. The adolescent subculture associates athletic participation with physical fitness, competitiveness, and social status (Savin-Williams & Berndt, 1990).

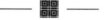

Exercise 5

Think back to your adolescent years. Describe your participation in leisure activities at that time. Which of these activities were relaxed leisure activities? Which of these activities were transitional leisure activities? How did these activities influence your experiences as an adolescent and your roles as an adult?

Young Adulthood

As persons transition from adolescence into adulthood, shifts in leisure activities occur as persons continue their education and begin their first real jobs. Many young adults move out of their family homes and enter a different world from that of their childhood and adolescence in which they shared living space with family members. This becomes a period of defining oneself outside of one's family of origin.

When young adults decide to go to college, they pursue courses of study that expand their base of knowledge into new areas. They may develop interests that they were previously unaware of and may come to find that the areas that they were originally interested in are less compelling than new academic areas that they have discovered. The college environment provides numerous new opportunities for leisure activities with new persons to befriend. Many young adults who enter college continue to have a great deal of leisure time. Living independently on a college campus with roommates presents opportunities to explore and experiment. New leisure opportunities may be available at college that were not available in students' communities of origin. Young adults from a large city may find themselves in areas that provide opportunities for outdoor activities such as bike riding, canoeing, hiking, or skiing. Young adults from rural areas may find themselves in a major metropolitan area and discover a love for live music and theater that they had never experienced. New friends may come from different backgrounds and expose young adults to new social opportunities. Additionally, activities that were chores of adolescence may now become valued leisure activities. Preparing a meal in one's own apartment for friends may be a way of expressing one's identity and a way of relaxing. Painting and decorating a dorm room or apartment may be a work of self-expression that a young adult can enjoy for long periods.

For young adults who enter the work force, their leisure activities may likewise change. Young adults entering the work force are entering a new cultural forum in which ethnicity, culture, and gender may be minimized because one is present to perform a job. Pressure may exist to conform to the majority culture, and young adults must learn to adjust their personal values and conduct in the work environment. Leisure is a critical occupational area for workers to explore so that they may find activities that reaffirm their sense of identity, allow them to develop areas of interest and talent, reaffirm a sense of belonging to specific cultural groups, and rejuvenate the soul and spirit. Workers may continue some of the leisure activities of their school years, such as participating in local adult sports leagues, participating in music bands, and attending spectator sports, movies, or live music events. These adults may remain in the same geographical area and may socialize with the same or similar friends. The major change in their lives is going to work full-time, which results in a notable decrease in their amount of leisure time compared with high school. Their leisure time is now limited to the weekends or to days off from work.

For all young adults, a considerable amount of leisure time may focus on establishing relationships with a significant other. Sharing leisure activities is a central part of courtship in Western culture. Through these activities, young persons socialize in a nonthreatening, neutral environment in which there is a mutually interesting activity such as dinner, a movie, a sporting event, or a bike ride. Such activities allow a relationship to develop in a relaxed manner. When like-minded persons share leisure activities, a bond of friendship may develop. Sharing an activity or adventure with another provides situations in which one learns about himself or herself and the other person. Persons may reflect their pleasure in the joint activity by having a positive regard for each other and may develop greater interest in learning more about the other as a person. As a meaningful relationship with a significant other develops, young adults adjust their time commitments to fit the other person's leisure interests. Couples negotiate how much leisure time they will spend together, especially when they have different individual leisure interests and pursuits. Each person in a couple adjusts leisure expectations in the interest of the relationship. One person may give up socializing in a bar or participating in a league sport to please a partner. Another person may adjust to a partner's hobby by developing an interest in that hobby to increase shared leisure time. Both partners may take up a new activity together such as ballroom dancing to deepen their bond. Persons may participate individually or with friends in some activities that are particularly rejuvenating, such as spectator sports or physical activities. Couples begin to share holidays and family traditions and events. They begin entertaining friends and family members together. A young woman may accommodate by learning to participate in her husband's traditional Italian family dinner every Sunday.

In healthy young adulthood, persons maintain solitary or group leisure interests that have developed during the life span. Certain activities are part of one's persona, support self-esteem, and rejuvenate the person. Some persons may have a longstanding interest in cars that develops into restoring vintage cars. Sewing, knitting, or jewelry making may be a way of expressing one's artistic side, even though one may work as a store clerk. Others may join adult community sports leagues or coach children's sport activities. Many young adults who enjoyed biking as children and teenagers join biking clubs to maintain physical fitness and rejuvenate their physical beings.

Drinking alcohol as part of social events is often part of the passage from childhood to adulthood in Western culture. The use of substances such as drugs and alcohol may stem from a search for pleasurable feelings that substances can induce (Kraus, 1994). Alcohol can lower one's inhibitions and make socialization easier. When drinking dominates how persons spend their leisure time, enjoyment of this activity (as well as other activities) diminishes.

Middle Adulthood

Whether adults choose to marry, remain single, or decide to have children influences how they conceptualize and use leisure time at middle age. Persons who marry are likely to change how they use some of their leisure time to include their spouses and extended family members. Taking care of children and sharing leisure pursuits with children occupy a large amount of the leisure time of most parents. Single adults continue to seek, establish, and maintain long-term relationships with significant others, but they are likely to pursue and further develop their skills in hobbies and activities in which they have engaged across the life span. Single adults are likely to be settled in their careers and have adjusted to single adulthood, so they have time to devote to enhancing skills in lifelong leisure activities and to pursue new interests. In the process, they discover more about themselves as persons and their potential to contribute to society in ways other than caring for children. In mid-life, some persons may become more reflective about community issues or politics and now decide that they have the personal skills and resources to have a positive effect on their community. Others may turn past hobbies into part-time careers; they may write, buy and sell antiques, or design jewelry, for example.

In some ways, single life presents a greater challenge but more opportunity for the development of a rich adult leisure life. Single persons confront expanses of unstructured time unencumbered by responsibilities to children or to a spouse. Persons may perceive this as freedom or as a burden. They can pursue interests without the restraint of the needs or disapproval of immediate family members. Without an active approach to leisure participation, a single person may experience isolation and discontent. Having solitary leisure interests can be helpful to a single adult because others may not be immediately available for interaction. Finding companions for joint leisure activities is a more active process for single adults than for persons with families or spouses. For some, a lack of companionship can present a serious barrier to leisure participation. For others, it is an opportunity to develop new relationships, deepen older relationships, and expand their leisure opportunities through varied companions. Single adults are more likely to participate in group travel or adult leisure organizations than persons with families or spouses. Single adults may be more independent and willing to take risks to participate in activities that interest them. Single women may not experience the retreat from exploration of their own abilities and personal interests that many married women do during their childbearing years.

Single adults may use some of their leisure time caring for and participating in leisure activities with children. They may be involved with the children of their siblings or close friends, or they may participate as volunteers in community organizations for children. Similarly, married adults who choose not to have children may have the opportunity to pursue their own interests and develop their sense of themselves as persons. They may participate in adult-focused leisure activities similar to those of single adults.

Adults who have children typically experience a dramatic change in their leisure life once children are born. As the adult's identity shifts to include the identity of a parent, leisure interests shift from individual and adult activities to family-oriented activities. Parent–child play optimally becomes a central leisure interest. Former leisure interests of new parents may be put aside because of time or financial constraints. Parents reorganize their activities to conform to the children's or family members' schedules. The additional constraints of child care, children's sleep schedules, and the appropriateness of activities for children are factors that influence parents' choice of leisure activities. The types of television shows that adults watch while children are awake change greatly because they now view many shows that were formerly favorite ones as inappropriate for family viewing.

Becoming a parent results in particularly notable role changes for women. Parenting changes a woman's work life or career to a greater extent than men experience, even if a woman continues to work after childbirth. Although more men share in child care and home maintenance activities, most mothers fulfill the role of primary caregiver. Women's former leisure experiences tend to decrease more notably than their husbands' experiences do. Men may share equally in leisure activities with children, but women typically provide more instrumental child care.

Leisure activities of parents who do not work outside the home are usually home centered. Activities may include gardening, sewing, home crafts, cooking, and parent–child play. These parents intersperse these activities among house and child maintenance chores. In families in which both parents work outside the home, family leisure activities are often limited to evenings and weekends. These activities are special because time together is rare. Eating a family meal, reading a book together, and playing a game may be more important than household maintenance activities.

The leisure activities of a family undergo many transitions as children grow. When the children are infants, they may greatly curtail parents' leisure activities as parents adjust to parenthood. Leisure may revolve around playful interaction with the infant or sharing parenting experiences with other young parents or with older adults who can provide support and guidance to the young parents. Satisfying leisure with infants and young children requires effort on the part of adults. In addition to home-based leisure activities, young parents often visit parks and other public places where other parents and children congregate. They may attend religious functions, parent–child drop-in centers, or gym activities designed to facilitate parent–child interaction and interaction with other families. These community activities provide parents with an opportunity to interact with their children in the proximity of other parents, which allows adults to share their parenting joys and frustrations. In these activities, children have the opportunity to meet other adults and children.

Some parents make connections to their children by sharing their leisure passions (Figure 8). Parents may teach their children sports, begin to take them to sporting events, and share the experience of cheering on their favorite team. If children show an interest in learning a sport that interests a parent, the sport may provide a means through which the parent and children relate. Positive feelings about the activity become closely associated with positive feelings toward one another, and the sport can bring the two closer together. Parents may return to the leisure activities of their youth as part of their role as parent. A parent may have loved soccer as a child and now coaches his or her child's soccer team.

When children reach adolescence, family-focused leisure time may occur less frequently. Although adolescents may still participate in selected family, religious, or cultural activities, they tend to begin to move beyond their immediate family for leisure pursuits. Parents may feel loss, abandonment, or a new sense of freedom as their adolescent children's leisure increasingly focuses on activities outside the family unit. Parents may experience jealousy as their teenagers' leisure activities become more exciting than their own activities. Some parents report that their amount of fun decreases as their adolescents' fun increases. For parents, activities in adolescence are very different from watching young children participate in the leisure activities of scouting or sports. This change may lead parents to question and reevaluate their own leisure activities.

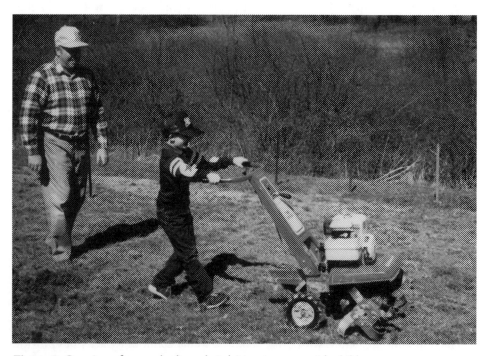

Figure 8. Caregivers frequently share their leisure interests with children.

The leisure triumphs of an adolescent may facilitate parents' positive moods and interests in activity participation (Steinberg & Steinberg, 1994).

As children grow into adults, parental satisfaction in activities outside of their role as parents provides a buffer to the experience of turmoil with the transition. In Steinberg and Steinberg's qualitative study (1994), parents who were not engaged in satisfying activities beyond that of parenthood were vulnerable to severe distress as their children became adolescents. Steinberg and Steinberg (1994) interpreted their findings as suggesting that activities such as individual hobbies or community service provide a distraction and support parents' sense of personal competence and self-worth.

When children move on to their own adult lives, middle-aged adults must refocus their leisure pursuits. Although women are more likely to experience psychological turmoil during their offspring's adolescence before the children leave home, women adjust more easily to the "empty nest syndrome" than fathers do (Steinberg & Steinberg, 1994). Women are more engaged in exploring new careers, new interests, or community activities than men typically are. Some believe that change may occur because young women may surrender their own desires in the interest of their husbands and growing family; once their children are grown, women may seek to reclaim their sense of individuality and pursue activities that provide personal satisfaction (Labouvie-Vief, 1994; Niemela & Linto, 1994).

During later middle age, a couple may pursue new joint activities. A parent may reinvest his or her newly acquired time in individual hobbies. Work demands may have lessened so that time that persons focused on career building is now available for leisure pursuits. Leisure travel may become more frequent because the parents' financial situation may be better now that children are independent and parents have few demands on their children's time. Middle to older adulthood can be a time to do some of the activities that one has always wanted to do but never did. One begins to see a time limit to one's opportunity to participate in those activities. Some persons run their first marathon at 50 years of age. Others use late middle age to challenge themselves intellectually in ways that they wished that they had done as younger adults. Some adults reenter education to finish a high school degree, pursue a college degree for the sake of knowledge, or pursue another career that they expect may be more fulfilling than their first career. For others, late middle adulthood is an opportunity to connect with other adults in ways that were not possible when they were raising children or focusing on their career. They may develop new or revived passions for activities such as gourmet cooking, golf, bridge, traveling, or book clubs.

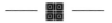

Exercise 6

Interview a parent. Discuss the effect of children on his or her participation in leisure activities. What does the parent value in his or her leisure time? How much leisure time does he or she have per day or per week? How does he or she spend it? What leisure activities does he or she participate in alone, with children, with other adults? Compare his or her leisure experiences with that of a single adult that you know.

Older Adulthood

Besides successfully avoiding disease and disability, successful aging requires the maintenance of physical and cognitive function and engagement in social and productive activities (Rowe & Kahn, 1997). Participating in leisure is the most important predictor of well-being among older adults (Zimmer, Hickey, & Searle, 1997).

When older adults retire from paid employment, they have a new opportunity to explore their interests, who they have been during their lifetime, and who they would like to be for the remainder of their lives. If they have maintained some leisure interests throughout their lives, retirement may allow them to expand on those interests and devote more time to the activities that they love. For others, retirement leads to depression or a crisis as they attempt to adjust to a new way of life. Past participation in leisure activities typically determines the activities that a retiree seeks out. Optimally, persons who have neglected developing leisure occupations throughout the earlier part of their lives will begin to explore leisure activities within their community and learn what they really like to do and care about beyond the daily routine of their life's work. Volunteer work in hospitals, schools, or community organizations can provide a structure that organizes daily life in similar ways that paid employment did and may offer the older adult an opportunity to find a new life purpose, enhance self-worth, and increase social contact with others (Singleton, 1996).

Persons' bodies and minds respond differently to the aging process. Although many elderly persons may seek out more solitary and sedentary leisure activities, many well elderly persons are gregarious and seek out regular exercise. They may swim a few miles every week, in-line skate, enter marathons, or bicycle ride. Others maintain an interest in and regularly participate in outdoor activities. Some older adults actually increase their involvement because they have greater discretionary time. Many persons retain solitary interests that have sustained their spirits throughout their lifetimes, including writing, playing an instrument, or painting. As their social obligations lessen, elderly persons may become more focused on these activities (Figure 9).

Leisure pursuits may markedly change when adults become grandparents, especially when grandchildren live nearby. Time spent with family members may now revolve around entertaining and engaging grandchildren. Grandchildren can bring out a more relaxed ability to nurture and play that may not have been possible with one's own children. Grandparents may have increased discretionary time and have the wisdom of experience to be able to enjoy the time they spend with their grandchildren (Figure 10).

Older adults living alone report fluctuations between extremes of involvement with others and projects and periods of isolation (Siegel, 1993). An issue for these

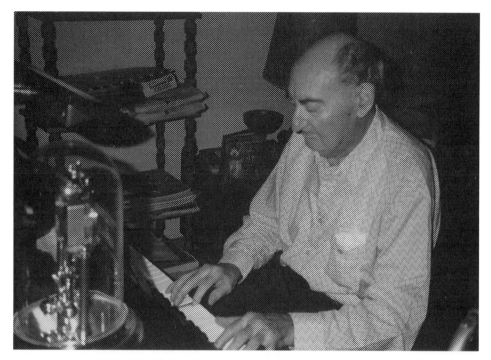

Figure 9. Lifetime solitary pursuits gain greater importance in defining the self and in providing leisure satisfaction in old age.

adults is how to find a balance in their time and to make the time that they have left to live more valuable and meaningful for themselves. Some persons may have difficulty managing this life stage; others seek and find creative aspects of themselves that they have not recognized during the years.

For some mature adults, senior citizens centers become important places of social interaction. Regularly attending meetings and activities may provide the structure and support that some persons need to deal with the loss of their jobs and former roles at retirement or with the loss of spouses and friends to death. Activities such as bingo, weekly card games, and day trips with local organizations demonstrate a shift from independent activity to activities that are more interdependent or involve dependence on others. Within the structure of these centers, older adults may find new ways to contribute to their communities; for example, they may make blankets for infants or participate in making products for nonprofit fundraising.

Older adults experience the loss of lifelong partners and close friends, which may result in feelings of isolation and disconnection. Because much of the daily activity of elderly persons is voluntary and is not required work, some persons may retreat from activity participation. Support groups with other adults experiencing similar losses often help these persons in coming to terms with these experiences and in finding a way to reconstruct meaningful lives. In summarizing the experiences of 56 older

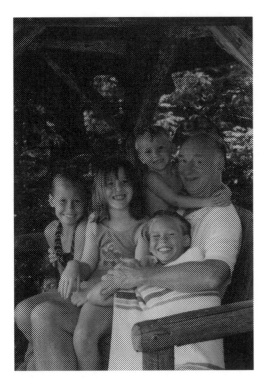

Figure 10. Children and their grandparents often treasure their shared leisure experiences.

women who participated in her qualitative study on aging, Siegel (1993) stated that

> With each death of a loved one, . . . we learn something more about who we were within that relationship and who we are without the presence of that person. With each loss, we also learn more about death and dying and about how to cope and survive. (p. 184)

As persons near the end of their lives, they will likely be unable to participate in some past leisure activities because of the infirmities of old age. Some persons may cease participation and not seek new activities that interest them, but many older adults replace physically active pursuits with more passive ones in which they can readily participate (Zimmer et al., 1997). Older adults who are likely to feel most in control of their lives will adapt their former interests to their bodies' changes in old age and will work to improve their bodies' functioning for participation through regular exercise, good nutrition, and mental activity (Baltes & Baltes, 1990).

Frail elderly persons may become homebound and lose gradual interest in many leisure activities, including social ones. They may spend more time reflecting on the past and become dependent on adult children or community services for social interaction. In some situations, the adult may require adaptations or assistive devices (e.g., a magnifier to read a book or newspaper, adaptations to a telephone to amplify sound) to participate in desired leisure activities.

Exercise 7

Talk with a healthy retired person who is more than 60 years of age. Discuss his or her leisure experiences. Talk to a person who is more than 80 years of age. How do these persons experience leisure? What do they value relative to leisure? How have their activities changed during the past 10 or 20 years? Do any barriers exist to what they would consider optimal leisure participation at their ages? If so, describe these barriers.

Occupational Therapy and Leisure Activities

In occupational therapy practice, leisure may be the focus of therapy, or the practitioner may use leisure activities to develop other life skills. This section addresses practice in which leisure as an occupation is the focus of intervention. Occupational therapy practitioners use various frames of reference and related intervention strategies to deal with the leisure needs of our clients. In this short section, we do not specifically address frames of reference because we believe that leisure is a key aspect of many frames of reference. Leisure is a critical aspect of occupational therapy's domain of concern. In addition, occupational therapy practitioners use leisure activities, one type of purposeful activity, as an important therapeutic tool. We use leisure activities individually with clients to address specific component deficits and with groups to address others. Historically, occupational therapy practitioners used leisure activities with clients because the focus for the client was on performing the activity versus the actions themselves. Today, however, we recognize that leisure activities are an important aspect of life; as an occupation, leisure is a primary concern for occupational therapy practitioners with all clients.

In the past, occupational therapists have consistently administered leisure interest checklists to explore what a person's interests are and how frequently he or she pursues them. What occupational therapists explore less frequently are what those leisure interests and related activities mean to a client. Meaning is central to occupational therapy practice, but meaning may be lost because of the pressures of today's health care system. If we explore the meaning behind activity for individual clients, we will more effectively engage clients in pursuing a rich leisure life. As previously noted, leisure participation may relate to a generalized sense of well-being, independence, and personal control. If we understand which needs persons have met through past leisure activities or which needs potential leisure interests may meet for individual clients, then we can help each client seek out meaningful leisure activities when limited personal or external resources block participation in activities of choice.

Practitioners must be cognizant of clients' temperament, personality style, physical stamina and abilities, cognitive skills, sociocultural views, and external resources to assist them in improving the quality of their leisure experiences. Persons who are slow to adapt to changes may need more support at any life stage when they attempt to pursue new leisure activities. Persons who adapt rapidly may not require any support when they approach new situations. Extroverted persons may be lonely and dissatisfied when they participate in solitary activities and may be most content when they spend most of their leisure time in the company of others. Other persons may need guidance in developing satisfying activity interests for their solitary time. These persons may want much smaller amounts of interactive leisure activities. Finally, some persons spend most of their time in passive leisure activities.

Effective and appropriate occupational therapy results from our understanding of the client's underlying abilities and needs. We use the client's personal circumstances, abilities, needs, and desires to help us guide him or her to rediscover the joys of using physical skills in leisure pursuits. Some children with disabilities may become frustrated by their physical skill level when they play with other children. A therapist may help them to discover different gross motor activities that may offer them greater satisfaction. We can guide children with a strong interest in sports in developing the necessary bilateral motor coordination and ball skills to enjoy playing sports with peers. Chronic physical or mental illness in a family may severely weaken marital and parent–child relationships, which reduces the amount and quality of emotional support that children receive from their parents or that spouses receive from each other. Joint leisure activities may be the first activities that the family members sacrifice as stress increases. Playful and relaxed interaction may be minimal or nonexistent. Reexperiencing positive family leisure activities can have a major positive effect on each family member's mood and on the overall emotional atmosphere of the family. Occupational therapy practitioners can help family members to alter their joint leisure activities in response to the effect of the illness and the change in family activities.

When a child has a learning disability or other cognitive disabilities, parents may struggle with interacting with the child in leisure activities. The child may avoid or be unable to attend to learning the typical leisure activities that parents teach and share with the child. The child may stay focused on familiar and repetitive activities or may be emotionally labile or withdrawn when confronted with leisure experiences that are pleasurable to other children. This may result in power struggles between parent and child or a more distant parent–child relationship with parent and child mutually feeling sad, frustrated, and angry. Occupational therapy practitioners can help parents guide their children in discovering individual and family leisure activities that are meaningful to both the parents and the child. The therapist may guide parents in learning how to provide support and assistance to their children in confronting new activities or new challenges in old activities. Parents may learn how to modify and adapt activities to foster their children's participation. Parental engagement in helping children in this way facilitates children's development of attentional and coping capacities necessary for future engagement in independent leisure activities. At the same time, satisfying parent–child leisure interaction has positive effects on both the parents' and the children's sense of competence and mood.

Whether it is a primary disability or a secondary one related to a physical disability, depression can have devastating effects on the everyday functioning of persons. Developing leisure interests and experiencing successful participation in them may lessen the negative effect of difficult life situations and give persons a new perspective on their lives and their ability to exert control over everyday activities. New interests may reduce a sense of alienation and make persons more available for interaction with others. Others may need to find leisure outlets to express strong emotions that they cannot express in other everyday activities. Actively participating in sports or games or watching spectator sports may provide a socially acceptable outlet for aggressive impulses.

Adolescents with behavior disorders may have little awareness of their own individual interests and talents and their potential to develop as a contributing member of society. They may be solely focused on their role within a negative peer group. Therapists may engage such adolescents in exploring leisure activities and discovering individual interests and talents. For example, one adolescent may find that he really enjoys the solitary experience of baking; baking may give the adolescent time to relax away from peers and to think about his own life issues. Baking may lead to more prosocial individual action on the part of the teen at other times of the day. In addition, he may become aware that he has a talent for baking, be motivated to participate in baking activities regularly, and may begin thinking about education or employment in food services.

Occupational therapy practitioners typically work with many persons with varied disabilities on an individual basis. Many clients are isolated from others and experience great dissatisfaction about how they use their leisure time. Some clients may experience little joy or freedom; leisure may be an alienating experience. Adolescents with disabilities may be isolated from their mainstream peer group and believe that they have few options for activity outside of school. Adults with brain injury may lose previous friendships and the ability to participate in some leisure pursuits resulting from reduced cognitive functioning. These life situations related to leisure can have a major effect on every area of life functioning; the person may become depressed, passive, and dependent. Participating in a group that focuses on the occupation of leisure may help the person explore potential leisure interests; develop activity, social, and time management skills for leisure participation; learn how to reduce barriers to leisure participation; and develop a network of similar persons who are interested in joint leisure activities. Developing a personally meaningful leisure life is likely to result in a generalized sense of well-being, independence, and personal control.

When a practitioner finds that a person has strong interest in particular leisure activities but does not participate in those activities, the practitioner must explore what the barriers are to participation. Occupational therapy practitioners help persons develop the necessary physical and cognitive skills that make client participation more likely in activities that interest them. A practitioner may help a child develop sufficient balance and bilateral coordination so that the child can ride a bicycle or in-line skate. Another practitioner may help persons with hand injuries redevelop their fine motor skills so that they can again participate in leisure activities such as sewing, cooking, card playing, or playing a musical instrument. Some clients may need to develop compensatory strategies to participate in leisure activities resulting from a congenital or recent disability. Persons with spinal cord injuries still enjoy many sports when adapted equipment is available. They may ski, scuba dive, or play basketball. Guiding clients to adapt their environment so that they can readily participate in activities is a treatment strategy that an occupational therapy practitioner may use. A parent may need to simplify game instructions so that a child with a learning disability can play with his or her family members. Reducing extraneous visual or auditory stimuli in the environment may greatly improve the ability of a person with developmental disabilities to participate in a leisure activity. Other clients may have or may develop sufficient skill during the course of therapy but may lack sufficient external resources for regular participation in activities that interest them. A therapist may then need to evaluate a client's present and required levels of resources necessary for satisfying leisure. A single adult with a physical disability may be interested in travel, or a senior citizen may be interested in finding partners for playing bridge. Helping clients find community resources or connecting them to another professional or agency that can find the appropriate external resources for clients are important interventions.

The leisure needs of our clients are critical to address despite all of the pressures to meet the other rehabilitation needs of our clients and the high demands of our health care system. Certainly we can address some needs simultaneously, but remember that helping clients to develop a rich and personally meaningful leisure life may facilitate clients' achievement of all of the other goals of intervention that our society values more than leisure.

Summary

Although leisure is a "second thought" that one may consider only after completing required and routine activities of daily living, leisure can be a powerful buffer for the stresses and negative events of other occupations. Leisure can facilitate relationships and help persons to discover their true vocation or life purpose. Through activities that help us express our full emotional range in socially acceptable activities, we maintain emotional equilibrium. One can only experience the benefits of leisure by truly engaging in activities that engage one's interest and possibly one's soul. Leisure is a challenge and requires as much focused energy as other human occupations. Without active pursuit of the development of a leisure life, free time may be a burden; free time may become a time of passivity, boredom, unconnectedness, unhappiness, confusion, or loneliness. ■

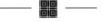

Exercise 8

Compare the leisure values and experiences of all of the persons of different ages with whom you spoke or thought about while studying this chapter. What did you learn about leisure across the life span?

_____

References

Aristotle. (1943). *Politics II: The treatises* (B. Jowett, Trans.). New York: Modern Library.

Baltes, P. B., & Baltes, M. M. (1990). Psychological perspectives on successful aging: The model of selective optimization with compensation. In P. B. Baltes & M. M. Baltes

(Eds.), *Successful aging: Perspectives from the behavioral sciences* (pp. 1–34). London: Cambridge University Press.

Brown, B. B. (1990). Peer groups and peer culture. In S. S. Feldman, & G. R. Elliot (Eds.), *At the threshold: The developing adolescent* (pp. 171–196). Cambridge, MA: Harvard University Press.

Bundy, A. C. (1997). Play and playfulness: What to look for. In L. D. Parham & L. S. Fazio (Eds.), *Play in occupational therapy for children* (pp. 52–66). St. Louis: Mosby.

Chess, S., & Thomas, A. (1984). *Origins and evolutions of behavior disorders: From infancy to early adult life.* New York: Brunner & Mazel.

Cotton, N. (1984). Childhood play as an analog to adult capacity to work. *Child Psychology and Human Development, 14,* 135–144.

Csikszentmihalyi, M. (1992). A theoretical model for enjoyment. In M. T. Allison (Ed.), *Play, leisure and quality of life: Social scientific perspectives* (pp. 11–23). Dubuque, IA: Kendall/Hunt.

Csikszentmihalyi, M., & Larson, R. (1984). *Being adolescent.* New York: Basic Books.

Csikszentmihalyi, M., Rathunde, K., & Whalen, S. (1993). *Talented teenagers: The roots of success & failure.* New York: Cambridge University Press.

Elias, N., & Dunning, E. (1986). *Quest for excitement: Sport and leisure in the civilizing process.* New York: Basil Blackwell.

Erikson, E. H. (1963). *Childhood and society* (2nd ed.). New York: Norton.

Fine, G. A., Mortimer, J. T., & Roberts, D. F. (1990). Leisure, work, and the mass media. In S. S. Feldman & G. R. Elliot (Eds.), *At the threshold: The developing adolescent* (pp. 225–253). Cambridge, MA: Harvard University Press.

Gulick, A. (1998, July/August). Project tide. *Alert Diver,* 39–43.

John-Steiner, V. (1985). *Notebooks of the mind: Explorations of thinking.* New York: Harper & Row.

Kleiber, D. A., Larson, R., & Csikszentmihalyi, M. (1986). The experience of leisure in adolescence. *Journal of Leisure Research, 18,* 169–176.

Kraus, R. (1994). *Leisure in a changing America: Multicultural perspectives.* New York: Macmillan College.

Labouvie-Vief, G. (1994). Women's creativity and images of gender. In B. F. Turner & L. E. Trol (Eds.), *Women growing older: Psychological perspectives* (pp. 140–165). Thousand Oaks, CA: Sage.

Manuele, E. (1998). My rebirth. *NARHA Strides, 4,* 2.

Murphy, L. B., & Moriarity, A. E. (1976). *Vulnerability, coping and growth: From infancy to adolescence.* New Haven, CT: Yale University Press.

Neulinger, J. (1981). *The psychology of leisure.* Springfield, IL: Charles C. Thomas.

Niemela, P., & Linto, R. (1994). The significance of the 50th birthday for women's individuation. In B. F. Turner & L. E. Trol (Eds.), *Women growing older: Psychological perspectives* (pp. 117–127). Thousand Oaks, CA: Sage.

Pieper, J. (1963). *Leisure: The basis of culture.* New York: Random House.

Rowe, J. W., & Kahn, R. L. (1997). Successful aging. *The Gerontologist, 37,* 433–440.

Savin-Williams, R. C., & Berndt, T. J. (1990). Friendship and peer relations. In S. S. Feldman & G. R. Elliot (Eds.), *At the threshold: The developing adolescent* (pp. 277–307). Cambridge, MA: Harvard University Press.

Siegel, R. J. (1993). Between midlife and old age: Never too old to learn. In N. D. Davis, E. Cole, & E. D. Rothblum (Eds.), *Faces of women and aging* (pp. 173–185). Binghamton, NY: Harrington Park Press.

Singleton, J. F. (1996). Leisure skills. In C. B. Lewis (Ed.), *Aging: The health care challenge* (3rd ed., pp. 106–125). Philadelphia: F. A. Davis.

Sloan, L. R. (1979). The function and impact of sports for fans: A review of theory and contemporary research. In J. II. Goldstein (Ed.), *Sports, games and play: Social and psychological viewpoints* (pp. 219–262). Hillsdale, NJ: Lawrence Erlbaum.

Steinberg, L., & Steinberg, W. (1994). *Crossing paths: How your child's adolescence can be an opportunity for your own personal growth.* New York: Simon & Schuster.

Storr, A. (1988). *Solitude: A return to the self.* New York: Ballantine Books.

Zillman, D., Sapolsky, B. S., & Bryant, J. (1979). The enjoyment of watching sport contests. In J. H. Goldstein (Ed.), *Sports, games and play: Social and psychological viewpoints* (pp. 297–336). Hillsdale, NJ: Lawrence Erlbaum.

Zimmer, Z., Hickey, T., & Searle, M. S. (1997). The pattern of change in leisure activity Behavior among older adults with arthritis. *The Gerontologist, 37,* 384–392.

13

Range of Human Activity: Work Activities

Jane Miller, MA, OTR/L

All work, even cotton-spinning, is noble; work is alone noble . . . A life of ease is not for any man, nor for any god. (Thomas Carlyle as cited in Beck, 1980, p. 474:4)

S ay the word "work," and many positive and negative thoughts come to mind. Throughout the world, people are working: children work during play, at school, and in the home during chores; adults have jobs, homemaking tasks, and hobbies. Whether engaged in job seeking, paid employment, volunteer activities, or retirement activities, most persons are working.

A job, an occupation, a vocation, a trade, employment, labor, a business, a calling, or a pursuit—work and work-related terms are very much a part of our lives and vocabulary. Work implies an activity of the body, mind, machine, or nature itself. Usually a sustained physical or cognitive effort, work applies to purposeful activity, especially earning one's livelihood.

The performance area of work, a major aspect of occupational therapy's domain of concern, is germane to occupational therapy. Briefly, work and productive activities are the purposeful activities of self-development, social contribution, and livelihood. In the American Occupational Therapy Association's (AOTA) Uniform Terminology (AOTA, 1994), work and productive activities include home management (e.g., clothing care, cleaning, meal preparation or cleanup, shopping, money management, household maintenance, safety procedures), care of others, educational activities, and vocational activities.

This chapter concentrates on the latter set of vocational activities. Participation in work-related activities encompasses vocational exploration, job acquisition, work or job performance, retirement planning, and volunteer participation. Vocational exploration is the determination of aptitudes, development of interests and skills, and the selection of appropriate vocational pursuits. Job acquisition consists of the identification and selection of work opportunities and the completion of the application and interview processes. Work or job performance is the timely and effective performance of job tasks and the acquisition and incorporation of work behaviors. Retirement planning involves the determination of aptitudes, the development of interests and skills, and the selection of appropriate avocational pursuits. Volunteer participation is the performance of unpaid activities for the benefit of selected persons, groups, or causes. This chapter does not explore retirement planning and volunteer participation.

Evolutionary Origins and the History of Work

Instinctively and via learned behaviors, animals work to acquire or construct shelter, obtain food, and protect and care for their young. Humans do the same: food gathering (albeit via the neighborhood grocery store or from a backyard garden), acquiring clothing and housing, defending themselves from enemies and protecting territory, and child rearing. Through the ages, from the Stone Age hunter-gatherers until recent times, persons have engaged in these activities because the work was necessary. Unless persons performed the task themselves, either independently or cooperatively with members of their family or community, they would not likely survive.

Colonial America consisted of farmers, artisans, and craftsmen. Potters, leather workers, silversmiths, glassblowers, masons, and blacksmiths were at the heart of small industries. Work centered around the home and the horse. Along the coast and lakes, maritime activities evolved such as shipbuilding and fishing.

With the emerging factory system, unskilled and semiskilled labor swelled the ranks of workers along with thousands of former agricultural workers. The factory system often exploited women, children, and minorities. Technological advances introduced during the Industrial Revolution began to make the world of work easier in some respects and more difficult in others. The horse gave way to the automobile, and McCormick's reaper performed tasks once completed by hand. The "machine [became] sacrosanct; the worker was [now] expendable" (Fraser, 1992, p. 2). Society paid little attention to the worker's health, safety, or social conditions. The plight of the factory worker, as dramatized in the writings of Charles Dickens and others, heightened the public's awareness of dangerous industrial working conditions. One's willingness to perform the task and the apparent lack of any limiting disability were sufficient criteria for evaluating one's fitness for the job.

Farmers comprised 60% of the working population in 1850 (Morris, 1976). By 1996, only 1.7% of the American workforce was employed in agriculture (JIST Works, 1998–1999). Air travel, the Internet, and the global market are just a few of the factors affecting today's work in the Information Age. Computerization and robotics have forever changed the ways in which we receive, process, and use information; perform tasks; and conduct business.

Noted author Studs Terkel's books, *My American Century* (1997) and *Working: People Talk About What They Do All Day and How They Feel About What They Do* (1971), further explore the historical development of and changes in work in the United States. Terkel has created an intimate portrait of work, life, and the American people.

Learning How To Work

Life grants nothing to us mortals without hard work. (Horace as cited in Beck, 1980, p. 106:17)

In primitive societies, work is clearly visible to children: sowing, threshing, grinding, kneading, dyeing, hunting, kindling, and carrying. Children learn basic work skills and help in adult tasks as soon as they are able. In developed areas, like the United States, children may not actually see their parents or community engaged in work. Children spend their time at play and going to school. Childhood games often mimic adult activities. These play experiences may later affect occupational choice and work behaviors (Argyle, 1972).

Persons establish the basic components of their work personality in childhood. Concentrating on a task, cooperating or competing with peers, developing appropriate responses to authority, and associating meaning and values with work and achievement will prepare the person for future work. During adolescence, teens usually try various kinds of work through home, school, and neighborhood employment. One difficulty inherent in orienting young persons in our modern society is the enormity of occupational choice. Several studies (Argyle, 1972; Steele & Morgan, 1991) have shown that adolescents are attracted to jobs that are similar to their self-image or require skills that they believe they possess. By the time the person has completed his or her formal education (e.g., high school, vocational program, college, or graduate school), society deems him or her to be ready to embark on a life's work.

Our society tends to look askance at persons who are idle and believes that hard work will pay off in the long term. These culturally bound tenets of Judeo-Christian tradition are still evident today. How many times have you heard the expression, "Idle hands are the devil's workshop"? This work ethic is evident throughout American history and literature.

When men are employed, they are best contented for on the days they worked they were good-natured and cheerful, and, with the consciousness of having done a good day's work, they spent the evening jollily; but on our idle days they were mutinous and quarrelsome. (Benjamin Franklin as cited in Beck, 1980, p. 348:21)

Reich (1970) wrote that "work and function are basic to man. They fulfill him, they establish his identity, they give him his place in the human community" (pp. 367–368).

More recently, Bellman (1996) reiterated the theme that work is central to our lives and is key to living with meaning. He stated that work feeds our need for growth and accomplishment and allows us to demonstrate skill, get attention, exercise discipline, and experience mastery. The benefits of steady employment are psychologically important, along with monetary rewards of a steady income, paid vacations, medical and unemployment insurance, discounts on products, reduced or paid tuition, and other fringe benefits.

Trends and Forecasts in Employment

> In order that people may be happy in their work, these three things are needed: they must be fit for it; they must not do too much of it; and they must have a sense of success in it. (John Ruskin as cited in Beck, 1980, p. 572:13)

As a result of new technology and economic and political developments, the job market in various occupational fields is constantly changing. According to the U.S. Department of Labor's Bureau of Labor Statistics (BLS, 1999b), a total of 143.2 million persons (70% of the working-age population 16 years of age and older in the United States) worked at some time during 1997. Moreover, 79% of all employed persons worked full-time (35 hr or more weekly). Increasing numbers of persons are working at home either as wage-earning or salaried workers, or they are self-employed. Many of these persons are in white collar occupations, and about 62% use a computer for the work they accomplish at home.

In early December 1997, BLS issued new projections for the American workforce for 1996 to 2006 (U.S. Department of Labor, BLS, 1999a). These projections of economic growth, the labor force, and employment by industry are useful for developing career information, planning education and training programs, and forecasting employment trends. According to the BLS report, the labor force will increase by 11% (up 15 million from 134 to 149 million). The demographic composition of the cohort of workers 45 to 64 years of age is changing more rapidly as the "baby boomer" generation continues to age. Projected declines in workers 25 to 34 years of age result from decreased birth rates during the late 1960s and early 1970s. Service-producing industries such as health, business, social services, engineering, management, and related services are expected to account for almost half of the growth. The fastest growing occupations include six health services and four computer-related occupations (see Table 1 and Figure 1). Through the year 2006, service and professional specialty occupations will provide about two out of five job openings.

The Balanced Budget Act of 1997 (Pub. L. 105–33) has dramatically changed the employment outlook for health care providers such as occupational therapists. The current health care system is fraught with mergers, downsizing, restructuring, reorganizing, and consolidation. In the light of the recent changes in health care, the BLS's report needs modification or an addendum. The BLS is currently updating its projections for the next 10 years. Occupations in the American labor market respond to global, societal, scientific, commercial, and legislative developments.

Table 1
The 10 Occupations With the Fastest Employment Growth, 1996–2006

	Employment		Change (1996–2006)	
Occupation	*1996*	*2006*	*n*	*%*
Database administrators, computer support specialists, and all other computer scientists	212	461	249	118
Computer engineers	216	451	235	109
Systems analysts	506	1,025	520	103
Personal and home care aides	202	374	171	85
Physical and corrective therapy assistants and aides	84	151	66	79
Home health aides	495	873	378	76
Medical assistants	225	391	166	74
Desktop publishing specialists	30	53	22	74
Physical therapists	115	196	81	71
Occupational therapy assistants and aides	16	26	11	69

Note. Numbers in thousands of jobs. From the online resource of the Bureau of Labor Statistics available at http://stats.bls.gov/ecopro.table6.htm

Vocational Exploration

> . . . the workplace is always in flux, always in transition, always in turmoil—it always has been, and it always will be. (Bolles, 1998, p. 11)

Today's typical college student will be engaged in approximately 100,000 working hours after graduating (Steele & Morgan, 1991). A person's work influences his or her way of life. Our career choices actually determine who our friends will be, the attitudes and values we develop, the geographical area where we will live, the patterns we will adopt, and how we will spend our leisure time. Work shapes and molds our identity and gives purpose and meaning to our lives. Work confers status in one's field of employment, among friends, in families, and most important, to oneself.

Society classifies the world of work in various ways. Some classifications list occupations according to their prestige. In this system, judges, physicians, and high government officials rank at the top, whereas janitors and garbage collectors generally rank at the bottom. Another method of classifying work is according to

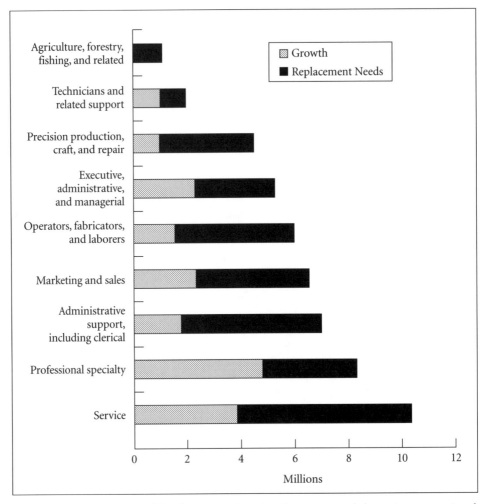

Figure 1. Job openings resulting from growth and replacement needs by major occupational group. *Note.* From the online resource of the Bureau of Labor Statistics. Available at http://ststs.bls.gov/images/ocotj07.gif

socioeconomic factors or the degree of intelligence, education, and skills required. Holland's RIASEC (Realistic, Investigative, Artistic, Social, Enterprising, Conventional) theory of careers is the basis for many inventories today (Holland, 1997). By using a typology of personality and environments, Holland characterized persons and their work into six groups.

1.   Realistic—concrete and practical activity involving machines, tools, or materials

2.   Investigative—analytical or intellectual activity aimed at problem-solving or creation and use of knowledge

3.   Artistic—creative work in the arts or unstructured and intellectual endeavors

4. Social—working with persons in a helpful or facilitative way

5. Enterprising—working with persons in a supervisory or persuasive way to achieve some organizational goal

6. Conventional—working with objects, numbers, or machines in an orderly way to meet regular and predictable needs of an organization or to meet specified standards

Holland's model provides a framework for which specific personal and environmental characteristics lead to satisfying and stable career decisions.

Another agency of the government has a different method of classifying work. The *Guide for Occupational Exploration* (GOE), produced by the U.S. Employment Service (1979), groups work according to interests, abilities, and traits necessary for successful performance. Persons can identify and explore types of work that closely relate to their own skills and interests. The GOC organizes data into interest areas, work groups, and subgroups. The 12 interest areas correspond to the following broad categories.

1. Artistic—creative expression of feelings or ideas

2. Scientific—discovering, collecting, and analyzing information about the natural world and applying scientific research findings to problems in medicine, life sciences, and natural sciences

3. Plants and animals—activities involving plants and animals, usually in an outdoor setting

4. Protective—use of authority to protect persons and property

5. Mechanical—applying mechanical principles to practical situations by using machines, hand tools, or techniques

6. Industrial—repetitive, concrete, organized activities in a factory setting

7. Business detail—organized, clearly defined activities requiring accuracy and attention to detail, primarily in office settings

8. Selling—convincing others of a particular point of view through personal persuasion by using sales and promotion techniques

9. Accommodating—catering to the desires of others, usually on a one-to-one basis

10. Humanitarian—helping others with their mental, spiritual, social, physical, or vocational needs

11. Leading and influencing—leading and influencing others through activities involving high-level verbal or numerical abilities

12. Physical performing—physical activities performed before an audience

Case Scenario 1

The broad Humanitarian interest area (10) lists occupational therapists as a subgroup (10.02–02 Therapy and Rehabilitation) in the work group of Nursing, Therapy, and Specialized Teaching Services (10.02).

Exercise 1

Think about why you decided to enter the profession of occupational therapy. How did you discover this area of work? Did you have a role model or a personal experience? Where did you go to obtain more information? If you could, how would you do go about this process differently?

Exercise 2

Read Richard Bolles' (1998) *What Color is Your Parachute?* It provides excellent tips and suggestions for analyzing your vocational interests and strengths and obtaining employment.

Exercise 3

On the World Wide Web, check out the Internet links and find information related to job seeking for special populations. Visit http://www.tenspeed.com/parachute.

The Socratic method of "knowing thyself" consists of asking probing questions, defining terms, and analyzing opinions to reveal their consistency or inconsistency. Career and life planning begins with similar steps. One of the best places to start research and reading is the *Occupational Outlook Handbook* (U.S. Department of Labor, BLS, 1998) and its special edition, the *Occupational Outlook for College Graduates* (U.S. Department of Labor, BLS, 1991). Published by the BLS, these books are guides to career opportunities.

The *Occupational Outlook Handbook*, which is revised every 2 years, describes approximately 250 occupations, specifically what the worker does on the job, working conditions, education and training needed, and the anticipated job prospects and earnings. The Internet version is available at http://stats.bls.gov/ocohome.htm. Each job title has a unique number, as stipulated in the *Dictionary of Occupational Titles* (DOT; U.S. Department of Labor, BLS, 1991). The nine-digit code identifies occupations uniquely within the related occupational group and according to worker functions. State employment service offices and other agencies use these title codes, which were defined more than 60 years ago, to classify applicants and job openings. The Department of Labor has recently replaced the DOT with an updated, Internet-based Web site, O*NET: The Occupational Information Network (U.S. Department of Labor, Office of Policy and Research, 1998). Along with the descriptions of the various job titles and many links to other sites (e.g., America's Job Bank, America's Labor Market Information System, BLS, National Skill Standards Board), this computerized database describes job requirements and worker competencies for approximately 1,100 current occupations: what the worker does; what equipment he or she uses; how closely the worker is supervised; how the duties of the worker vary by industry, establishment, and the size of the company; how the responsibilities of entry-level workers differ from those of experienced, supervisory, or self-employed workers; how technological innovations affect what workers do and how they do it; and emerging specialties. Additionally included are typical working and environmental conditions for workers in the occupation; typical hours worked; workplace environment; susceptibility to injury, illness, and job-related stress; necessary protective clothing and safety equipment; basic clothing required; and travel required (Figure 2).

Case Scenario 2

The Occupational Outlook Handbook describes an occupational therapist as follows. "Occupational Therapists (DOT 076.121-010) . . . are among the fastest growing occupations. The high demand, good job opportunities, and high pay are spurred on by a rapidly aging population with increased demand for therapeutic services and the survival of medically critical" (U.S. Department of Labor, BLS, 1998). The book (and Web-based handbook) elaborates on both the pros and cons of a particular occupation. For example, occupational therapy can be tiring because therapists are on their feet much of the time. Persons employed in home health may spend hours driving to and from appointments. Occupational therapists face job-related hazards such as back strain from lifting clients and equipment. Some of the qualifications for occupational therapists are patience, strong interpersonal skills to inspire trust and respect, ingenuity, and imagination in adapting activities and environments.

Role of Occupational Therapy in Work and Work Activities

Historically, work was a modality of treatment rather than the goal of treatment. "Occupational therapy took root in a rich soil of work activities for the mentally ill. In the early 1920's, the first occupational therapists documented steps for a uniform program of curative activity" (Marshall, 1985, p. 297). Today, work and work activities are both the treatment approach and the end goal. These applications include, but are not limited to, work-related games for children, welfare-to-work programs, work-hardening and work-conditioning programs, transition from school to work, supported employment, work readiness, vocational exploration, injury reduction, stress management, tool modification, and job accommodation.

Occupational therapists are uniquely qualified to synthesize the information for the design and implementation of a safe work environment; are able to establish appropriate productivity levels for homebound, sheltered, modified, or competitive

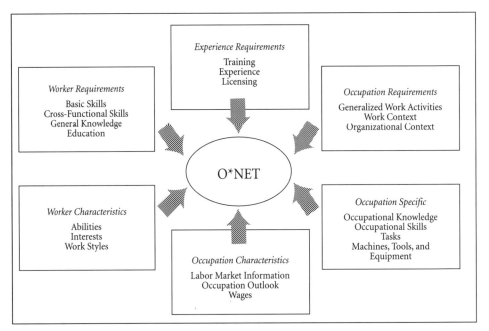

Figure 2. The O*NET database identifies, defines, and describes the comprehensive elements of job performance in the changing world of work. It contains hundreds of information units on job requirements, worker attributes, and the content and context of work, capturing what pople do as functions of their roles within organization. By examining and measuring the processes of work, O*NET data allow users to profile similarities and differences across occupations and anticipate skill changes now and into the 21st century. The framework that organizes O*NET data is a skills-based structure called the Content Model. The Content Model classifies data into six domains, or "windows" that look into all aspects of the workplace, from the attributes of occupations to the characteristics of people who do the job. The graphic illustrates how the Content Model structures information put into the O*NET database.

With comprehensive terms designed to incorporate occupational descriptions across all sectors of the economy, the O*NET structure standardizes the way that occupational information is defined and described. Creating a common ground of understanding on which public and private workforce initiatives can work together, O*NET data become a communication link to help integrate learning, training and work. *Note.* From: O*NET: The Occupational Information Network, U.S. Department of Labor, BLS, 1998. Available at www.doleta.gov/programs/onet/database.htm

work; and are able to implement tool or job site evaluations and modifications. The therapist develops and guides job-specific programs of graded activity for the worker, performs job task analysis and workstation and tool modification, and identifies and remediates behaviors inappropriate to the work environment. The benefits to the worker, employer, and the work environment include increased productivity, decreased worker's compensation insurance claims and lost work days, and prevention or reduction of injury.

Occupational therapy practitioners may collaborate with professionals who specialize in ergonomics. Ergonomics, the science of work, is the matching of human abilities or capabilities and job requirements within the context of the physical and social work environment. Also called *human factors* or *human engineering*, ergonomics interacts closely with other applied and life sciences such as engineering, medicine, and psychology to preserve health, prevent injury, and maximize work efficiency. The role of ergonomics in rehabilitation is in the redesigning of the external environment to accommodate the worker with disabilities or injuries, thereby enabling the person to contribute fully and independently (Rader Smith, 1989; Figure 3). In disability prevention, ergonomists examine human factors relevant to the job, human capabilities, and the human–machine interaction or interface under given environmental conditions. Ergonomic design is the application of this knowledge to tool, machine, system, job, and environmental design for safe, comfortable, and effective human use. Ergonomists are often engineers (e.g., safety, mechanical) and therapists (e.g., occupational and physical) who have undergone specific educational experiences.

Examining the Workplace and the Worker

Job analysis and worker evaluation is a multiphase process: job description (which includes an objective record of job and components similar to those in the DOT or O*NET), task or job analysis (which includes evaluation of selected tasks or activities in terms of human demands such as vision, hearing, cognitive processes, and muscle recruitment), and identification of worker capabilities. These phases do not always proceed in a neat and orderly sequence.

Activity analysis is at the core of conducting a job analysis evaluation. The process of job analysis examines the physical demands; cognitive factors; specific tasks, tools, and machines; the environment; and the psychological and physical hazards of the work. The following techniques are useful in conducting a job evaluation: interviews with employer and employees, questionnaires, photographic documentation (still photographs and videorecordings), anthropometric data collection, and functional and specific work assessments. The examiner identifies potentially hazardous or inadequate work habits, equipment, and environments. After analysis of the data, recommendations include reducing the risk of work-related injury, providing workers with guidelines for safe and efficient task completion, and suggesting possible workstation modifications.

Functional capacity evaluation (FCE) is a procedure to evaluate a person's level of physical ability to perform basic work tasks. This protocol may be useful in litigation, preemployment screens, the return to work, and work capacity evaluations. The FCE measures tasks such as lifting, pulling, pushing, and climbing. An FCE includes numerous standardized and nonstandardized assessments. Readers should refer to the bibliography for additional information.

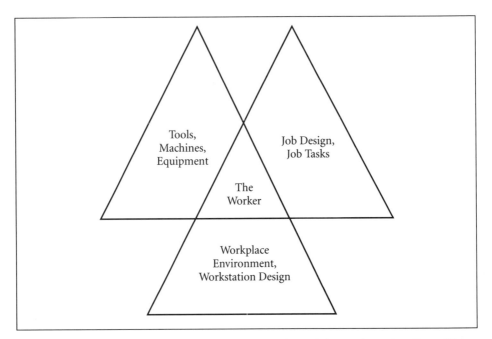

Figure 3. Interactions between the workplace, the job, and the worker. *Note.* From "Ergonomics and the Occupational Therapist," by E. Rader Smith. In S. Hertfelder & C. Gwin (Eds.), *Work in Progress: Occupational Therapy in Work Programs*, 1989, p. 129, Rockville, MD: American Occupational Therapy Association. Copyright 1989 by the American Occupational Therapy Association. Reprinted with permission.

Case Scenario 3

Let us examine the work of a typical office worker. According to the U.S. Department of Labor, U.S. Employment Services (1991), the job title of Administrative Secretary (DOT Code 169.167-014) involves the physical demands of sedentary work (maximum lift of 10 lbs.) and the abilities to talk, hear, reach, handle, finger, and feel. The job requires a limited amount of walking, standing, and carrying light objects. The worker must be able to extend the arms in any direction and seize, hold, grasp, turn, pick, pinch, and perceive the size, shape, temperature, or texture of objects. Working conditions are inside (75% or more, with protection from weather conditions but not necessarily from temperature changes). This job title involves overseeing and carrying out office operations; applying clerical skills including planning own or others' work program; using reasoning; using hands and fingers in typing; recording data; obtaining and safeguarding confidential information; recognizing and proofing copy to correct errors in spelling, grammar, and punctuation; speaking distinctly; and making decisions involving policy (U.S. Department of Labor, U.S. Employment Services, 1991).

An administrative secretary, a woman 52 years of age with a 2-year employment history with Happy Socks Unlimited, was interviewed regarding her job tasks and responsibilities and work-related health concerns. She has a below-average sick leave usage rate (i.e., less than half of the allotted 12 days per year). Absences are usually because of seasonal allergies and sinus headaches. During periods of high keyboarding activity, she reports stiffness in her neck, pain accompanying neck rotation to right, radiating pain down both arms, and nocturnal numbness and tingling in both hands.

The administrative secretary oversees the general functioning of the office and supervises full- and part-time clerical personnel. The specific job duties and tasks are as follows.

Cognitive tasks

- Gathers and develops information

- Stores and retrieves information

- Reads

- Proofreads and edits

- Calculates and analyzes data

- Orders supplies

- Inspects supplies and compares invoices

- Plans and schedules

- Makes decisions

Social tasks

- Answers and uses telephone and routes calls

- Confers and meets with persons

- Works with other persons

Physical tasks

- Stores and retrieves documents and files

- Writes with a pen, pencil, or marker

- Handles mail

- Collates and sorts

- Photocopies documents

- Types documents from handwritten drafts or typed matter

- Maintains calendar

- Maintains and conducts minor repairs of equipment (e.g., fixes paper jams in photocopier, loads paper, changes printer toner)

- Uses equipment (e.g., pencil, computer, photocopier, printer, telephone)

The physical demands, consistent with the DOT description, include the following.

- Standing

- Walking

- Sitting (75% of the time [sedentary work])

- Lifting and carrying (light objects less than 10 kg)

- Reaching and grasping

- Handling and fingering

- Stair or step climbing (infrequently)

- Balancing, stooping, and kneeling (infrequently)

- Communicating (talking)

- Hearing

- Vision (near, midrange, far vision, visual accommodation, and color vision)

By using the guidelines and standards that Grandjean (1988) listed, an evaluator takes anthropometric measurements with a tape measure and then compares these external bodily dimensions (e.g., standing height, forward reach, arm span, foot to popliteal length) with group norms. A goniometer measures range of motion (ROM). A dynamometer and pinch gauge measure hand strength, specifically grasp and pinch. A full upper-extremity evaluation was completed and evaluated overall coordination, sensation, and functional abilities. The evaluation confirmed that the worker was within normal limits in all areas (for age and gender).

Work sampling is conducted. The secretary sits at her desk in an upright posture. The computer, monitor, and printer are on. The examiner evaluates the task of keyboarding a brief memorandum from a two-page, handwritten draft in detail. The steps include the following.

- Takes draft out of "to do" box on the desk or receives draft from the originator or courier

- Puts draft on copy stand

- Selects word processing icon (software loads)

- Creates document file (input via typing on keyboard and mouse clicking)

- Proofreads, edits, and spell checks document

- Clicks on print icon

- May need to walk to printer location, retrieve paper from storage bin, and load paper

- Walks to printer location and retrieves document

- Completes final proofreading

- Puts finished memorandum in "out" box

Time studies determine the approximate hourly keystroke rate. The secretary completed three trials by using a keyboarding assessment. She produced documents that were well formatted, error free, and edited for content, style, spelling, and grammar. The secretary's preferred rate allows for simultaneous conversation with others and does not appear to result in any physical complaints. If the workload warrants, she is able to perform two to three times faster than this rate; however, upper-extremity problems usually result with prolonged exertion.

The work site is housed in a newly renovated facility. The space includes company offices, secretarial areas, reception, and storage. A fully equipped lounge with a kitchen area (e.g., sink, refrigerator, microwave oven, coffee and hot water system, table, chairs) is available for mealtime and snacks. Accessible restrooms are located in the building.

Secretarial workstations contain standard office desks, lateral filing cabinets, shelving, an adjustable desk chair, and guest chairs. All enclosed offices are soundproof within an acceptable level. Except for the hallways, kitchen, restrooms, and storage areas, all floors have carpeting. The heating ventilation air conditioning (HVAC) system is reportedly a source of irritation: it is noisy, drafty at certain locations, and does not regulate the temperature well throughout the office. The secretary usually sits 24 in. (61 cm) from her monitor and maintains a viewing angle of 18°. Seat height, back angle, elbow angle, keyboard height, and screen height are within acceptable ranges.

Regarding the findings and recommendations of the evaluation, overall, the flexibility inherent in her job allows the secretary to pace the work. Although the work site is not perfect (e.g., the HVAC system), and job demands are more stressful at times, the job is usually manageable. Her capabilities and work requirements are normally balanced. The following suggestions will further enhance performance, reduce work-related injury, and increase worker comfort.

- Modify the workstation by adding task lighting, adding a keyboard wrist rest, adding an angled adjustable footrest (as well as clearing the area under the desk to allow for more leg room), adding a chair mat, changing shelf spacing to improve arrangement of work materials, and changing the desk if possible to a reduced-length, rounded D-shaped work surface.

- Reduce repetitive components as much as possible by incorporating varied job tasks, increasing freedom of motion in the workstation area (by ridding area of nonessential storage material), taking frequent "micro breaks" (stretch and exercise periods), and using autosuggestive techniques to relax the body during activity.

■   Encourage the worker to avoid excessive extension, flexion, and deviation
of the wrist and constrained postures.

■   Encourage the worker to vary and alternate tasks to reduce the amount of
sedentary work.

■   Maintain a comfortable environmental temperature and relative humidity
and minimize static electricity and drafts.

An Epidemiological Approach

An epidemiological study of a work-related disease is particularly subject to inherent
difficulties, especially in providing evidence for causality of observed phenomena
(World Health Organization [WHO], 1989). Causative factors often have a complex
etiology, and confounding variables of lifestyle, work habits, and individual capabilities influence these factors. A disorder requiring a long exposure time or repeated
injuries such as repetitive strain injury (RSI) is more difficult to identify with a specific work activity and onset. The Person–Environment Fit Model, on the basis of
McGarth's work (Van Harrison, 1978), depicts the tenuous balance (often an imbal-
ance) between the job demands and the abilities of the person to satisfy those
demands. The National Institute for Occupational Safety and Health (NIOSH), the
federal agency that provides recommendations to prevent work-related illness and
injury, agrees that exposure to stressful working conditions can have a direct influence on worker safety and health. Psychological and physiological strain results when
demands and abilities are not matched well (U.S. Department of Health and Human
Services, NIOSH, 1999; Van Harrison, 1978; Figure 4 and Table 2).

Case Scenario 4

Traditionally, workers in food processing, health services, manufacturing, and
craft industries have incurred work-related injuries secondary to repetitive, manual exertions. The increased use of the computer in the workplace has introduced
another source of work-related concerns. The work of a computer keyboard user
may involve rapid, repetitive movements of the upper extremities and static load-
ing (i.e., wrists and shoulders held in same position for extended periods). RSI,
also known as cumulative trauma disorder, occupational overuse syndrome, or
repetitive motion disorder, is a generic label for various painful, debilitating, soft-
tissue conditions that result from repetitive movements of the hands or arms.
Activities such as stooping, sedentary work, and constrained postures and bio-
physiological factors such as physical size, strength, fitness, ROM, and work
endurance likely contribute to RSI. Psychological stressors from the job structure
(e.g., scheduling, machine pacing), job content (e.g., time pressures and overload, underload, lack of control), and organization (e.g., role ambiguity, competition) can further compound the situation with anxiety, dissatisfaction,
psychogenic illness, and absenteeism. Various conditions, many of them not well
defined, comprise RSI. Tenosynovitis, shoulder pain, tension neck, tendinitis,

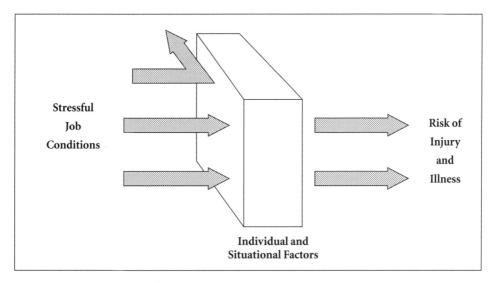

Figure 4. NIOSH model of job stress. *Note.* From *Stress at Work* by the U.S. Department of Health and Human Services, National Institute for Occupational Safety and Health, 1999 (DHHS Publication No. 99-101), Cincinnati, OH: Publications Dissemination EID.

and carpal tunnel syndrome are but a few of the many musculotendinous conditions involved in this disorder. Persons often list many complaints such as tenderness, pain, swelling, cramping, and tingling sensations.

Health in the Workplace

In the United States, more than 39 million persons are hospitalized or receive emergency services because of accidental injuries. More than 3 million persons sustain disabling injuries on the job. Escalating costs from loss of productivity, absenteeism, retraining, and medical and disability insurance have focused attention on the concern for a healthy worker and a healthy work environment. The traditional approach of treating illnesses has changed to a health maintenance or preventive medical focus. The role of employees' health services has become more comprehensive in many settings. In addition to providing medical care, industrial safety, and compliance with state and federal regulations, the employer may provide

■ preplacement examinations (baseline medical profiles that protect both the company and the worker),

■ periodic health and medical surveillance examinations (preventive early detection screenings),

Table 2
Job Conditions That May Lead to Stress

Condition	*Example*
The design of tasks Heavy workload; infrequent rest breaks; long work hours and shift-work; hectic and routine tasks that have little inherent meaning, do not use workers' skills, and provide little sense of control.	David works to the point of exhaustion. Theresa is tied to the computer, allowing little room for flexibility, self-initiative, or rest.
Management style Lack of participation by workers in decision making, poor communication in the organization, lack of family-friendly policies.	Theresa needs to get the boss's approval for everything, and the company is insensitive to her family needs.
Interpersonal relationships Poor social environment and lack of support or help from coworkers and supervisors.	Theresa's physical isolation reduces her opportunities to interact with other workers or receive help from them.
Work roles Conflicting or uncertain job expectations, too much responsibility, "too many hats to wear."	Theresa is often caught in a difficult situation trying to satisfy both the customer's needs and the company's expectations.
Career concerns Job insecurity and a lack of opportunity for growth, advancement, or promotion; rapid changes for which workers are unprepared.	Since the reorganization at David's plant, everyone is worried about their future with the company and what will happen next.
Environmental conditions Unpleasant or dangerous physical conditions such as crowding, noise, air pollution, or ergonomic problems.	David is exposed to constant noise at work.

Note. From *Stress at Work* by the U.S. Department of Health and Human Services, National Institute for Occupational Safety and Health, 1999 (DHHS Publication No. 99-101), Cincinnati, OH: Publications Dissemination EID.

- return-to-work and disability management (to prevent accidents, reinjury, or spread of illness and to provide proper care and rehabilitation to minimize duration of injury) (Figure 5), and

- wellness and fitness programs (to promote fitness such as smoking cessation, general nutrition, weight reduction, and stress reduction).

> The most important element for control is prevention through environmental protection in the workplace, safety education of workers and managers, the application of appropriate and safe work practices, and the application of basic ergonomic principles. (WHO, 1989, p. 7)

Work injury management and prevention is a multidisciplinary effort (Isernhagen, 1995). Medical, legal, vocational, and insurance professionals and employers and employees must communicate and cooperate to safeguard the worker and prevent job-related injuries. Work evaluation consists of evaluating the injured worker (or potential worker), the type and method of work, and the unique capabilities and interests of the employee. Each professional contributes to the worker's success at the work site, including occupational therapists and physical therapists, vocational counselors, physicians, and psychologists. Depending on the situation, occupational health and safety engineers, industrial psychologists, ergonomists, kinesiologists, personnel and human resources staff members, attorneys, insurance adjusters, and workers' compensation insurance judges may be involved in the return-to-work process. The resulting documentation must be readable, devoid of jargon and highly technical wording, and understandable to a wide audience. To ensure competitiveness in the world market, employers must maintain a healthy workforce. Providing ongoing safety training and ensuring timely rehabilitation of sick and injured workers are sound practices.

Case Scenario 5

The Nut Factory Worker

Presenting Problem. An injured worker was offered immediate employment. The job, checking the quality of pecan nuts in a candy factory, is light work and is within the employee's capabilities. The worker, subsequent to a back injury sustained while unloading packaging materials from the delivery trucks, had orthopedic surgery in which surgeons fused his L5 and S1 vertebrae. The worker was familiar with the job but was not sure whether he would be able to cope with the demands of the work.

Job Description. Employees either sit or stand in front of a slow-moving conveyor belt carrying pecans. Employees must identify imperfect and broken nuts, pick them by hand, and place them on another belt (located 10 in. behind the first belt). Placing the rejected nuts on the second belt requires forward reaching. Most workers prefer to stand (little room is available for their legs) and lean forward over the belt with their forearms resting on the edge of the conveyor belt. If the employee sat, he or she would need to twist sideways to reach the belts.

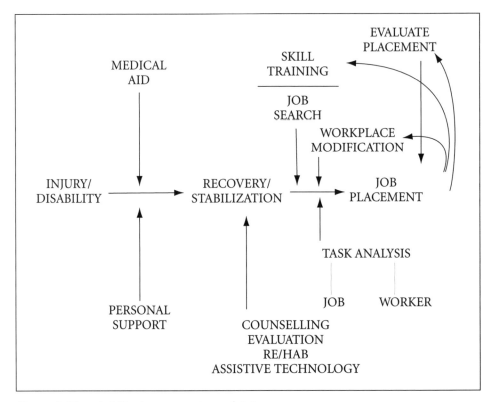

Figure 5. The rehabilitation process in work injury.

Conclusion. Both positions available (standing with a stooped posture or seated with a rotated spine) cause considerable load on the lower back. The employee was able to return to work after the candy manufacturer changed the workplace. The modifications included removal of storage bins below conveyor belts, provision of raised stools for sitting, and provision of a foot bar for support while standing. Although these changes required an outlay of capital, they allowed all workers to sit comfortably without rotation. As a secondary benefit to the employer, complaints of neck and low back pain from other workers, absenteeism, and sick leave greatly declined.

Case Scenario 6

The Tire Factory Worker

Presenting Problem. In another example of an injured factory worker, the worker experienced a lumbosacral sprain, right knee sprain, and ringing in the ears. The factory has continuous, high-volume background noise and a slight but noticeable floor vibration.

Job Description. The job involves identifying and marking defective tires transported through the area by an overhead carrier. Employees accomplish this partly by sight and partly by touch while walking slowly behind the moving tire. Workers remove surplus rubber left by the molding process with a sharp knife. Employees remove rejected tires from the overhead carrier and place them in wheeled carts for reprocessing. The job requires standing and walking through-out the work shift. Lifting a tire weighing approximately 13.62 to 20 kg occurs once every 4 to 5 min.

Conclusions. The lifting requirements are in excess of the employee's capabilities and will likely exacerbate the back condition. Prolonged standing and walking combined with floor vibration are likely to worsen both the knee and back. Because of the high noise level, communication with coworkers is difficult and is a source of stress. The worker should consider alternative employment. This job and work site environment have numerous problems that may affect other workers in terms of work postures, work rate, vibration, and other stressors. A thorough ergonomic evaluation is necessary.

Compliance With State and Federal Regulations

The Occupational Safety and Health Act of 1970 established the Occupational Safety and Health Administration (OSHA) in the U.S. Department of Labor to "disseminate and enforce safety and health standards to protect employees at work" (Career Information Center, 1990, p. 55). Places of employment should be free of recognized hazards. A work site with 11 or more employees must maintain records of work-related injuries and illness and provide medical surveillance and protective equipment. Specifically, the employer must identify chemical, physical, biological, and ergonomic hazards in the workplace. The employer must provide medical monitoring for exposure to toxic elements such as asbestos, noise, and lead along with protective equipment such as safety shoes, helmets, safety glasses, respirators, and hearing protectors.

Hazard communication, or right-to-know compliance enacted by OSHA in 1983 further requires that all employers notify workers if they are exposed to or have contact with hazardous materials. Employers must identify and label all hazardous chemicals. Employees must obtain material safety data sheets from the manufacturer or supplier. These technical bulletins describe a chemical, its characteristics, its health and safety hazards, and precautions. Employees must receive training in the safe handling of the chemical.

The Older Worker

Increasing life expectancy, low birth rate (which has reduced the numbers of younger replacement workers available), and an aging labor force are changing the age composition of the workplace. The amendments to Age Discrimination in Employment

Act (ADEA; Pub. L. 99–592) of 1986 abolished a mandatory retirement age. The ADEA safeguards the older worker (i.e., more than 40 years of age) from age-based distinctions in hiring, salary, promotions, and training. Cost projections of retirement to the individual worker and society are staggering. Legislators have proposed and implemented actions and policies to extend one's working career. Some programs include

- expanding work opportunities and alternative work schedules via job redesign, phased retirement, job sharing, and part-time jobs;

- outlawing age discrimination in employment;

- retraining and second (third, etc.) career opportunities;

- subsidized employment; and

- pension reforms that raise the age of eligibility.

Physical changes occur with age. As work capabilities vary, every older worker requires individual evaluation. Common deficits and limitations are as follows.

- Functional capacity, the ability to perform tasks or physiological activities, declines with age. Between 30 and 65 years of age, maximum breathing capacity reduces by 40%, nerve conduction velocity reduces by 20%, and cardiac function reduces by 25%.

- Homeostasis, the body's ability to maintain operation, also changes as one ages. Age may affect body temperature and glucose regulation. Temperature extremes more easily incapacitate older workers than younger workers.

- Cardiovascular changes are likewise a part of aging. The resting heart rate decreases from 72 beats/min at 25 years of age to 50 beats/min at 65 years of age. Maximum heart rate likewise drops from 190 to 200 beats/min at 30 years of age to 150 to 160 beats/min at 70 years of age. Cardiac output, the volume of blood that the heart pumps with each beat, lowers annually by 1%. Risk of hypertension (secondary to elevated blood pressure), cerebrovascular accidents (resulting from reduced elasticity of the veins and arteries), and arteriosclerosis (hardening of arterial walls associated with accumulation of fatty deposits) are more frequent in the older worker.

- Hearing losses common to older adults include the inability to distinguish low-volume and high-pitched sounds (e.g., consonants f, g, s, t, and z). Older persons may have difficulty filtering out extraneous noises and may need increased volume to hear.

- Other changes in skin (e.g., loss of underlying fatty tissue and skin elasticity), gastrointestinal systems, and body composition (e.g., reduced muscle mass, loss of calcium in bone) seem less likely to influence work performance but may increase the risk of disease and reduce optimal functional capacity. Despite these naturally occurring physiological changes, the older worker is not necessarily an unhealthy or unproductive employee. Age is a poor predictor of the person, work capabilities, and performance.

Productivity may not decline with age. Life experiences enhance decision-making abilities. Reaction time slows with age. The older worker tends to be less apt to engage in risk-taking behavior, which results in lower accident rates. Declines in memory are slight and have little influence on performance. Intellectual functioning does not appear to alter with aging itself but rather alters with changes in perception, attention, health status, and motivation associated with aging.

The older worker may be a valuable asset to the workplace. In terms of overall health, the older population displays wide variation. Because ill employees tend to leave the work force voluntarily, the employed older worker tends to be physically healthy. Poor work performance, absenteeism, and turnover (often associated with poor health) are less common with older workers. Employers must use caution when fitting the right person to the specific job. This caveat, however, concerns all employees regardless of age.

The Worker With Disabilities

Work site accessibility is one's ability to overcome barriers to arrive at his or her workstation. A common simplifying assumption is to equate accessibility issues only with wheelchair use. Many issues may restrict access such as reduced endurance for walking, visual impairment, amputation, incontinence, hearing loss, and worker or peer attitudes. A successful job placement depends on surmounting all "barriers" along relevant access routes (see Figure 6).

Although this chapter does not discuss specific disabilities, the chapter does list guidelines for optimizing workstations and the general work environment for the worker with disabilities. Application of these principles will enhance work productivity and performance for both employees with disabilities and those without. Designing workstations that enhance user capabilities contributes to user comfort, motivation, and productivity. Poor designs result in fatigue, discomfort, and stress.

Case Scenario 7

Work site analysis involves identifying jobs and workstations that contain, cause, or pose risk factors for hazards. This includes identification of symptoms, especially musculoskeletal symptoms, and associated risk factors such as awkward posture, repetitiveness, sustained exertions, extreme temperatures, and vibration.

Case Scenario 8

Employees can prevent injury and hazard via job modification; changing job assignments, tools, or the environment to eliminate risk factors through alterations in method or strength necessary to complete the task; changing the location and position of equipment or tools; changing the speed or frequency of task

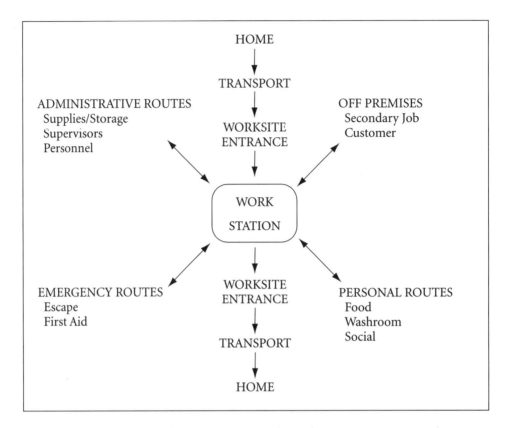

Figure 6. Primary and secondary access routes to the work site.

performance; and changing ambient factors such as light, noise, and air quality. Common workstation changes include layout, seating, and materials handling that promote adjustability for the worker and neutral postures.

Case Scenario 9

Training and education of employees and management staff members in ergonomics principles and safety are effective means to prevent injury and facilitate a safe working environment.

With increased computer usage and automated equipment in many industries, assistive technology can increase ease of use. Some of these end-user tools may be as simple as a glare protection screen on a computer monitor to minimize visual fatigue, a large monitor to increase character size in proportion to monitor dimensions, and voice recognition software to eliminate the need for keyboard data entry. Once thought to be costly and impossible dreams, today's computer systems (hardware and software) incorporate many energy-efficient, accessible features.

Computers and robots are now commonplace in routine tasks that are dangerous, boring, or tedious for the human worker. Robotic devices are now capable of skills far beyond simple addition. Sophisticated programming has enabled these aids to imitate the way persons solve problems, judge between different courses of action, and make "smart" decisions. The use of robotic aids for persons with disabilities has many benefits: cost-effectiveness (e.g., lessening dependence on attendant care), improved reliability (i.e., they are always available), and increased environmental control and quality of life. Robotic aids, like a robotic arm, are useful in a workstation. A worker with no or limited arm function can control the robotic arm via switches (e.g., puff-and-sip, chin control, eye gaze).

Accommodation refers to the application of ergonomic principles to maximize the capabilities of all users and thus provide an optimal interface. The Job Accommodation Network (JAN; 1999) is a federally funded operation that assists employers in accommodating workers with disabilities. JAN provides information about the employability of persons with disabilities.

The Americans with Disabilities Act of 1990 (ADA; Pub. L. 101–336) is perhaps the most far-reaching legislation of our time. The ADA's protection applies primarily but not exclusively to persons with disabilities by including persons with a current or prior history of a physical or mental impairment that substantially limits one or more major life activities. Intended to make our society more accessible, the ADA has five specific parts: employment (e.g., employers must provide reasonable accommodations such as modifying equipment or restructuring jobs), public services, public accommodations, telecommunications, and a miscellaneous category prohibiting retaliation against persons with disabilities. Employers can accommodate workers with disabilities through the use of enlarged and raised signage, assistive listening devices, audiotapes, computers, and sign-language interpreters.

Summary

The sum of wisdom is, that the time is never lost that is devoted to work. (Emerson, as cited in Bohle, 1967, p. 453:14)

The performance area of work is a major aspect of occupational therapy's scope of practice. Work activities include an infinite number of purposeful activities that occupational therapy practitioners use as part of interventions. Ultimately, for many clients, the goal of occupational therapy intervention is the ability to return to work or to engage in vocational occupations. ■

References

American Occupational Therapy Association. (1994). Uniform terminology for occupational therapy—Third edition. *American Journal of Occupational Therapy, 48,* 1047–1054.

Argyle, M. (1972). *The social psychology of work.* New York: Taplinger.

Beck, E. M. (Ed.). (1980). *John Bartlett/Bartlett's familiar quotations* (15th ed.). Boston: Little, Brown.

Bellman, G. M. (1996). *Your signature path: Gaining new perspectives on life and work.* San Francisco: Berrett-Koehler.

Bohle, B. (1967). *The home book of American quotations.* New York: Dodd Mead.

Bolles, R. N. (1998). *What color is your parachute? A practical manual for job hunters and career-changers.* Berkeley, CA: Ten Speed Press.

Career Information Center. (1990). *Employment trends and master index* (4th ed.). Mission Hills, CA: Glencoe.

Fraser, T. M. (1992). *Fitness for work.* London: Taylor & Francis.

Grandjean, E. (1988). *Fitting the task to the man: An ergonomic approach.* London: Taylor & Francis.

Hertfelder, S., & Gwin, C. (Eds.). (1989). *Work in progress: Occupational therapy in work programs.* Bethesda, MD: American Occupational Therapy Association.

Holland, J. L. (1997). *Making vocational choices: A theory of vocational personalities and work environments* (3rd ed.). Odessa, FL: Psychological Assessment Resources.

Isernhagen, S. J. (Ed.). (1995). *The comprehensive guide to work injury management.* Gaithersburg, MD: Aspen Publishers.

JIST Works. (1998–1999). *Career guide to America's top industries.* Indianapolis, IN: Author.

Job Accommodation Network. (1999). Available: http://janweb.icdi.wvu.edu/

Marshall, E. (1985). Looking back. *American Journal of Occupational Therapy, 39,* 297–300.

Morris, R. B. (Ed.). (1976). *United States Department of Labor bicentennial history of the American worker.* Washington, DC: U.S. Government Printing Office.

Rader Smith, E. (1989). Ergonomics and the occupational therapist. In S. Hertfelder & C. Gwin (Eds.), *Work in progress: Occupational therapy in work programs* (pp. 127–156). Bethesda, MD: American Occupational Therapy Association.

Reich, C. A. (1970). *The greening of America.* New York: Random House.

Steele, J. E., & Morgan, M. S. (1991). *Career planning and development for college students and recent graduates.* Lincolnwood, IL: VGM Career Horizons.

Terkel, S. (1971). *Working: People talk about what they do all day and how they feel about what they do.* New York: Pantheon Books.

Terkel, S. (1997). *My American century.* New York: New Press.

U.S. Department of Health and Human Services, National Institute for Occupational Safety and Health. (1999). *Stress at work* (DHHS Publication No. 99-101). Cincinnati, OH: Publications Dissemination EID.

U.S. Department of Labor, Bureau of Labor Statistics. (1991). *Occupational outlook for college graduates* (Bulletin 2076). Washington, DC: U.S. Government Printing Office.

U.S. Department of Labor, Bureau of Labor Statistics. (1998). *Occupational outlook handbook, 1998–99 edition* (Bulletin 2500). Washington, DC: U.S. Government Printing Office.

U.S. Department of Labor, Bureau of Labor Statistics. (1999a). *Employment projections* [On-line]. Available: http://stats.bls.gov/news.release/ecopro.nws.htm

U.S. Department of Labor, Bureau of Labor Statistics. (1999b). *News release* [On-line]. Available: http://stats.bls.gov/newsrels.htm

U.S. Department of Labor, Office of Policy and Research. (1998). *The nation's new resources of occupational information: O*Net: The occupational information network* [On-line]. Available: http://www.doleta.gov/programs/onet

United States Department of Labor, U. S. Employment Service. (1979). *Guide for occupational exploration.* Washington, DC: U. S. Government Printing Office.

United States Department of Labor, U. S. Employment Service. (1991). *Dictionary of occupational titles* (4th rev. ed.). Lanham, MD: Bernan Press.

Van Harrison, R. (1978). Person–environment fit and job stress. In C. L. Cooper & R. Payne (Eds.), *Stress at work.* Chichester, UK: Wiley.

World Health Organization. (1989). *Epidemiology of work-related diseases and accidents: Tenth report of the Joint ILO/WHO Committee on Occupational Health* (Technical Report Series No. 777). Geneva: Author.

14

Range of Human Activity: Self-Care

Beverly Bain, EdD, OT, FAOTA

Self-care is part of an intimate, ego invested portrait, a powerful narrative of one's self and one's relationship with others. (Fidler, 1994, p. v)

Self-care encompasses the total human being. Although self-care includes the various activities and tasks that persons engage in to maintain their personal physical needs, self-care additionally exemplifies our psychological and social selves. Self-care is grounded in the person's culture, values, and his or her unique personality. Self-care has always been an important area of concern for occupational therapy practitioners. We believe that caring for ourselves is part of being human. We believe that all persons value and want to be independent in self-care. We believe that independence in self-care contributes to a person's sense of self-dignity and self-esteem. We believe that participating in basic human self-care activities such as feeding, toileting, bathing, dressing, communicating, moving around one's environment, and sexual expression are the foundation on which persons become functional members of society.

Performance Areas in Occupational Therapy's Domain of Concern

A profession's domain of concern specifies its areas of expertise. As described earlier in this book, occupational therapy's domain of concern consists of performance components, performance areas, and performance contexts. The activities of daily living (ADL) performance area contains 15 categories of self-care activities: grooming, oral hygiene, bathing or showering, toilet hygiene, personal device care, dressing, feeding and eating, medication routine, health maintenance, socialization, functional communication, functional mobility, community mobility, emergency response, and sexual expression (American Occupational Therapy Association [AOTA], 1994).

When self-care occurs in a natural setting, that person is engaging in an occupation. The occupation of self-care consists of many activities. For example, for an American man who lives in an apartment, the occupation of showering may include getting into the shower, washing his body, getting out of the shower, and drying himself. This occupation is grounded in the man's needs, values, culture, and environment. Self-care as an occupation consists of several distinct purposeful activities. Each activity is purposeful because it is meaningful to the person and is goal directed. Each occupation includes a range of purposeful activities that are included in that specific occupation for that person.

This chapter presents how occupational therapy practitioners use specific self-care activities in treatment as purposeful activities. The end goal of occupational therapy is often the client's ability to complete specific self-care activities. When the end goal of occupational therapy is the client's ability to perform various self-care activities in a natural setting, the goal is the client's ability to engage in a self-care occupation, not the performance of individual purposeful activities. Whenever practitioners use self-care activities therapeutically as purposeful activities for a client in treatment, they must keep the client's self-care occupations in mind. The reason that we select self-care purposeful activities is so that the client will be able to engage in self-care occupations (AOTA, 1997).

Determinants of Self-Care Activities

Persons of all ages and cultures carry out and perform various self-care activities. A wide range of factors including age, gender, culture, occupational roles, skills, and abilities determines which activities we participate in and what we choose to do.

Self-Care Activities Specific to Age

We have a wide range of purposeful activities that we include in our ADL that evolve and change as we grow, mature, develop skills, and assume different responsibilities within our social groups. Although the general categories of basic self-care activities (e.g., eating, dressing, personal hygiene, communicating, and independent mobility) may remain the same, our life tasks and goals change. Although presenting an in-depth discussion of self-care activities during life is beyond the scope of this chapter, the following section provides a brief overview of the various purposeful self-care activities and goals as they evolve throughout life.

We are born dependent in all areas of self-care. Although we can suck and swallow, we cannot feed ourselves and, instead, depend on adults for our survival. Slowly, we develop self-care skills as we interact with our human and nonhuman environments. We begin to develop self-care skills related to survival functions of feeding and resting. To use feeding as an example, as we develop underlying abilities, we begin to want to feed ourselves. This desire to participate in our world is evident in many areas of self-care. As we develop into social beings, we participate more, interact more, and demand to take care of ourselves. Early childhood involves learning how to eat, toilet, dress, walk, and talk. Mastery of these basic self-care skills provides the foundation for later, more advanced self-care activities.

During the preschool period, as we develop our personalities and begin to relate to other children, we become more independent in selected areas of self-care. Developing motor, cognitive, and psychosocial skills provides us with new skills and abilities. During feeding, we not only feed ourselves but also decide what we want to eat. We want to make choices about what we wear. Self-care hygiene and toileting become more important as we relate to other children and adults.

The development of cognitive skills and the ability to talk to other children and adults means that we are ready for school. As school-aged children, we must be independent in basic self-care personal hygiene. We must be able to dress ourselves, tie our shoes, put on coats, and communicate our needs. New self-care skills that we must master include the abilities to eat in groups in the school cafeteria, to move around safely in our communities (e.g., cross streets, manage school buses, use public transportation), and to write.

Adolescence provides us with many new opportunities. As we refine our own personalities and begin to spend more time with our peer group, we assume more responsibilities for our own self-care activities and the way that we will perform them. Peer pressure and personal changes in our bodies may mean that we spend more time managing what we eat. Some of our self-care activities are related to gender (e.g., managing personal hygiene during menstrual periods, shaving). Our peers influence what we wear, how we dress, and how we act.

When we enter young adulthood, we begin to adjust our behaviors, dressing styles, and personal hygiene practices to reflect our roles as college students, employed adults, parents, and so forth. Now independent in all areas of self-care, we assume responsibility for all aspects of our daily lives. We accept additional responsibilities when we drive cars, perform employment duties, and establish a sexual relationship with another person. We must now be able to manage money and time, and we may begin to assume some self-care responsibilities for others (e.g., children, parents).

As we move into older adulthood, our self-care concerns may shift to balancing our diets, managing medications, and adapting to changes in our bodies. These changes may require that we use visual and auditory devices, use public transportation, and seek help from others for managing some daily tasks. We may need to customize our home environments to allow us to continue to be independent in specific self-care activities. We may need adaptive devices and mobility aides.

Exercise 1

Reflect on your childhood. What self-care activities did you participate in? Which self-care activities were important to you? Why were they important? How do you think that mastery of these skills contributed to who you are today?

Exercise 2

Think back to your adolescent years. Describe your self-care activities. Which self-care activities influenced your experiences as an adolescent? How do you think these self-care activities influence your roles as an adult? How did your peer group influence your self-care activities?

Gender

Some self-care activities are gender specific, such as shaving for men and personal hygiene for women during menstrual periods, pregnancy, and menopause. Most persons in the United States are concerned with their weight, and physical appearance can affect the way we eat, dress, and care for skin and hair.

Cultural Factors

Culture is an important factor in self-care activities. For example, one's culture determines the way that persons self-feed. For example, Asian cultures typically use chopsticks, near Eastern cultures use thin bread, Mexicans use tortillas, and Europeans use forks and spoons. Dressing likewise varies from culture to culture in determining what a person wears and how he or she wears it. Culture influences how persons in that culture view or value self-care activities. For example, in some cultures, a child must accomplish toilet training at a very young age, whereas other cultures wait until the child is ready. Additionally, culture influences one's gender roles regarding specific self-care activities. Some cultures expect women to learn to prepare food and clean homes, whereas in other cultures, men and women share these responsibilities.

Socioeconomic Considerations

Like culture, socioeconomic factors may influence self-care activities. A person with a great deal of resources may have a personal attendant and a maid to take care of personal needs. The person may need to learn prescribed etiquette for eating in special social situations. On the other hand, a person with limited resources may have to do different self-care tasks. A person who does not have running water in the home may have to include "carry and store water in the home" as a self-care activity.

Intervention Approaches

> The outcome of occupational therapy intervention is to enable a way of living that allows persons to develop and bring into harmony a configuration of daily living activities that have personal, social, and cultural relevance for them and their significant others. (Fidler, 1996, p. 141)

Historically, occupational therapy practitioners used self-care activities as purposeful activities with clients (Brett, 1960; Fields, 1956; Lowman & Liphum, 1947; Lucci, 1958; Richert, 1950; Wellerson, 1951). They recognized participation in self-care as a basic way that humans occupy their time. Today, clients' abilities to perform self-care activities are important functional outcomes of intervention (Holm, Rogers, & James, 1998; Reed & Sanderson, 1993). Third-party payers and the consumers themselves often determine the effectiveness of therapy by how independent the client is in performing his or her own self-care. Unfortunately, the measurement of the functional outcome is commonly the ability to perform the specific self-care activity physically and does not consider the psychological, social, or personal meaning of the performance for the client, which practitioners view as critical to self-care as an occupation.

Occupational therapy practitioners use a frame of reference, paradigm, or model that is appropriate to the client to guide which self-care activity to use in intervention. Three common broad classifications of intervention approaches are remediation, compensation, and education (teaching and learning) (Holm et al., 1998). These broad classifications show how occupational therapy practitioners approach intervention regarding the use of self-care activities. These classifications are not specific frames of reference, paradigms, or models.

Remediation Approaches

Remediation approaches focus intervention at the performance component level to restore the performance components that are necessary for functional tasks, such as increasing endurance, motor learning, improving figure–ground perception, and enhancing problem-solving abilities (Trombly, 1995). Thus, when selecting purposeful activities, the focus is on enhancing skills and abilities in specific performance components. Occupational therapy practitioners select activities because of their therapeutic value in relation to the client's performance component deficits.

Case Scenario 1

Maria is a young woman 24 years of age with a history of depression and suicide attempts. An occupational therapy evaluation determines that Maria has a poor self-concept and is unable to manage personal care and medication routine because of poor organizational skills. The occupational therapy practitioner selects various activities that require Maria to organize and plan. During a cooking group, the occupational therapy practitioner requires Maria to develop a shopping list and to check off each item that she buys at the store. Later, when preparing a meal, she must make a list and check off her accomplishments. Finally, Maria develops a plan and a schedule for managing her medications that involves preparing a list and checking off items as she completes them.

Compensation Approaches

Compensation approaches, which are commonly used in rehabilitation, require learning new tasks such as using a computer for writing and learning new ways to do a familiar task such as one-handed dressing or learning to shower while sitting down. Adapting equipment and adapting the environment are important aspects of this approach. For example, a client who has had a cerebrovascular accident (CVA) may need to learn one-handed wheelchair mobility for daily use in the hospital environment while receiving gait training for use when he or she returns home. In this approach, occupational therapy practitioners focus on using existing skills and abilities to enhance a client's ability to complete a particular self-care activity. Some compensation approaches base their intervention techniques on biomechanical principles. For example, practitioners commonly use work simplification and energy conservation with clients who have physical disabilities (Holm et al., 1998). An example of a compensatory approach would be giving a person with limited shoulder range of motion (ROM) an extended long-handled comb to comb his or her hair. Another compensatory strategy would be to raise the dressing table to conserve energy and allow the client to use the surface of the table to support his or her arm during combing.

To continue with the previous example of Maria, the compensatory approach would involve providing Maria with strategies or techniques to counter her lack of organizational skills. The occupational therapy practitioner would give Maria a pill box with a timer that will remind her to take her pills.

Teaching and Learning

The teaching and learning approach (or acquisitional frame of reference) relates to learning the "specific skills needed for successful interaction in the environment" (Mosey, 1986, p. 433). After an injury, with increasing age, or because of a congenital disability, a person may need to learn or relearn self-care activities. Clients may need to learn how to use adaptive equipment or aids to complete self-care tasks. Additionally, occupational therapy practitioners must instruct clients or caregivers in the maintenance of the equipment or devices. Because teaching and learning theories are the basis of acquisitional approaches, occupational therapy practitioners must select the appropriate frame of reference for the teaching and learning that must take place. For example, one client may have an easier time learning a self-care activity if the intervention uses a frame of reference that includes operant conditioning. Another client may more easily learn if the frame of reference involves social learning theory. This interdependence between the client, the activity, and the therapeutic approach is likewise important when teaching caregivers (Bain, 1998).

Again with the example of Maria, the teaching and learning approach would focus on teaching Maria new skills and how to work with others to manage her daily routines. Maria would receive instruction on developing routines with handouts and homework assignments. Additionally, the occupational therapy practitioner could work with Maria so that she could use a computer to plan her day and organize her medication routines.

Selection of the Appropriate Approach

Rarely in real practice does a therapist use only one approach with a particular client. In the real world of practice, occupational therapists develop therapeutic goals after a comprehensive evaluation. On the basis of the evaluation and the frame of reference, the occupational therapy practitioner selects specific activities that are relevant given the client's total program. An occupational therapy practitioner then selects appropriate tools that are consistent with that frame of reference, paradigm, or model. When a client's needs are in the area of ADL, the occupational therapy practitioner uses a frame of reference, paradigm, or model that guides the selection of specific purposeful activities (self-care activities) that he or she may use as part of the intervention. For example, an evaluation of a child 5 years of age with cerebral palsy resulting in spastic diplegia indicates that the child needs to develop the ability to drink from a cup. The practitioner decides to begin by using a straw and provides the child with an adapted straw and cup. In this example, drinking with a straw is a purposeful self-care activity.

Another scenario is evident when the client does not have specific deficits in ADL, but the therapist determines that self-care activities are appropriate for developing particular skills. In this case, a therapist selects an appropriate frame of reference, paradigm, or model and, on the basis of the guidelines for intervention, chooses to use specific self-care activities. For example, a child 11 years of age with learning disabilities is independent in self-care but needs to develop visual discrimination and organizational skills. The therapist decides to use a cooking activity to work on visual discrimination and organizational skills. As part of therapy, the child must select a recipe, plan for a shopping trip, buy the items, and prepare the dish. In this case, the self-care activity is a purposeful activity that does not directly relate to the child's deficits but rather addresses underlying deficits.

As a client's needs change, the intervention approach may shift. When a client has multiple needs, the therapist may use a combination of approaches to meet those needs. Some therapists assert that combining remedial and compensatory approaches is necessary in the teaching and learning approach to learn functional activities (Trombly, 1995).

Evaluation

Selecting an appropriate intervention approach requires that an occupational thera-pist conduct a comprehensive evaluation of the client and his or her situation. This evaluation includes evaluating the client's capabilities, needs, and goals. A compre-hensive evaluation requires that the therapist consider the client's goals and wishes in the present and future environments in which he or she will perform the activities (Bain, 1997). Each aspect is important, and each depends on the other.

A comprehensive self-care evaluation of a client's performance components includes evaluation of his or her physical or motor abilities (e.g., strength, ROM, coordination), cognitive abilities (e.g., memory, following directions), sensory pro-cessing and perceptual-motor skills (e.g., figure–ground perception, motor planning, spatial relations), and psychosocial abilities (e.g., motivation, social interaction with others). The self-care activities that a person needs to complete or perform each day are personal care, verbal and written communication, and functional mobility.

Evaluation of performance. A client's actual performance is an important aspect of any evaluation. Evaluation must include the self-care activities that the client needs and wants to be able to do. This evaluation begins by completing a mental activity analy-sis of each task in the activity. On the basis of this knowledge, the occupational ther-apist asks the client to do various related tasks. As the client performs more complex tasks, the therapist judges the client's performance of each task. During this aspect of the evaluation, the therapist uses real-life activities, often in a simulated situation. If possible, the therapist asks the client to complete specific activities. For example, the therapist may ask the client to doff a shoe and then don it. During the client's per-formance of the activity, the therapist may suggest specific strategies to see if the client's performance improves. On the basis of the client's overall performance of the given activities, the therapist determines that the client needs assistance such as assis-tive or adaptive device or environmental modification. For example, after a therapist observes a person with a hearing impairment and motor coordination problems try-ing to type into teletypewriters or telecommunication devices for the deaf (TDDs), he or she may suggest that the client write letters. Other alternative suggestions for this client may be use of a computer to write letters, write and send faxes, and write e-mail messages. Alternatively, a therapist may notice that the client's performance improves when he or she types while standing. In this case, the therapist may rec-ommend a standing table so that the client can stand while typing. Observing actual performance is a critical aspect of the client's self-care evaluation.

Whenever evaluating self-care performance, the occupational therapist consid-ers safety factors. For example, when the occupational therapist evaluates a client's functional mobility, he or she gives special attention to safety. Safety is relative to the client's physical endurance and the accessibility of the multiple environments in which the client must be mobile. In evaluating functional mobility, cognitive, psy-chological, social, and cultural factors are as important as the client's physical ability.

Evaluation of environments. For an occupational therapy evaluation to be comprehensive and relevant to the client's occupations, the occupational therapist considers all present and possible future environments in where the client will engage in self-care activities. Given the scope of self-care activities, this is not simple. A client must be able to perform activities in his or her home, school, work, community, or play environments, not only in the occupational therapy clinic. For example, an evaluation of a person who had a CVA would be different if he or she were returning home to live alone or to a nursing home where he or she will have 24-hr attendant care. A person who uses a wheelchair must be able to move around the home, get into bed, and transfer to the toilet. The person must be able to accomplish personal hygiene in the home as well as in a public restroom. Thus, during the evaluation, the occupational therapy practitioner evaluates a client's performance by ascertaining the effect of the environment on the client's performance of self-care activities. Again, the occupational therapist must consider the psychosocial influence on a client's performance. An important aspect of the environment is people; their presence can have a direct influence on a person's ability and willingness to complete a self-care activity.

Evaluation of psychological factors. Psychosocial factors to consider when conducting a self-care evaluation include the person's personality, cultural background, motivation to perform self-care activities, and willingness to accept assistance or assistive equipment. A person's personality influences his or her participation in the intervention process and the ways in which he or she interacts with others. Personality is part of the complex human being. Occupational therapists draw from their knowledge and expertise in the area of psychosocial development and its influence on behavior to evaluate this area.

Understanding the client's psychosocial status requires that the occupational therapist consider and learn about the client's culture. Although family members may overprotect and wait on a person with a disability in some cultures, in other cultures, family members may abandon the person or hire attendants to care for the person. The culture's beliefs about disability will influence how the client and his or her family members will respond to the disability and the intervention. Furthermore, one's culture strongly affects the area of self-care. Culture often directly determines the manner in which one carries out a self-care routine and the activities in which one chooses to engage. Accordingly, the occupational therapist must obtain information from the client and his or her family members about beliefs and values. These basic views provide information on which the therapist develops an appropriate intervention plan for the client.

Motivation to care for oneself in some activities and not in others is an important psychological factor to consider during the evaluation and when planning the client-centered intervention. Persons with low self-esteem may not care about their personal hygiene but may be highly motivated to eat and be mobile. Some clients may reject assistive or adaptive devices because they perceive the device to be making them dependent on equipment rather than improving physically and becoming independent of any devices.

Other evaluation information. A team approach to any self-care evaluation should include the client, all caregivers, and other members of the team (e.g., physical therapist, social worker, physician, speech pathologist). Team members' attitudes regarding which and how self-care activities are to be accomplished are equally as important as their knowledge. An evaluation is an ongoing aspect of an intervention program.

When completing a comprehensive evaluation, a therapist uses observations, interviews, checklists, and formal testing. Table 1 includes a list of some assessments and the areas they evaluate. Whenever using a standardized instrument, the occupational therapist must comply with standardized procedures and be competent in the administration and interpretation of the assessment, which involves an understanding of the psychometrics of the test, including the reliability and validity of the assessment (Asher, 1996; Crist, 1998; Law, 1997; Rogers & Holm, 1989). Some self-care evaluation instruments are specific for certain conditions (e.g., arthritis, spinal cord injury), and others are specific for the type of treatment center (e.g., acute hospital, rehabilitation center). Some assessments may be equipment related (e.g., wheelchair, computers), and others may be task specific (e.g., dressing, driving) (Bain, 1997; Galvin & Sherer, 1996).

When evaluating a client's performance, the practitioner often rates his or her level of independence according to the following.

■   How much physical assistance the client requires

■   How many verbal cues are necessary

■   Where the task is completed (in bed, in a wheelchair, in the bathroom)

■   What equipment is necessary

■   How much time, energy, and endurance is necessary (Trombly & Quintana, 1989)

On the basis of the performance, Trombly and Quintana (1989) suggested a seven-point rating scale.

1   Independent—client can complete the task with or without equipment

2   Independent with setup—client can complete the task once someone has applied adaptive equipment

3   Supervision—client needs supervision because of cognitive deficits or poor balance

4   Minimal assistance—client requires physical help or verbal cues 25% of the time

5   Moderate assistance—client requires help 50% of the time

6   Maximum assistance—client requires help 75% of the time

Table 1
Self-Care Assessments

Assessment	Communication and Emergency Response	Grooming and Hygiene	Feeding and Eating	Mobility Transfer	Dressing	Other
Arnadottir OT-ADL Neurobehavioral Evaluation (A-One; Arnadottir, 1990)	X	X	X	X	X	
Assessment of Living Skills and Resources (ALSAR; Williams et al., 1991)	Reading Telephone					Medication management
OT FACT (Smith, 1990)	X	X	X	X	X	Computer driven
Functional Independence Measure (FIM™; Jette et al., 1986)	X	X	X	X	X	Cognitive function
Klein-Bell ADL Scale (Klein & Bell, 1979)	X	X	X	X	X	
Kohlman Evaluation of Living Skills (KELS; Kohlman Thompson, 1992)	Telephone	X		X		Safety Money management
Milwaukee Evaluation of Daily Living Skills (MEDLS; Leonardelli, 1988)	X	X		X	X	Money management Medication management
Performance Assessment of Self-Care Skills (PASS, version 3.1; Rogers & Holm, 1994)		X		X		Home management
Routine Task Intervention (RTI; Heinemann, Allen, & Yerxa, 1989)	X	X			X	Money management Time management

Areas/Domains

7   Dependent—client is unable to do any part of the task

Another instrument to evaluate the client's level of independence is the Functional Independence Measure (FIM™) (Jette et al., 1986). The FIM uses a seven-point scale. The seven-point system includes the following.

7   Completely independent

6   Requires modified assistance

5   Needs some supervision

4   Minimal assistance is necessary for the client to achieve 75% independence

3   Moderate assistance is necessary for the client to achieve 50% independence

2   Client is able to achieve 25% independence

1   Total dependence

This seven-point scale converts to a four-point scale as (7) = 4, (6) = 3, (5, 4, 3) = 2, (2, 1) = 1, or complete dependence (Uniform Data System for Medical Rehabilitation, 1993).

Intervention

Occupational therapy practitioners often consider the client's ability to complete self-care activities as an indicator of improved functional performance. In occupational therapy, performances of self-care activities are both the goals of intervention and a key aspect of treatment. As described previously, three common approaches to intervention in the area of self-care are remediation, compensation, and teaching and learning (Rogers & Holm, 1989; Trombly, 1989). The remediation approach is more time consuming than the compensatory approach, which focuses on adapting the activity, changing the environment, using adaptive equipment, and altering the method of doing the task. Although remediation is frequently a primary concern of many occupational therapy practitioners, practitioners most often use a combination of approaches.

The teaching and learning approach involves the occupational therapy practitioner's use of the teaching and learning process to provide instruction and learning experiences to the client and caregivers. Individualized instructions are appropriate for tasks that are personal such as bathing, toileting, and grooming. Group instruction can be effective for a homogeneous group because group instruction can foster peer interaction (e.g., eating, applying makeup, and practicing wheelchair controls). Group instructions can be cost effective. In a teaching and learning approach, practitioners teach clients self-care activities by using demonstrations and verbal cues. Other methods of instruction that are valuable both in the clinic and after discharge are written instructions, manuals, videotapes, audiotapes, and the Internet (e.g., peer support groups and chat rooms). Education of all caregivers is important, especially for family members who are not familiar with the disability, special equipment, and different methods of performing familiar tasks and who are emotionally affected by the situation. The practitioner must consider the learning style (cognitive abilities) of the client and caregiver and their physical abilities. The caregiver may need to learn proper body mechanics, and occupational therapy practitioners must reinforce safety measures in the teaching process.

Guidelines and Parameters

Purposeful activities in self-care are quite individualized. The following is a list of general guidelines to use whenever self-care activities are part of an intervention program.

- Occupational therapy practitioners must respect the client's desires and wishes concerning his or her accepted level of independence.

- Occupational therapy practitioners must recognize a client's capabilities and limitations.

- Safety is always a consideration whenever practicing a technique, participating in an activity, or providing adaptive equipment. The occupational therapy practitioner must address future safety issues.

- The client's values, beliefs, and desires determine the value of any activity.

- When the practitioner presents self-care activities at the level of the client's abilities, the client will be better able to learn and enjoy the activity.

- When selecting and using self-care activities, the occupational therapy practitioner must consider the environments in which the client will ultimately perform the activities (Bain, 1997; Holm et al., 1998; Trombly, 1993).

Value of the Activity to the Client

The value the client places on the activity is proportional to the effort that the client places on learning. The first question a practitioner should ask a client is "What do you want to learn to care for your self?" Some persons may be more concerned with their hair than with writing their name. Age, gender, culture, social status, physical well-being, and emotional state are factors that determine the value of the activity to the clients. Furthermore, the relative value of these factors to the client may vary from treatment session to treatment session (Holm et al., 1998; Trombly, 1993).

Safety While Performing an Activity

Safety is an important consideration in all situations. When working in the area of self-care, occupational therapy practitioners must ensure that the client can do the activity safely. The client and the person helping the client must be able to do the activity in a safe manner that will not cause physical injury. Devices and equipment must be well constructed and durable. The environment should be accessible and hazard free. The practitioner and the client must be confident that the client can do all procedures, methods, and techniques safely. For example, in the situation in which a client has poor balance, toileting activities are not appropriate until the client has the physical ability to perform the task, safety bars are in place, rugs have been removed, and the client has learned the safe steps in the procedure.

Safety is likewise a concern for the practitioner. A practitioner should not attempt a task independently until he or she is competent and safe in doing the activity. Additionally, the practitioner should not provide equipment or adaptive equipment until he or she is knowledgeable about all aspects of the equipment. Another aspect of safety that is important to all clients and practitioners is personal protection from infection. All occupational therapy practitioners are responsible for knowing and following universal precautions in all situations. These procedures protect the practitioner and the clients with whom he or she works.

Client's Ability To Learn

When planning purposeful self-care activities, the occupational therapist considers the cognitive abilities of the client and the requirements of the various tasks that the client must complete to accomplish the activity. After determining the sequencing, long- and short-term memory requirements, and precautions that the client must follow, the practitioner matches each task to the client's cognitive skills and abilities. By using an appropriate teaching method (i.e., demonstration, verbal instruction), the practitioner creates a learning environment that supports the client's ability to learn. For some clients, visual and verbal cueing and memory notebooks or checklists are effective (Parente & Herrman, 1996).

Time Factors

Time factors, including the time for intervention, time to introduce self-care activities, and the time necessary to complete self-care tasks, are important concerns when addressing a client's needs. The practice setting and available funding support often regulate the occupational therapy practitioner's, the client's, and the caregiver's time. With the demands of today's health care system, payers have reduced the amount of time for intervention or rehabilitation, which often means that occupational therapy practitioners do not have adequate time to establish an optimal rapport with clients to deal with personal self-care concerns. Shortened time to implement and carry out interventions may limit treatment goals, and practitioners may only select intervention approaches that support expeditious results. Because of time constraints, clients may not learn proper methods for independence in self-care. Sometimes practitioners provide devices or adaptive equipment rather than working on developing skills. Therefore, occupational therapists must be resourceful and efficient. Use of electronic managerial aids, such as computers, is effective in improving documentation and managing tasks to provide additional time for clients.

When a client is unable to develop or is not developing skills that will lead to independent performance of a particular self-care task, the occupational therapy practitioner must work in collaboration with the client to consider alternatives. A common alternative is to explore adaptation of the particular task or to try adaptive devices or equipment. When adapting a method of doing a task or providing equipment, the practitioner must meet the client's needs, expectations, and aspirations. Studies have supported matching the equipment with the client's needs and have suggested that many clients abandon devices once they are home (Batavia & Hammer, 1990; Phillips & Zhao, 1993; Scherer, 1993). Another situation in which a client may not be ready to accept modified methods or adaptive equipment is when a client is still grieving after a traumatic injury. In this situation, a client may believe that, if he or she accepts adaptations, he or she will not improve. At a later time, when the client is ready, the occupational therapy practitioner will introduce the adaptations and equipment.

Timing is an important element when treating persons with progressive diseases or elderly persons. Often these persons are not ready to accept modified methods or equipment either. They may not want to use a wheelchair or a walker outside the home. In these cases, occupational therapy practitioners must work slowly with clients by providing real-life experiences that allow them to experience how to use the equipment or to practice a different method. With experience, the client may come to appreciate the increased safety, energy conservation, and improved efficiency that come from using the equipment or methods. Timing and experience are key factors in the client's acceptance or rejection of any adaptation.

When working with children, practitioners may introduce specific self-care activities such as dressing, eating, and toileting at the appropriate time in their development, for example, teaching a child who is 2 years of age to don a hat, use a spoon, or use the toilet.

"Saving time" is often the reason caregivers give for doing self-care tasks for the client rather than having the client laboriously try to do the activity independently. Often this is necessary at times when clients are on a tight schedule or when the client is exhausted after a full day of activity. Assisting may be necessary when the caregiver has limited time and many clients to assist. Occupational therapy practitioners have the responsibility to explain the physical and emotional therapeutic value of independent self-care activity to the caregiver and client. Asking the caregiver if he or she would take the client's medication may emphasize the importance of the caregiver not doing the client's self-care activities. In cases in which physical limitations (e.g., persons with high-level spinal cord injuries) require that clients conserve their energy to be able to do their jobs, a caregiver may need to handle the client's personal care activity in the morning and at bedtime.

Performance Context

As stated above, the practitioner should consider the expected environment in which the client performs the self-care activity during evaluation, planning, and intervention. Societal, cultural, and personal values and expectations often determine the acceptable and unacceptable performance of self-care. Understanding that the way one eats, dresses, cares for personal hygiene, and communicates varies from culture to culture is necessary in our global society in which the client's standards may be different from those of the occupational therapy practitioner. Think of how a person from Asia eats, how a person from India might dress, how a person may attend to personal hygiene if he or she is from a country where water is scarce, or how we all differ in the ways we communicate.

The physical (climate, space, location), psychological (attitudes, motivation), and cultural contexts are parameters that guide intervention, in other words, the development of goals and selection of activities. Physical and cultural contexts are the easiest to address because they are more concrete, and the client or caregivers can describe them. Practitioners must interpret what clients and caregivers say and do to learn about the client's psychosocial environment. One way of obtaining information is to discuss with clients and caregivers their perceptions and views during interventions and follow-up appointments.

Adjustments to a disability and the way that some clients adapt fall into four common patterns. The first category includes clients who accept their disabilities and learn to modify methods to perform self-care activities and use adaptive equipment. The second category involves clients who use the modifications and equipment but are not satisfied because they believe the modification does not meet their needs. The third category includes clients who use the modifications and adaptive equipment in the clinic but abandon them at home (these persons are again dependent). The fourth category involves clients who try other equipment and devise their own methods (Phillips, 1992). This pattern can result from a client not having input into the selection of the equipment or from a client having his or her own habitual method to complete a task and not being willing to accept the modified method. For a self-care activity to be purposeful, the activity must meet clients' needs and occur in the appropriate context in the most efficient manner.

Examples of Purposeful Self-Care Activities

The following scenarios illustrate how occupational therapy practitioners use self-care activities as part of their interventions. The organization of self-care activities according to impairments is for learning purposes, is not conclusive, and does not reflect best practice. Impairment is the loss or abnormality of cognitive, communicative, physical, emotional, physiological, or anatomical structure or function (National Center for Medical Rehabilitation and Research, 1991). Many clients may have more than one impairment, such as an elderly person who has had a CVA may have poor vision or hearing loss. Likewise, clients with cerebral palsy or traumatic brain injury may be nonverbal, have poor vision, and have physical deficits on only one side of their body. Table 2 serves as a quick reference, but for additional treatment strategies, refer to the detailed charts in chapter 19 of *Willard and Spackman's Occupational Therapy* (Holm et al., 1998).

This section presents case scenarios for persons with five types of impairments: unilateral (upper and lower extremities on the same side), lower extremities, all four extremities, low or absence of vision, and low or absence of hearing. Because no set rules exist stating which specific activity is purposeful or meaningful to any given client, each scenario highlights only pertinent occupational therapy intervention issues in the areas of communication, mobility, and personal self-care.

Persons With Unilateral Impairments

For persons who have functional use of one upper and one lower extremity, usually on the same side (e.g., CVA, cerebral palsy, traumatic brain injury), the occupational therapy goal is often to teach clients to use their affected upper extremity to assist or stabilize objects for bilateral activities. For communication tasks, practitioners teach clients to hold the paper down when writing. For personal hygiene tasks, clients learn to stabilize bottles when opening or closing them. When appropriate, the occupational therapy practitioner encourages the client to use commonly available devices such as clipboards to hold paper and pump-action containers for soap or toothpaste to accomplish tasks. Purposeful activities in these situations are the real-life activities that a person must do. The occupational therapy practitioner provides opportunities for the client to practice the activity and facilitates active problem solving while the client is engaged in the various tasks. During these tasks, occupational therapy practitioners focus on performance and the clients' other needs (e.g., psychosocial, cognitive). After the practitioner is confident that the client can do the task and can perform specific activities, the practitioner will have the client complete specific self-care activities in the home environment.

When persons have injuries resulting in unilateral impairment on the dominant side, the goal of intervention is often to develop skills in the nondominant hand. These clients must learn new ways to write for communication, to shave, to comb their hair, and to manipulate objects. Safety is a crucial factor in teaching these activities. As in the previous discussion, the occupational therapy practitioner provides opportunities for the client to practice while doing the activity and facilitates active problem solving while engaged in the various tasks. Occupational therapy practitioners attend to clients' other needs (e.g., psychosocial, cognitive). Again, once the practitioner is confident that the client can do the task and can perform specific activities, the practitioner will have the client complete specific self-care activities in the home environment.

Table 2
Examples of Self-Care Tasks, Goals, and Purposeful Activities

Impairments	*Activity*	*Purposeful Activity*
Unilateral (cerebral vascular accident, traumatic brain injury, cerebral palsy, hemiplegia)	Communication Mobility Personal care	Change hand dominance for writing Transfers and one-handed wheelchair control One-handed shoe lacing, eating, grooming, and dressing
Bilateral lower extremity (paraplegia, amputation, burns)	Communication Mobility Personal care	Use e-mail Transfers and hand controls for driving Dressing lower extremities while sitting and shower and bathtub care
Upper extremity and lower extremity (quadriplegia, multiple sclerosis, traumatic brain injury, cerebral palsy, arthritis, burns)	Communication Mobility Personal care	Adapted pencils, telephones, computers Transfers, powered wheelchair training, walker, cane, and scooter Adapted equipment for eating, grooming, and dressing
Low or absence of vision (diabetic retinopathy, macular degeneration, glaucoma, congenital blindness, stroke)	Communication Mobility Personal care	Writing with large black markers Voice-activated computers and telephones Safety, auditory, and tactile skills cues Organizational skills for eating Grooming and dressing Money management
Low or absence of hearing (congenital deafness, traumatic brain injury, aging)	Communication	Telephone, message pad writing Awareness of fire alarms and traffic

Impairments of the Lower Extremities

Persons who have impairments of one or both lower extremities (e.g., persons with spinal cord injuries, amputations, burns, hip fractures, or other orthopedic injuries) will depend on their upper extremities for self-care activities. Occupational therapy focuses on the clients' development of performance skills and on providing equipment that clients will need to be able to dress and care for themselves. During therapy sessions, occupational therapy practitioners provide clients with opportunities to learn new ways to use equipment for dressing, showering (while sitting), using a wheelchair or walker, and driving with hand controls. Practitioners teach clients energy conservation techniques, proper body mechanics, and how to inspect and care for their skin. In this situation, practicing the actual self-care activities is important for the client.

Impairments in All Extremities

Clients who have impairments in all four extremities may be the most challenging for the occupational therapy practitioner. These impairments may be the result of birth defects (cerebral palsy), spinal cord injuries, arthritis, multiple sclerosis, traumatic brain injury, or orthopedic trauma. Most of these clients need to learn to perform self-care activities in different ways and when and how to use adaptive equipment. The occupational therapy practitioner must complete a holistic evaluation, including the psychological and cognitive components and not just the physical components. These clients may have poor coordination, decreased muscle strength, low endurance, and limited ROM. Some clients may have poor self-esteem and may have limited cognitive abilities. When the limitations are severe, caregivers may perform most self-care activities (e.g., feeding, personal hygiene, mobility, and communication). When developing and carrying out an intervention plan, practitioners must include caregivers. Occupational therapy involves educating the caregivers about the most efficient and effective way of doing specific self-care activities. Observing and working closely with caregivers provides the practitioner with the information that he or she needs to make appropriate and sensitive suggestions.

Occupational therapy practitioners provide assistive devices to these clients so that these persons are independent to the extent that they can be. Providing the appropriate device and training clients to use the assistive devices may be a lengthy process. Augmentative communication devices may provide effective communication. Functional mobility becomes possible with powered wheelchairs and adapted vans. Environmental control systems allow clients to manipulate tasks such as turning the lights and the television on and off and opening doors. Many assistive devices are expensive and are not available to all clients (Bain, 1997). Before providing assistive devices, clients should try to do the activity as independently as possible. Sometimes introducing assistive devices to clients early in their rehabilitation can contribute to learned helplessness that can be prevalent in this population.

Case Scenario 2

Five years ago, Craig had a high-level spinal cord injury resulting from a diving accident. He was unable to feed himself, be mobile, use the telephone to communicate with his family members and friends, or turn his television on and off. During his rehabilitation, an occupational therapy practitioner provided and taught Craig how to use a sip-and-puff switch to turn on his television, use a telephone, drive a powered wheelchair, and use a computer. Today, Craig is a computer programmer, drives his own van to work, prepares simple meals, and controls his television and other appliances. When you ask him about his new independence, he will tell you what he thought as he was lying in the hospital bed. "I will never be able to do anything again. Being taught to do one simple task such as turning on the TV was a breakthrough which led to my trying other activities."

Low Vision or Legally Blind

Before developing an intervention plan for a person with low vision, the occupational therapy practitioner must determine how much the person can see. Can he or she see shadows or shapes or nothing at all? This information is often in the client's file. Another important factor in selecting the most appropriate activities is whether the visual impairment is congenital, acquired, or progressive. Information on home, school, and work environments is important in planning activities. Additionally, the therapist should determine how much and when assistance is available. As with any intervention program, the therapist should select self-care activities on the basis of what clients want or need to increase their independence. The following suggestions are guidelines, and, as such, their application will vary with each person.

Eating. Initially, some clients learn the "clock pattern" as a way of organizing food on their plates in a consistent pattern (e.g., meat and fish or main entree at 12 o'clock, vegetable at 3 o'clock, bread at 6 o'clock, and dessert at 9 o'clock). In addition, in the beginning, hot beverages should be half full with sugar or milk stirred in and served at a lukewarm temperature. For small children, commercially available weighted, two-handled, spill-proof straws attached to cups and glasses are helpful. Training, consistency, and incorporation of the client's own abilities are the keys to developing independence and self-confidence. Eventually, most clients will develop their own approaches to preparing and serving food.

Personal hygiene. Safety sensory enhancement (touch and smell) and routines or patterns are crucial. Safety factors include the following: keep doors and drawers closed; store sharp objects (razors, hair dryers, nail clippers, etc.) properly and use them with caution; eliminate rugs and sharp objects; and mark stove and oven controls with tactile indicators. As with eating patterns, clients usually develop methods that work for them as they learn about and organize their home environment.

Dressing. This activity may require assistance from a caregiver to establish a routine and pattern, but gradually the client can achieve independence once he or she learns the pattern. To simplify color selection, hang coordinating clothing together, place coordinating clothing in the same drawer, or code the clothing with tactile labels. Clients may need the assistance of a caregiver to determine whether the clothing needs cleaning. For example, Sara is a legally blind dark room developer in the X-ray department of a hospital. At first, a friend came over once a week and checked her clothing for the next week, and, once a month, they shopped for clothing that they label with a method they designed together. Most of the time, however, Sara manages her clothing effectively by herself with her own system.

For persons who have low vision, increasing the amount of light, decreasing glare, using magnifying mirrors and glasses, and using contrasting colors are ways to compensate. For clients who have lateral neglect, placing clothing to the side of sight is necessary, and the use of compensation methods suggested above may increase dressing independence.

Toileting and personal grooming. Some clients need sensory training, especially after bowel movements. This is a delicate and personal task that the occupational therapy practitioner must be comfortable in teaching the client and caregiver. The use of moistened wipes in addition to toilet paper is helpful to many clients. Pocket-size packets of wipes and toilet seat covers are available in most pharmacies. The client should learn safety measures in the shower and bathroom. The client should pay special attention to safety with water temperatures and appropriate bottles or containers for soap, shampoo, and toothpaste. Persons with vision problems usually manage familiar spaces and objects quickly if they have no other disabilities and no cognitive problems.

Manipulation activities. Persons with visual impairments must learn safe management of medical supplies and equipment. All medication must be identifiable either by shape or tactile labels (rubber bands, Velcro® strips), or caregivers must place them in containers. Many clients with diabetic retinopathy need to test their urine each day. The occupational therapy practitioner must help clients learn to use the commercially available instruments to do so. Pillbox time reminders are available to assist persons with low vision or poor memory.

Telling time is an activity that clients with low vision can do by using large or magnifying watches. Clients who are blind may require "talking" watches. Purposeful activity related to time management is important to everyday living.

Using large black markers or increasing the font size on a computer may enhance written communication for persons with low vision. For persons who use computers, several affordable voice-activated computer programs are available in many college and public libraries. Computers are helpful in sending e-mail messages and faxes.

Using tape recorders for listening to books on tape, keeping notes, or listening to telephone messages can aid in reading. The occupational therapy practitioner must be familiar with resources that are available for persons who have low vision or are progressively losing their vision.

Functional mobility. Persons who have recently become legally blind will usually need an evaluation and training from a mobility specialist. Clients with low vision need sensory training, need to develop safety measures, and need to develop behavioral memory aids. Holding on to handrails when using stairs and listening to sounds around them are activities to increase their mobility. Safety measures such as wearing low flat shoes, having stair edges marked with a contrasting color, using proper lighting, and removing area rugs and furniture from traffic areas are necessary. Until clients master spatial orientation, they may need a caregiver to help them find their way.

When planning activities, the occupational therapy practitioner must be aware that many clients who have other conditions (multiple sclerosis, traumatic brain injury, cerebral palsy, CVA) may have visual impairments. Changing or altering the task method or modifying the environment can increase the independence of a person with vision impairments. When occupational therapy practitioners observe the client doing an activity in the natural environment, they can provide realistic, practical interventions.

Case Scenario 3

Tom, who has a traumatic brain injury after a motorcycle crash, is legally blind and has limited communication skills that cause him to receive and respond to verbal information extremely slowly. Visually, he can see large print. Although he has poor fine motor coordination, Tom has gross grasp and can touch a point with his index finger if he has adequate time. Tom wants to communicate with his friends by writing letters. The occupational therapy practitioner works with Tom so that he can use an adapted keyboard with large keys. Tom can walk and move around his environment. The occupational therapy practitioner works with him on safety and provides him with opportunities to move in real environments outside the clinic. The practitioner uses self-care grooming activities to develop Tom's fine motor control, increase his speed of actions, and increase his self-care independence. A consensus of which activities Tom needs and wants to do now and in future environments is the focus of therapy.

Hearing loss or deafness. Persons who have hearing loss or deafness often have difficulty in the self-care areas of mobility and verbal communication. While moving around, safety is a factor because these persons probably cannot hear environmental sounds such as doorbells, fire alarms, or oncoming traffic. Occupational therapy practitioners often teach clients awareness strategies before clients attempt to move around in the community by themselves. Because safety is an important concern, occupational therapy practitioners work with clients in the community to give them real-life practice experiences. The occupational therapy practitioner may work with clients to ensure that their home environments are safe with vibrating or flickering-light doorbells and lighted fire alarms.

Communicating with others outside the home is possible by using a telephone with a TDD (some are portable). The Americans With Disabilities Act of 1990 (Pub. L. 101–336) mandates that relay systems be available 24 hr a day, every day of the year, so that persons with hearing impairments can be independent in using the telephone. Other methods of enhancing communication are possible through the Internet, including e-mail messages and faxing.

Summary

Self-care is an important area of expertise for occupational therapy practitioners. Historically and in today's practice, the ability of a client to engage in self-care occupations is an ultimate goal. Likewise, the ability to engage in the many purposeful activities involved in self-care occupations is important in occupational therapy. The value of any self-care activity as a therapeutic medium is grounded in the client's values, needs, and goals. The artful occupational therapy practitioner selects self-care activities by understanding the client's future occupations. Through a clearly articulated frame of reference, the practitioner uses self-care activities to meet the client's needs and desires. ∎

References

American Occupational Therapy Association. (1994). Uniform terminology for occupational therapy—Third edition. *American Journal of Occupational Therapy, 48,* 1047–1059.

American Occupational Therapy Association. (1997). Statement—Fundamental concepts of occupational therapy: Occupation, purposeful activity, and function. *American Journal of Occupational Therapy, 51,* 864–866.

Arnadottir, G. (1990). *The brain and behavior: Assessing cortical dysfunction through tasks of daily living.* St. Louis: Mosby.

Asher, I. E. (1996). *Occupational therapy assessment tools: An annotated index* (2nd ed.). Bethesda, MD: American Occupational Therapy Association.

Bain, B. K. (1997). Rationale for using assistive technology in rehabilitation. In B. K. Bain & D. Leger (Eds.), *Assistive technology: An interdisciplinary approach* (pp. 9–16). New York: Churchill Livingstone.

Bain, B. K. (1998). Assistive technology in occupational therapy. In M. E. Neistadt & E. B. Crepeau (Eds.), *Willard & Spackman's occupational therapy* (9th ed., pp. 498–513). Philadelphia: Lippincott.

Batavia, A. J., & Hammer, G. S. (1990). Toward the development of consumer-based criteria for the evaluation of assistive devices. *Journal of Rehabilitation Research and Development, 7,* 425–436.

Brett, G. (1960). Dressing techniques for the severely involved hemiplegic patient. *American Journal of Occupational Therapy, 14,* 262–264.

Crist, P. (1998). Standardized assessments: Psychometric measurement and testing procedures. In J. Hinojosa & P. Kramer (Eds.), *Evaluation: Obtaining and interpreting data* (pp. 77–106). Bethesda, MD: American Occupational Therapy Association.

Fidler, G. S. (1994). Foreword. In C. Christiansen (Ed.), *Ways of living: Self-care strategies for special needs* (pp. v–vi). Bethesda, MD: American Occupational Therapy Association.

Fidler, G. S. (1996). Life-style performance: From profile to conceptual model. *American Journal of Occupational Therapy, 50,* 139–147.

Fields, B. (1956). What is realism in occupational therapy? *American Journal of Occupational Therapy, 10,* 9–10, 34.

Galvin, J. C., & Scherer, M. J. (Eds.). (1996). *Evaluating selecting, and using appropriate assistive technology.* Gaithersburg, MD: Aspen Publishers.

Heinemann, N. E., Allen, C. K., & Yerxa, E. J. (1989). The Routine Task Inventory: A tool for describing the functional behavior of the cognitively disabled. *Occupational Therapy Practice, 1,* 67–74.

Holm, M. B., Rogers, J. C., & James, A. B. (1998). Treatment of activities of daily living. In M. E. Neistadt, & E. B. Crepeau (Eds.), *Willard & Spackman's occupational therapy* (9th ed.) (pp. 323–364). Philadelphia: Lippincott.

Jette, A. M., Davis, A. R., Cleary, P. D., Calkins, D. R., Ruberstein, L. V., Fink, A., Kosecoft, S., Young, R. T., Brook, R. H., & Delbanco, T. L. (1986). The functional status questionnaire: Reliability and validity when used in primary care. *Journal of General Internal Medicine, 1,* 143–149.

Klein, R. M., & Bell, B. (1979). *The Klein-Bell ADL Scale manual.* Seattle, WA: Educational Resources, University of Washington.

Kohlman-Thompson, L. (1992). *Kohlman Evaluation of Living Skills (KELS)* (3rd ed.). Rockville, MD: American Occupational Therapy Association.

Law, M. (1997). Self-care. In J. Van Deusen & D. Brunt (Eds.), *Assessment in occupational therapy and physical therapy* (pp. 421–433). Philadelphia: Saunders.

Leonardelli, C. (1988). *Milwaukee Evaluation of Daily Living Skills (MEDLS).* Thorofare, NJ: Slack.

Lowman, E. W., & Liphum, F. (1947). An occupational therapy aid for paraplegics. *American Journal of Occupational Therapy, 1,* 148.

Lucci, J. A. (1958). Daily living achievements of the adult traumatic quadriplegic. *American Journal of Occupational Therapy, 12,* 144–147, 160.

Mosey, A. C. (1986). *Psychosocial components of occupational therapy.* New York: Raven Press.

National Center for Medical Rehabilitation and Research. (1991). *Report of the task force on medical rehabilitation research.* Bethesda, MD: Author.

Parente, R., & Herrman, D. (1996). *Retraining cognition: Techniques and applications.* Gaithersburg, MD: Aspen Publishers.

Phillips, B. (1992). Technology abandonment from the consumer's point of view. *National Rehabilitation Information Center Quarterly, 3,* 3–11.

Phillips B., & Zhao, H. (1993). Predictors of assistive technology abandonment. *Assistive Technology, 5,* 36–45.

Reed, K., & Sanderson, S. R. (1993). *Concepts of occupational therapy* (2nd ed.) Baltimore: Williams & Wilkins.

Richert, B. J. (1950). Occupational therapy for the quadriplegia patient. *American Journal of Occupational Therapy, 4,* 1–5.

Rogers, J. C., & Holm, M. B. (1989). The therapist's thinking behind functional assessment. In C. Royeen (Ed.), *Assessment of function: An action guide* (Lesson 1). Rockville, MD: American Occupational Therapy Association.

Rogers, J. C., & Holm, M. B. (1994). *Performance Assessment of Self-Care Skills—Revised (PASS)* (Version 3.1). Unpublished functional performance test, University of Pittsburgh, PA.

Scherer, M. J. (1993). *Living in the state of stuck: How technologies affect the lives of people with disabilities.* Cambridge, MA: Brookline Books.

Smith, R. (1990). *Occupational Therapy Functional Compilation Tool (OT FACT): Administration and tutorial manual.* Rockville, MD: American Occupational Therapy Association.

Trombly, C. A. (Ed.). (1989). *Occupational therapy for physical dysfunction.* Baltimore: Williams & Wilkins.

Trombly, C. A. (1993). Anticipating the future: Assessment of occupational function. *American Journal of Occupational Therapy, 47,* 253–257.

Trombly, C. A. (1995). Planning, guiding, and documenting therapy. In C. A. Trombly (Ed.), *Occupational therapy for physical dysfunction* (4th ed., pp. 29–40). Baltimore: Williams & Wilkins.

Trombly, C. A., & Quintana, L. A. (1989). Activities of daily living. In C. A. Trombly (Ed.), *Occupational therapy for physical dysfunction* (3rd ed., pp. 386–409). Baltimore: Williams & Wilkins.

Uniform Data System for Medical Rehabilitation (UDSMR). (1993). *Guide for the Uniform Data Set for Medical Rehabilitation (Adult FIM)* (Version 4.0). Buffalo, NY: State University of New York at Buffalo Foundation Activities.

Wellerson, T. L. (1951). Occupational therapy program for eye patients. *American Journal of Occupational Therapy, 5,* 140–145.

Williams, J. H., Drinka, T. J. K., Greenberg, J. R., Farrel-Holtan, J. Euhardy, R., & Schram, M. (1991). Development and testing of the Assessment of Living Skills and Resources (ALSAR) in elderly community-dwelling veterans. *Gerontologist, 31,* 84–91.

15

Range of Human Activity: Care of Others

Deborah R. Labovitz, PhD, OTR/L, FAOTA
Dalia Sachs, PhD, OT(I)R

Caring is a basic relationship between persons and is the activity that structures most of the primary and ongoing forms of connection between human beings. Caregiving directed toward appropriate care receivers is one of the important activities responsible for the survival of human beings and society. When they do not receive care, humans cannot survive during many critical periods of their lives, such as during infancy and childhood, during temporary or permanent illnesses or disabilities, and during extended old age. Without caring and being cared for, persons cannot have a fully meaningful day-to-day existence throughout their lives.

Caring for the self and caring for others are, therefore, essential activities of human existence and as such are part of the primordial structure of human life. We express these dual forms of caring, self-care, and caregiving to others in various ways, and these forms function at the physical, cognitive, interpersonal, psychological, emotional, and moral or spiritual levels.

We have not always clearly recognized caregiving as one of the activities that is immensely important to our own lives and to the lives of so many of our clients. But recently, with a focus on client-centered care that includes the environment, occupational therapy practitioners have focused on caregiving as part of the profession's domain of concern (Christiansen & Baum, 1997). We acknowledge that caregiving is an occupational role that not only involves care that clients receive from professionals but also includes the clients themselves, the clients' family members, and their formal and informal caregivers (Clark, Corcoran, & Gitlin, 1995; Gitlin, Corcoran, & Leinmiller-Eckhardt, 1995).

What Is Caregiving?

The primary human populations that require care are children, older adults, and persons whose acute or chronic physical, psychosocial, or cognitive conditions limit their daily activities. Caregiving, however, does not include only persons who need long-term assistance in their daily activities. Caregiving is appropriate for family members, other loved ones, and friends who have temporary needs for some kind of care. Think of instances when friends turned to you during difficult periods and asked you to help them do their shopping, clean their house, listen and advise them, or care for them in some way. How did you feel when you helped them? Was it a challenging, a difficult, or a satisfying activity, or was it some or all of these? Again, think of yourself when you had the flu or went through a personal crisis, and your mother or friend or partner prepared hot soup, a clean bed, and a warm bubble bath to comfort you. How did you feel when that person cared for you? Did the caring feel pleasant? Did it give you a sense of belonging?

We additionally take care of others who are not necessarily in crisis situations or who may not seem to be in immediate need of care in many small and large ways. We bake cakes for family members and friends to mark special occasions, we bring a cup of coffee as a thoughtful treat to someone immersed in studying, we bring a casserole for dinner to a family moving into the house next door, or we shop at the airport on our way home from a business trip for a gift to bring to a spouse or a child. But where and when do we learn to care and how to express our caring in appropriate ways?

Caregiving and care receiving are the two parts of caring, and caregivers and care receivers are the two (or more) parties involved. Both caregiving and care receiving are important for the survival of the persons in need, and caregiving and care receiving can be satisfying to both persons. At the same time, we must recognize the complexity of both roles and understand some confusion about the concept that forms their basis, caring. The word *caring* may describe many things, and, for some, the word involves some often seemingly contradictory concepts.

For example, caring for a child or a family member is supposedly a valuable activity, and society considers persons who do so to be loving and responsible; yet, in most companies, staying home from work to care for a sick child or to take an elderly parent to a medical appointment is not generally a legitimate excuse to receive pay for the day as a "sick day." Likewise, society highly values *curing* (i.e., what the physician does with drugs, surgery, or other medical means), but society does not as highly value *caring* (i.e., what the nurse and everyone else on the medical team does), an attitude that medical insurance companies reinforce by generally not reimbursing caring actions or by reimbursing caring actions only in limited ways.

Similarly, although we recognize that home health aides are vital to the survival of their clients and to the rest of a client's family members as well, insurance companies and government medical assistance programs do not pay for home health aides. Despite the fact that the work can be unpleasant, constantly demanding, physically taxing, and emotionally stressful, society considers the home health aide's work to be menial labor, and these jobs are available to persons who have no specific training for the work and receive minimum wages. Therefore, as is evident from these examples, caring connotes on the one hand a meritorious attitude and a virtue, whereas, on the other hand, caring denotes activities that sometimes earn little appreciation in society, that we associate with much burden, and that society may even negatively penalize.

Another quite common example of these contradictions is evident in descriptions of motherhood. Mothering is a role we associate with caring, as hundreds of popular songs, stories, and Mother's Day cards confirm. Women must mother correctly, with enthusiasm and love, because mothering is tremendously important to the health, well-being, and future development of our most important resource, our children. Mothering is an activity that society widely perceives to be an admirable one, a role that mothers value and a role that the rest of society, according to popular culture, greatly admires. Mothering is not only the most fundamental of caring relations, but also mothering represents, at least symbolically, an archetype of caring (Bowden, 1997). Similarly, in one study, female occupational therapists stated that they consider mothering to be the prototype of professional caring (Sachs, 1988), yet society often trivializes caregiving related to mothering, considers mothering to be less important than other careers available to women, and describes mothering as a burden and hardship (Cahn, 1975; Diemut Bubeck, 1995; Fisher & Tronto, 1990; Nieva & Gutek, 1981). In addition, like much of the work that takes place within the home, caregiving, done within and for the family, is usually unpaid labor. Few women receive formal education or training in how to be a good mother, but society expects them to do a good job nonetheless, "naturally." Yet we do not generally recognize or formally reward the skills and knowledge that are necessary to mother well. Similarly, society does not always appreciate the skills and knowledge necessary for formal, informal, and professional caregiving in the workplace, which we perceive possibly as an extension of women's activities at home with their families, and the pay is generally lower for those who do such work.

Nevertheless, the satisfaction related to caregiving is often immeasurable and priceless to those who engage in it. Caring is often part of a woman's self-definition (Gilligan, 1982). We discuss this aspect of caring later in this chapter. Occupational therapy practitioners recognize caring as a part of our clients' self-definitions, as an activity that may consume a large part of their time, and as a role that constitutes an important part of their self-images and provides meaning for their lives. An occupation this complex and long lasting certainly has definite value for the persons who do it, and they would sorely miss this occupation if they could not continue it because of an illness, injury, infirmity, or lack of opportunity. We believe that, for many women, as well as for some men, the decision in general to join a health care profession, and specifically to become an occupational therapy practitioner, is related to a strong caring commitment and to the sense of satisfaction that we derive from caregiving.

We are health care professionals, and as such, our perception of caring affects our role definition (Sachs & Labovitz, 1994). In the study of female occupational therapists (Sachs, 1988), the researcher found that, because female therapists acted on many levels and in many ways for their clients, they made themselves available to and felt responsible for those clients far beyond their perceived professional role definition. The broad scope of professional responsibility and this personal quality of caring, although sometimes overwhelming, gave the occupational therapists many advantages in working with clients. These therapists provided therapy that satisfied their own understanding of what was professionally and morally "right." Providing such care was deeply satisfying for the individual therapists and indeed was part of how they defined "doing a good job" as occupational therapists or "doing things right." These therapists informally assumed the role of "care manager" for their clients; doing so enabled them to provide total care to address the person's many needs. In many ways, these therapists acted like a mother in a household by never letting anything "fall between the cracks." They did this because they consider caring for all parts of the client a necessary aspect of competence and professionalism (Sachs & Labovitz, 1994).

Most of us give care to other living things such as household pets, which often become like members of our families. Many of us care for plants indoors in our homes and offices or outdoors in our gardens. These are caregiving activities that most persons find rewarding and enjoyable as hobbies and as vocations.

We care for larger groups in our communities as well when we volunteer to cook for the local Meals-on-Wheels program, volunteer at a homeless shelter, or help persons clean up a town. As a community, we provide education for our children, programs for persons with special needs, shelters for the homeless, transportation systems for persons with disabilities, and day centers for elderly persons as part of our governmental structure or our charitable agencies.

Thus, the concept of care and caring is interwoven with and forms the basis of our attitude toward responsibility and concern for other persons, nonhuman living things, social issues, and environmental concerns. Because caregiving as an activity between persons, however, falls within the scope of this book, and such caregiving generally involves actual doing for others, in this chapter, we confine our analysis mainly to caring for persons.

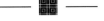

Exercise 1

Think about and write down a list of the occasions during the past month in which you gave and received care. What caring responsibilities do you have that many of your classmates probably share? What unique caring responsibilities do you have? How do these activities relate to your daily occupations? In what ways do they enhance your occupational therapy education, such as by providing you with case examples or by creating empathy? In what ways do they interfere with your occupational therapy education, such as by being time-consuming or by creating role conflict (e.g., having to choose between performing your child care responsibilities and studying for an examination)?

Definitions of Caregiving

Caring is a special relationship that encompasses a sense of attachment and of commitment to others' well-being. Caring, or as Graham (1983) termed it, "the labor of love," is "that range of human experiences that have to do with feeling concern for, and taking care of, the well-being of others" (p. 14). Caring includes feelings, knowledge, skills, and the sensitivity necessary to care for someone else. Caregiving is "providing services and support to those in need" (Moroney et al., 1998, p. 2). Caring is the spirit or the attitude of respect and concern in which we provide that service and support. Caring is the commitment that the persons receiving care can make their lives meaningful.

Caregiving thus consists of tending to the needs of others and includes physical activities such as feeding, washing, cleaning, dressing, shopping, and transporting; cognitive activities such as solving problems of finances, logistics, scheduling of services, and organization of the overall care plan; psychological activities such as understanding, protecting, comforting, and reassuring; emotional activities such as forming bonds with and worrying about the welfare of the care receivers; interpersonal activities such as helping care receivers and their family members to cope with their new or progressively worsening circumstances while maintaining their roles, relationships, and activities; and moral or spiritual activities such as ensuring that care receivers receive the sensitive and compassionate care they need in the light of the entire situation while not exploiting the resources and capabilities of the caregiver. Therefore, in addition to its instrumental aspects (i.e., doing for), caregiving has a relational, emotional component, that of connection with and love for other persons, concern for their welfare, and feelings of responsibility for their well-being.

Some of the physical activity necessary in caregiving can indeed be taxing and burdensome. On the other hand, doing the physical labor related to caregiving does not always signify that the activity is a burden to the caregiver. Conversely, some emotional and cognitive activities of caregiving do not require physical activity or exertion, such as when we sit and listen to persons and hold their hands, talk to them on the telephone, give them advice to help them organize their lives, or make telephone calls to arrange services for them. Yet these nonphysical activities can be burdensome to caregivers if caregivers perceive them to be excessively demanding, if they occur at a time of unusual and competing stress for the caregivers, or if caregivers are not positively emotionally connected to the persons requiring care. Therefore, determining when and under what circumstances persons joyously give care and when care is a burden is not always easy. Sometimes both feelings can be present sequentially in the same caregiving relationship, and sometimes ambivalent and contradictory feelings may be present simultaneously.

Case Scenario 1

Sometimes caring for a loved one with a chronic condition that becomes progressively more debilitating can start out as a labor of love and necessity. But over months or even years, providing care can become an overwhelming burden that taxes the physical and emotional strength of even the most loving family member. Although the positive feelings of love and respect for the care receiver may not change, as time goes on, the physical and psychological burden may increase beyond the endurance of the caregiver. In such situations, the occupational therapy practitioner or other medical professional may recognize that the well spouse or the adult son or daughter caregiver's physical or psychological health has deteriorated to the point that he or she or the entire family is in "dire straits." Such professional awareness can lead to support for seeking alternative care arrangements such as nursing homes or other long-term care facilities (Cohen, 1996).

Caregiving can embody the various components of caring in many different ways. We can give the care without the feelings associated with or seemingly necessary in the special caring relationship. For example, we can be skillful caregivers to our clients even if we do not always have the positive caring quality in our relationship with all of them (Grott, 1998). At the same time, we can love our grandparents positively and strongly and be intensely committed to their well-being, yet, because of our lack of skills and knowledge, geographical distance, or the fact that someone else (e.g., our parents, siblings, or a professional caregiver) has the primary caregiving responsibility on a daily basis, we may participate little in the actual instrumental activities required of daily caregiving. We can talk with our grandparents, be sensitive to their needs, feel responsible for them, and include them in family life, thus participating in the emotional or interpersonal level of caregiving (Piercy, 1998). Although caregiving in the personal sphere places more emphasis on feelings and relationships, and caregiving in the public sphere places more emphasis on skills and instrumental knowledge, the ultimate quality of caregiving relies much on the balance between all components of caring (Sachs, 1988).

By using these definitions, we can now analyze caregiving as an activity that involves many levels of performance. First and foremost, caring involves a moral or spiritual component related to a general sense of personal attachment and of moral commitment to the well-being of others. In addition, the action or doing part of caregiving involves physical, cognitive, psychological, emotional, and interpersonal components.

Literature in other professions such as nursing often strongly emphasizes the physical requirements of caregiving to children, elderly adults, and persons with disabilities, thus stressing the burden we associate with these activities. Although many of the activities that we associate with caregiving demand the use of motor skills such as lifting, cleaning, feeding, carrying, and transporting, caregiving as a total activity encompasses all of the components we describe in this chapter. Therefore, as occupational therapy practitioners, we must consider all of these aspects when analyzing caregiving activities and using them therapeutically.

Caregiving requires an ongoing cognitive process of thinking and of problem solving. To face the changing needs of others, caregivers must be involved in planning and problem solving while doing in the concrete world of real-life situations (Rudick, 1989). Sometimes finding ways of giving care that will both satisfy the caregiver's needs for effective action to resolve a situation or achieve a goal and fulfill the needs of the care receiver is difficult (Hasselkus, 1998).

Case Scenario 2

When your child does not want to go to bed on time and you have an examination the next day, you must identify the problem and determine whether he or she is having fears about the coming night or whether the child is testing boundaries. Analysis of the situation will help you in making the decision. Does your child need help and support, thus fulfilling the child's needs for security and reassurance, or do you need to insist on immediate bedtime to fulfill your child's needs for appropriate limits and your own need to study. This problem-solving process will direct your behavior with your child in the above situation.

Caregiving involves interpersonal relationships and therefore requires a special sensitivity and attentiveness to the care receiver's needs. The caregiving dyad can be intimate and, because of this, may require emotional and physical closeness. In certain caregiving situations, you may be devoted to fostering the care receiver's growth and development, and thus you may experience the other person "both as part of you and as apart from you" (Moroney et al., 1998, p. 8). On the surface level, the relationship is giving for one party and receiving for the other party. Accordingly, we must be aware of the possibility of the development of dependence and power relationships (Clement, 1996), and we must instead learn how to develop appropriate interdependence–codependence relationships. On the interpersonal level, caregiving is not only a skill but also an art. The art consists of developing a mutual interpersonal relationship with someone who needs our care and being sensitive to the verbal and nonverbal cues with which they communicate their emotional and physical needs. By examining the previous case scenario, we see that only an intimate knowledge of the child and an ability to understand his or her feelings and actions will help you to identify why he or she is refusing to go to bed at that moment. Empathic understanding of your child will enable you to use the problem-solving process and select the technique necessary for dealing appropriately with the situation.

A dimension of caregiving that we frequently neglect is that caregiving is a work of emotions. Caregiving is heavily engaging, partly because it involves the management of our own and of other persons' feelings (Hochschild, 1983; McRae, 1998). Often in personal caregiving, and many times in professional caregiving, we become emotionally attached to the care receiver and are thus more able to engage positively in the caregiving situation. In addition, when a child, an elderly person, or a person with disabilities does not want to cooperate with our caregiving, we may try to use our therapeutic selves to work to change their attitudes. This kind of engagement of emotions and the use of emotions to connect can produce much stress in the caregiver.

Caregiving can be even more stressful in complex situations and when success is difficult to define, such as in the case of giving care to persons who are dying (Hasselkus, 1993). On the other hand, however, sometimes caring for a person who is dying may be easier because the situation has a well-defined and anticipated finite end; conversely, the continuing responsibility to care for a child with disabilities or a young adult whose illness or disabilities are chronic and have no end in sight may cause a much higher level of stress precisely because the caregiver has no way no way to predict how long the caregiving situation will last (Cohen, 1996).

Despite all of our caution and attempts to change situations, sometimes the client, the caregiver or family members, and the therapist develop negative feelings about one another. Hate can be a powerful emotion in the therapeutic milieu, and hate can arise when clients project their anger and disappointment about having a disability or about not succeeding in achieving successes in the treatment process onto the caregiver or onto the practitioner. Conversely, the caregiver or practitioner may begin to dislike an uncooperative, unsuccessful, or unappreciative client such that the caregiving or therapeutic relationship is difficult to maintain (Abbot, 1990).

Exercise 2

Imagine that you are the caregiver in each of the following situations.

■ Situation 1: You are an adult caring for your dying father, with whom you have a warm and loving relationship. He lives by himself in his own apartment, which is a short distance from your home, and he has only a few months left to live because he is in an advanced stage of cancer.

■ Situation 2: You are an adult with responsibility for your father, from whom you have been estranged for most of your life. He lives alone in an apartment several hundred miles from your home and is becoming less able to take care of himself as his Alzheimer's disease progresses.

Describe how the various levels of caregiving above relate to your activities and responses as a caregiver in each scenario. What would you do, and how might you feel?

Caregiving and Human Occupation

When we examine how caregiving relates to human occupation, we develop a deeper understanding of the meaning of caregiving to persons. We must attempt to uncover how different persons ascribe meaning to caregiving and how gender, age, culture, physical and mental disability, class, and sexual orientation affect the form, process, context, and meanings of caregiving. If we want to understand caregiving as an important occupation that involves purposeful activities in the occupational therapy intervention process, we must demonstrate how personal, social, and environmental aspects influence caregiving's meanings to the individual client.

Exercise 3

Examine the possible meanings of caregiving in the following nine situations.

1. A single mother of three children who works outside the home and takes care of her elderly parents

2. A middle class grandmother who is retired and is caring for her only grandchild while her daughter, the child's mother, is at work

3. A paid aide who is taking care of a lonely and frustrated elderly man

4. An adult son who is helping his elderly mother who needs assistance in every-day life activities

5. A paid day care worker or babysitter caring for a young child during the day

6. A woman 37 years of age who has had total responsibility for the past 5 years for her husband, who is 40 years of age and to whom she has been married for 15 years, who has progressively more extensive permanent disabilities resulting from multiple sclerosis

7. An elderly man taking care of his dependent wife of 45 years

8. A daughter, 60 years of age, caring for her mother, 90 years of age, who is in a hospice facility dying of cancer

9. A religious leader who is taking care of his or her community

We can assume that, because of the different personal, social, and environmental circumstances, the meanings and the forms of caregiving for each of these persons will be quite different. Identify possible feelings for each scenario. See the Appendix for a short discussion.

As we can see from the foregoing exercise, many personal, social, and environmental variables affect the meanings of caregiving and the way persons carry it out.

Caring, Morality, and Gender Differences

Historically, and to a large extent today, in most Western societies, women assume responsibility for caring. Much of this caring occurs in the home as the unpaid work of wives, mothers, daughters, daughters-in-law, grandmothers, and granddaughters. Paid caring occurs in the workplace and consists mainly of female nurses, nurses' aides, teachers, teachers' aides, day care workers, social workers, and various health professionals, including occupational therapists. Society considers much of this caring activity to be the "natural" work of women, and these professions often require little or no formal training or skill, and women perform them for such reasons as helping others or to make themselves feel good because society believes that women enjoy the role of helper. Society and government undervalue and underpay these caring tasks of women (Diemut Bubeck, 1995; Fisher & Tronto, 1990).

Until the late 1960s, society perceived caring to be a natural instinct of women. Congruent with social stereotypes, some presented the caring role as an inferior psychological position and a biological destiny of women, whereas others described women's caring behavior as a natural maternal instinct (Williams, 1983). This belief was the basis for the dichotomy that developed between the caring of nurses and other women and the curing of medicine, which involved the valued role of physicians, who were then primarily men. For example, listening to a client who is depressed and who needs to have his or her hand held or a friendly hug are not reimbursable services. Staying with a client who needs empathy because, after her stroke, she can no longer take care of her own grooming needs is not generally a valid reason for changing treatment objectives during a therapeutic session or missing a staff meeting. Similarly, persons not involved in caregiving and even the health care team often at best do not appreciate and at worst ignore or trivialize the absolute burden of day-in, day-out, 24-hr care for a family member with disabilities.

Still, despite these attitudes, many women still find caregiving extremely rewarding and, in fact, consider caregiving to be one of the primary aspects of their lives. This relationship between women and caring is complex, and caring has different meanings for men and women. Although caregiving is at times hard labor, it is at the same time an activity that is not only satisfying but also greatly relates to the development of self. Moreover, because caregiving is an activity crucial for the survival of all persons, some segment of the population of future generations must consider caregiving worthwhile and therefore willingly and even eagerly do it.

Carol Gilligan (1982) demonstrated in her research that women define themselves through relationships and judge themselves on the basis of their caring ability. Her findings provided a new understanding of women's outlook regarding the connection between morality and care. She explained that, unlike men, who base their moral decision making on a rational model of "right and wrong" detached from context, women tend to view decision making in terms of the morality of relationships. Women's moral perspective focuses on caring, and women are concerned with the ultimate welfare of all persons involved.

Although women's commitment to care has not decreased, in recent years, more men are providing care to their family members (Chang & White-Means, 1991; Harris, 1998; Harris & Bichler, 1997). In a behavioral development that goes against traditional gender roles, men are participating in caregiving for their wives, children, and parents. Some of these men choose to accept the caring responsibility, whereas others do so out of necessity. Sons, husbands, and fathers become involved in caring out of a sense of commitment and love. Under these circumstances, men are emotionally absorbed in the situation and the task and experience both satisfaction and stress from the caregiver role and from doing the caregiving tasks (Harris, 1998; Harris & Bichler, 1997).

Closer examination of the participation of men in caregiving demonstrates how the division of caring labor by gender affects not only the meanings ascribed to caring but also the way in which women and men differ in their methods of caregiving. For example, when adult children provide care for their parents, daughters and daughters-in-law are generally the main or primary caregivers, with sons and sons-in-law helping them (Abel, 1991; Scharlach, Low, & Schneider, 1991). In addition, in the less common situations in which sons are the main caregivers, they are more likely than daughters to be involved in primarily instrumental tasks and in organizing outside help for their parents. Sons are less likely than daughters to be involved in providing hands-on caring, especially for personal needs, and in helping with routine household chores such as cooking, cleaning, shopping, and other errands. At the same time, sons are as much involved in providing financial and emotional support to their parents as are daughters (Dwyer & Coward, 1991; Harris, 1998; Horowitz, 1985).

Exercise 4

Reflect on your roles in caregiving with family members. Consider the situations that are relevant to you among the following list: How do you think that your gender influences what you do and what others expect you to do? Do you and your spouse share equally in child care activities and responsibilities? Do you share equally in caring for elderly parents or in-laws? Do you and your siblings of a different gender have equal responsibilities and roles in caring for your older parents? Which of you does more? For which types of care are each of you responsible? Do your children of different genders have different past experiences with and expectations for their future roles as caregivers? Do you have differing expectations for each of them? Who do you expect will care for you when you are old?

Caregivers and Care Receivers

As we have described, most human beings spend parts of their lifetimes performing the normal kinds of caring activities that make life possible. On an informal basis, parents care for children, children care for siblings and pets, persons care for family members and friends, adult sons and daughters care for elderly parents, and on a formal basis, professional paid caregivers care for persons in need of such attention.

An Internet site about caring (www.nfcacares.org/about.html) presents the preliminary results of their 1997 *NFCA/Fortis Report: Caregiving Across the Life Cycle* (National Family Caregivers Association, 1997). Results of the survey revealed some of the meanings of caregiving for respondents. Among the positive outcomes of caring were the following: "found inner strength I didn't have before," "developed a closer relationship with the person I help," and "learned proactive skills." The negative outcomes included the following: "more headaches," "more stomach disorders," "more back pains," "more sleeplessness," and "more depression." Caregiving emotions included frustration, compassion, sadness, and anxiety. Among the caregiving difficulties cited were a sense of isolation and a lack of understanding from others, having responsibility for making major life decisions for a loved one, loss of personal leisure time, and no consistent help from other family members. The caregiving responsibilities that take up the most time were activities of daily living (ADL) (e.g., feeding, dressing, housework, meals, laundry, groceries, emotional support), guardianship, legal responsibilities, financial management, health care tasks (e.g., bandaging, medication), and providing transportation. Many of the negative responses are indicative of the burdens we associate with caregiving by and for family members. As this survey confirmed, women generally provide most of the care (Brody & Lang, 1982).

Case Scenario 3

Recently, a new group of women have joined the list of caregivers: grandmothers with primary caring responsibility for young children as more younger women with children enter the workforce. More than 4 million American children live with grandparents, mainly women, and many do so under stressful circumstances (American Association of Retired Persons, 1999). A support network called Grandparents as Parents (GAP) facilitates the sharing of experiences and feelings between grandparents who are raising their grandchildren. GAP provides information and referrals, a telephone support network, a directory of group members, and assistance in starting groups ("Dear Abby," 1999).

Cultural and ethnic aspects are involved in the expectations for caregiving and care receiving. For example, caregiving is deeply imbedded in the culture of African-Americans, which dictates that family members will care for family members in need, and caregivers will receive care from family members when the caregiver needs it. Other cultures around the world have developed varying methods of providing care to those in need; some support the view that caregiving is family members' responsibility only. The absence of formal caregiving mechanisms in such societies may result from that orientation.

Case Scenario 4

Persons from the Philippines have a tradition of informal care for family members and elderly persons that results from, and results in, a society with no retirement or nursing homes. Children learn at an early age to respect elderly persons and to expect to help their family members and their neighbors. Their experiences with informal caregiving to their elderly family members translate into marketable formal caregiving skills in countries to which they emigrate in large numbers and seek jobs for economic advancement. Filipinas often work in other countries as caregivers, and they are in great demand as much for their dedication to their charges, which stems from their attitude of respect for caring, as for their well-developed instrumental caregiving skills. As reported in a recent issue of *Hadassah Magazine,* Eduardo de Vega, Philippine Consul in Israel, described their attitude toward their work as follows. "For the Filipina, [being a caregiver is] not simply an employee–employer relationship; [h]er employer becomes part of her family. It's important to ease his pain. It's important that he smile" (Mason, 1999, p. 80).

Other countries pride themselves on their elaborately designed social services that function as a "safety net" to take care of segments of their population who cannot live on their own in the economic or social system. Westernized, industrialized countries in which persons live in cities, in poverty, or far away from their families of origin tend to follow this pattern to a greater or lesser degree, depending on their blend of cultural and religious traditions that influence their attitudes toward helping others.

Case Scenario 5

Sweden has an extensively developed governmental social services system that provides universally available care for persons of all ages at public expense. The government supports universal access to such care in progressive formats such as combining housing for elderly persons with child care centers so that the generations can mix for their mutual benefit. In such facilities, children interact with many caring adults, and the seniors enjoy the stimulation and future orientation that comes from dealing with infants, toddlers, preschoolers, and their parents on a daily basis.

In American society, parents and other family members care for children on an informal basis. A parallel formal child care network of paid caregivers has expanded in response to the increase in families in which both parents are employed and in response to welfare reforms that stress reducing the welfare rolls by requiring mandatory employment. Paid babysitters and paid family day care providers provide formal child care for infants, toddlers, and preschool children in private homes. Day care centers for infants and toddlers, private preschools and nursery schools, and government programs employ day care staff members at various levels to care for and teach children.

Some employers provide on-site or other subsidized day care programs for the children of their workers. School-aged children receive care in afterschool programs, from private paid babysitters and care providers, and from older siblings.

Occupational therapy practitioners can be consultants for day care workers, preschool aides and teachers, and paid family day care providers who may need advice about using developmentally appropriate play and toys, using creative activities, reducing behavior problems, and identifying children at risk for physical, emotional, or social problems. Occupational therapy practitioners can provide therapeutic interventions in such settings for children already identified as needing these professional services.

Adults and elderly persons receive care from a plethora of paid and professional caregivers and care agencies. Paid companions provide attendant care on a one-to-one basis in homes and hospitals. Senior centers and other such facilities have day programs with activities and meals for persons who are mobile enough to attend. Home health aides and volunteers visit homebound persons to provide medical treatments, assist with self-care activities, and help with cleaning and household tasks. Agencies that supply such home caregivers are part of a growing care industry that includes agencies that provide care for relatives who live in different cities and that perform the day-to-day oversight functions for adult sons and daughters who live at a distance from their elderly parents. This approach is one of the roles currently called *case management*. Privately owned, for-profit independent living and assisted living residences and life care communities involving varying levels of care serve more affluent well or nearly well elderly persons, whereas persons who are too sick to live on their own at all or who are unable to afford other care live in nursing homes and in other kinds of long-term care institutions. In the not-for-profit group, community visiting nurse associations provide in-home caregivers, whereas hospice services in homes and in special residence facilities ease suffering and help direct caregiving toward death with dignity in persons who are terminally ill and in the process of dying.

Occupational therapy practitioners frequently instruct such formal caregivers and paid staff members in performing instrumental ADL in ergonomically sound ways. Practitioners likewise help caregivers understand the importance of meaningful activities in their clients' lives and assist them in helping clients use activities more successfully (Hasselkus, 1998). Occupational therapy practitioners can help clients and family members make transitions when necessary from one level of care to another.

Who Receives Care?

The population of care receivers varies widely. We have already noted that, in general, children, persons of all ages with disabilities, and elderly persons are the broadly identified target groups. Beginning in the early 1980s in the United States, a new working-age adult population needing care developed: persons with HIV and AIDS.

In many cases, foster parents care for infants and children born with HIV and AIDS, and friends and acquaintances of both genders care for adults with these conditions.

Case Scenario 6

Caregiving for persons with HIV and AIDS generally begins before major deterioration takes place and continues through progressive illness, debilitation, and ultimately death. Persons who often provide care under extremely difficult conditions may experience stress and may require help with the grieving and mourning process that follows the death of the loved one. Caregiver organizations have published how-to manuals, and family members have written about their experiences to help others know what to expect (Greif, 1994).

The Development of Caregiving Skills

As human beings, at first we receive caring, then we learn how to care for ourselves, and finally we discover how to care for others. How do we discover caring? Is caring part of our nature, is it a personal tendency, is it part of our gender, or do we learn it through training and modeling? As with most other human occupations, caring must be a combination of all of the above. The important questions are "How can we foster the acquisition of a caring attitude?" and "How can we facilitate the learning of the skills and the knowledge required for caregiving activities for both girls and boys as they grow?"

The development of prosocial behavior begins early in infants and toddlers as they become aware of their own selves and the presence of others in their environments. Smiling, which begins as a random reflexive behavior, soon becomes a valuable piece of social interaction as the baby finds responsive family members paying enthusiastic attention to every grin. The developing infant notices others in the environment, including his or her mother, father, babysitter, siblings, playmates, other family members and friends, and the family pet. Recognition that these are separate persons helps the baby begin to understand that not only do others exist, but also they have their own feelings and their own reactions to the baby's behavior. The beginnings of empathy, or a concern for the feelings of others, become the foundation for the ability to interact with others and to care about them. Caring about someone is a precursor to being able to care for someone. Through complex interactions with these and other persons, the infant, and later the toddler, learns social interaction skills that include caring about and caring for others. In early play experiences, and later in nursery schools, kindergartens, and elementary schools, growing children practice caregiving behaviors as they play with others and experience their world.

Young children, mainly girls, imitate their parents' caregiving behavior by playing with dolls or with younger siblings or friends. They feed and clean their dolls, play house, and role-play parenting with other children. In many cultures, and in large families, children may have some caregiving responsibilities while still quite young. In Western cultures, children generally take care of pets and plants. After they learn and can demonstrate the skills necessary for proper performance of these activities, children gradually receive more responsibility related to these duties. As school-aged children or as adolescents, they may share a few caregiving responsibilities for their younger siblings, such as feeding them, helping them with homework, playing with or otherwise occupying them, ensuring that they come home from school safely, babysitting for them in the afternoon while the parents are at work or in the evening while the parents are out, or, when they are old enough, driving them or accompanying them on public transportation to afterschool activities.

Case Scenario 7

Educating Children for Parenting (ECP), which is headquartered in Philadelphia, brings infants and parents into preschool and elementary school classrooms to teach young children about caring for babies. Through the ECP program, once a month, a parent and a real baby visit in classrooms. Students observe the parent and baby closely and ask questions to deepen their understanding of the awesome responsibility of parenthood. The parent demonstrates parenting skills and child development right before the students' eyes. Children discuss their own home situations with their teachers, and this has led to opportunities for counseling and parent education.

In families that take care of grandparents who need assistance in their daily occupations, school-age children and adolescents may share some activities of caregiving, such as talking with their grandparents, reading to them, bringing them newspapers or meals, helping them to walk safely or to perform some self-care activities, or taking them to medical appointments. Later, children may practice their caring skills by taking care of each other. In families with children with special needs, with adult family members with disabilities, or in which certain parental pathologies such as alcoholism, drug abuse, mental illness, domestic abuse, or traumatic experiences including stress, unemployment, or extreme poverty are present, children may need to assume parental caregiving responsibilities at an even earlier age. In such families, children may take on the role of parenting siblings or, in some situations, even parenting their parents.

Case Scenario 8

Adolescents can learn to care for children as babysitters or mothers' helpers in short courses at schools, churches, and community centers. Such courses include overview information on child development, play and toys, discipline, and routine safety procedures relative to supervision, prevention of household accidents, and who to call in emergencies. Occupational therapy practitioners can organize, present, or contribute their expertise to these courses, and in communities in which these courses are not available, practitioners can advocate with parents or health agencies for the development of such courses.

We must teach, encourage, and provide opportunities for children and adolescents to develop their caregiving roles. In research that drew on the testimony of youths involved in community services, Wuthnow (1995) concluded that caring itself and caring behavior are not innate but rather that children learn caring from both experiencing a warm and caring family life and from having the opportunity or finding the right place to learn such caregiving skills and attitudes. Sometimes sheer necessity draws adolescents into caregiving because they have a sibling with a disability, a parent with a problem, or a grandparent in their home. In such situations, training for the teenagers and other family members and support are critical to prevent the stress levels from becoming so high that burnout occurs. Beach (1997) concluded that sharing caregiving responsibilities for grandparents resulted not only in the development of greater empathy on the part of the teenagers for older adults but also resulted in improving sibling relationships and strengthening the adolescents' bonding with their mothers. Apparently caring for grandparents when mothers are the main caregivers is not too much of a burden on the adolescents and allows them to experience the positive effects of integral involvement in family caregiving activities.

Adolescents' involvement in caregiving encompasses the gamut of life experiences that includes burden, stress, sensitivity to others, responsibility, wage-earning opportunities, changing attitudes, sharing, and developing intimate relationships. In addition, when the burden and stress of caregiving is not too overwhelming, such as with grandparents and community projects, caregiving can be an enriching role that contributes to adolescent growth and development. Caregiving prepares the adolescent to enter adulthood as a person with enhanced responsiveness to the needs of others.

Case Scenario 9

Even adults need instruction in caring when specialized situations occur. Hospitals and community agencies routinely hold classes for new parents. These classes include information on specifics such as feeding, bathing, and caring for the new infant, child development and safety procedures, and dealing with issues such as the changes in family life that caring for an infant can cause. Courses for new grandparents help them transition to a new role and to redefine their relationships with their adult children and their new grandchild. Courses help parents and family members deal with the birth of a child with special needs or with caring for a child who develops problems after illness or an accident.

Similarly, the development of social caring and community responsibility relates to early experiences with caring and with positive role models of caregiving. Persons who respond to community needs by becoming adult volunteers on projects to help the less fortunate in their communities or in religious and charitable organizations tend to have learned these values earlier in their lives. Performance of good deeds and acts of kindness and charity are linked to a strong sense of empathy for others, which is a basic foundation of the caring relationship. Even the ability to act morally when faced with difficult decisions in extenuating circumstances such as wartime has its roots in a well-developed commitment to caring. In extreme situations, the willingness to risk one's own life to save another is inextricably tied to a strong sense of caring. Research about German civilians and citizens of Nazi-dominated countries who helped save Jews during the Holocaust of World War II shows that these ordinary people who behaved heroically came from families in which altruism and care of others were strong values (Fogelman, 1994; Oliner & Oliner, 1988).

Caregiving: A Human Activity in Occupational Therapy

Clearly, caregiving involves purposeful activities, and the caregiver is a role that is important and necessary in the lives of many of our clients and in the lives of their family members. In addition, the valuing of and active engagement in caregiving are essential to the development of an emotional and moral commitment to the well-being of others and to enhancing one's ability to acquire the skills necessary to perform the tasks involved. At the same time, and sometimes for the same persons, caregiving can be hard and stressful labor, especially for persons responsible for the daily functioning of children, elderly persons, or persons with severe disabilities. Accordingly, we now examine the different ways in which occupational therapy practitioners can help clients engage in caregiving as a purposeful activity that includes so many dimensions and so many levels of performance.

Occupational therapy practitioners work with both informal and formal caregivers who are engaged in giving care to others. Interventions with these clients involve helping to develop successful and satisfying ways of giving care and helping them to prevent or deal with stress. Because occupational therapy practitioners themselves work as professional caregivers, they can consider themselves to be clients as well, particularly regarding using meaningful activities with clients and preventing caregiver stress. Another group of clients is potential caregivers whom we can help to develop caring attitudes or who can learn caregiving skills. These persons include children, persons with developmental disabilities, persons with mental illness, or new teenage mothers. A final set of clients includes persons who are or who have been caregivers and have lost their caregiving roles. To elderly persons; persons with newly acquired, chronic, or progressively worsening disabilities; or anyone whose opportunities for caregiving are reduced or eliminated, occupational therapy practitioners can offer guidance in relearning lost caregiving skills or in finding alternative ways to fulfill caregiving needs.

Occupational Therapy for Family Members and Other Informal Caregivers

Occupational therapy can be valuable for family members, friends, or paid helpers who participate in caregiving for persons who cannot live independently because of cognitive, developmental, or physical disabilities. Because occupational therapy is involved in nontraditional community and home-based settings, and most caregiving for the frail population occurs in the home, informal caregivers have become a major group of clients needing and receiving professional services. These caregivers may include family members who are the main caregivers for their spouse, parents, and children; neighbors and friends who share only a few caregiving responsibilities; or paid caregivers in the home or in day care facilities and nursing homes. The stress, hard labor, and skills necessary to provide quality care on an ongoing, daily basis transforms these caregivers into an important group needing occupational therapy services. Understanding the multiple meanings of caregiving for these caregivers and analyzing the way that they provide care can help us design appropriate occupational therapy intervention strategies with these clients (Dougherty & Radomski, 1990).

Research on the interaction between family members and occupational therapy practitioners has revealed that one of the first difficulties that practitioners encounter in working with family caregivers is accepting them as the ones responsible for the well-being of the care receivers and respecting their knowledge (Gitlin et al., 1995). Hasselkus (1988) found that occupational therapy practitioners differ from family caregivers in their values, beliefs, and ethics. For example, occupational therapy goals are not always compatible with family caregiver priorities. Although occupational therapy practitioners focus on enhancing a care receiver's independence in ADL, family members are more concerned with care receiver safety and sense of identity and with maintaining a daily routine (Gitlin et al., 1995; Hasselkus, 1991). As a result, family caregivers do not always cooperate fully with occupational therapy programs. At the same time, occupational therapy practitioners perceived family caregivers to be obstacles to their own intervention (Gitlin & Corcoran, 1993). This research demonstrates the importance of understanding the meanings of caregiving to individual caregivers, of considering their knowledge and skills, and of respecting their personal and cultural values when designing caregiver interventions.

Gender, cultural background, age, and family relationships result in differences in the experience of caregiving. Family members or other nonformal caregivers may vary in their attitudes toward their caregiving role, in their knowledge, and in the way they practice its tasks; nevertheless, they may need guidance, support, and instruction to improve their skills to provide efficient caring for their loved ones. Caregivers may need to master some treatment techniques such as transferring, feeding, dressing, and teaching independence. First and foremost, they may need to learn management strategies to organize caregiving around the sometimes extensive and changing needs of care receivers (Corcoran & Gitlin, 1992). Caregivers may need support and may need to learn how to deal with their own stress. Participating in support and stress management groups may help them to deal with the burden and extended demands of caregiving (Cohen, 1996; Peiffer & Crooker, 1990). Occupational therapy practitioners can organize and run such support groups and can inform family members about such groups at local hospitals, agencies, or volunteer organizations devoted to various illnesses. Recognizing the limits of family caregiving, providing professional advice about alternatives, and supporting difficult decisions that family members face surrounding the need to institutionalize their loved ones can be part of the occupational therapy practitioner's treatment responsibility because he or she can offer valuable insight to the family members regarding evaluating nursing homes and other long-term care facilities. Therapists who are familiar with the family members and with the caregivers can help them in the transition to a care facility and can design ways to continue treatments and maintain achievements and levels of function in the new setting by acting as consultants to family members and to the residence or long-term care facility staff members.

Some caregivers are frail elderly persons themselves and thus may need medical and physical support. They and others, including paid caregivers in the home, in day care centers, or in nursing homes, may need an improved ergonomic environment to reduce the chances of injury to themselves or to the person for whom they are caring. Discovering and learning to implement successful ways to involve clients in activities meaningful to them can be extremely satisfying to such daily caregivers and can help prevent burnout. Caregivers may need enhanced knowledge in engaging care receivers in purposeful activities. Therefore, to design efficient interventions for caregiving clients, we must consider programs that fit each person in his or her own unique caregiving situation and will provide caregivers with the knowledge, skills, and support they need (Dougherty & Radomski, 1990; Hasselkus, 1998).

Certain situations present particularly stressful conditions for family members and individual caregivers. For example, the birth of a child with disabilities can be traumatic for the entire family. Bringing home a high-risk infant and adapting the home setting to accommodate the needs of the baby can challenge the patience and the emotional resilience of even the strongest and most stable families. Major stress may result from fear of the frail physical condition of the infant, uncertainty about how to perform medical or other procedures that the infant needs, and the amount of time needed for and the inconvenience of repeating such daily routine tasks as feeding, changing, dressing, and transporting the baby. Moreover, the inability to give attention simultaneously to other children or to respond to their and other family members' needs can cause major distress for the entire family. The realization that this may be a lifelong problem that will require major reorientation of the family members' patterns of functioning can be a shock. Furthermore, the financial burden of special equipment, repeated medical consultations or procedures, and specialized babysitters or paid caregivers, coupled with the possible loss of income if one of the parents must leave paid employment to assume caregiving tasks, may prove impossible for the family to handle (Vergara & Angley, 1990).

Case Scenario 10

Raising a child with special needs changes the dynamics of family life and places demands on the parents and siblings that can either cause major difficulties or conversely provide opportunities for growth and family cohesion. Family members must work out their own accommodations to the needs of their special member. To do this, they may need help with the psychological tasks of accepting the disappointment and anger they feel regarding the disability, adjusting to their altered roles and perceptions of themselves as parents and family members, and recognizing their uncertainties about the future expectations for their child with disabilities. They must deal with the disappointments and those of other extended family members and the reaction of friends, neighbors, and colleagues who may or may not be helpful in their responses to the situation. Family members may need guidance and reassurance about the physical procedures and adaptations that they will need to learn to participate in the various treatments that their child will need. They will have to learn to cope with the parade of therapists and medical personnel who will become a part of their households on a daily or periodic basis. Moreover, family members may require help to find the resources to deal with the financial burdens that dealing with the child with disabilities will impose (Humphry & Case-Smith, 1996).

Siblings, especially, may worry about their future responsibilities for caring for a brother or sister when their parents become too old to do so (Humphry & Case-Smith, 1996). At the same time, various family members in addition to the parents, such as siblings and extended family members (particularly grandparents) may find satisfaction in caring for the special needs of the child with disabilities as part of the family's cohesive support system.

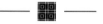

Exercise 5

Imagine that you are an occupational therapy practitioner working as part of an interdisciplinary health team with a family who has a child for whom providing care is difficult. You are to provide the therapeutic handling that is the focus of the occupational therapy intervention, but you realize that the family is not cooperating with the child's treatment program. What are the contextual and psychosocial aspects of the caregiving situation that you would analyze to understand the family's attitude? What are your responsibilities to the family members? How would you try to enlist their cooperation?

In this situation, the practitioner must be sensitive to the family's priorities and the other children's needs and must be sure to include both parents in discussions. The therapist and parents should jointly negotiate and agree to treatment priorities. The therapist should develop goals and activities cooperatively so that the therapy fits the family's needs, goals, and schedules. Ascertain with the parents how much time and energy they are able to invest in the care of this child, and take the family seriously as the ones who know the child best. The occupational therapy practitioner may coordinate services with all the other team members and be aware of everything they are doing and what their goals are. The therapist should schedule treatments to be sensitive to the family's time constraints (i.e., do not make the parents take time from work to meet with you, and do not allow treatment to take up room in the family's house or to come at mealtimes that can disrupt the family's routine). The therapist should suggest ways to make the daily chores easier if possible. Teach the family members care strategies. Listen to their feedback, and act on it.

Because, as we have indicated, all caregivers are different, and all care receivers are different, the caregiving situation will vary immensely. Hasselkus (1990) described the process of ethnographic interviewing to ascertain exactly what the caregiving experience means to each person in the situation. This knowledge can aid the occupational therapy practitioner in designing the proper intervention strategy on the basis of the variables in the situation at hand. Smalley (1990) clarified the difference in the meanings of *caretaking* versus *caregiving*, particularly regarding how the distinction affects the interpretation of what is taking place for the caregiver, the care recipient, and the family members.

On the basis of human occupation, Gitlin and colleagues (1995) provided an approach for occupational therapists to use to develop a plan for intervention. Although the specific example below concerns caregiving for elderly persons, the principles are applicable to all caregiving situations. Four principles represent four stages of intervention. We briefly present the principles with case examples to demonstrate how to translate the understanding of caregiving as a human occupation into an effective intervention program in occupational therapy.

Stage 1

The first stage involves identifying the main person responsible for providing the care. When we make a home visit, we must recognize that the home already has an organization of caregiving. Out of necessity, the family members have probably already developed their own strategies, practices, and skills of caregiving. Therefore, we first must identify the main caregivers who can give us the information about the unique caregiving situation of the family members. For example, we can determine in the initial home visit that the elderly wife is the primary caregiver for her husband with dementia and that she is responsible for managing the care and provides most of it by herself with some help from her children. Identifying her as a key person will enable us to get the necessary information about the caregiving situation.

Stage 2

The second stage involves attempting to understand the caregiver's unique perspective that shapes his or her caregiving practice. At this stage, we observe the caregiving situation and pay attention to how caregivers organize the environment, we listen to caregivers' stories of their daily routines and their past experiences, and we ask them questions that will help us understand their attitudes, beliefs, concerns, and priorities. In the example, during the following visits, we can observe while the woman helps her husband dress, walk to the dining room, eat, and sit to watch television. We can listen to her describe what she does on a typical day and ask her about her concerns regarding her caregiving activities. We can ask her how she perceives her husband's situation, what his main difficulties are, how he was in the past, how would she like to plan their future, and in what areas would she like us to help her.

Stage 3

The third stage involves self-questioning and self-evaluation of how much insight we, the occupational therapists, received regarding the caregiver's perspectives and the caregiving situation and to what extent our professional and personal goals, beliefs, and values are congruent with those of the caregiver. At this stage, we can ask ourselves how much we know about the caregiving situation; whether we gained an understanding of the caregiver's values, beliefs, and goals; and whether our intervention goals are congruent with those of the caregiver. In the example, we can ask some of the following questions: Do we know what the wife's main physical and psychological difficulties are in providing the care? Whom does she trust and consult when she encounters difficulties? To what degree are the grown children accessible, and in what ways do they participate in providing the care for their father (and mother)? How would the wife like to organize her daily activities? How does she perceive her husband's situation, and what does dementia mean to her? Furthermore, we should then examine ourselves and ask whether we could accept the wife's priority to dress her husband so that he appears well groomed rather than taking the time to let him dress independently and refraining from helping if independent dressing is time consuming and tiring for both of them and ultimately produces less successful results.

Stage 4

On the basis of the previous stages, the occupational therapist in the fourth stage analyzes and interprets the caregiver's point of view to design an intervention that will best suit the unique caregiving situation. In this example, we can plan, on the basis of our understanding and interpretation of the caregiving situation, to teach the wife grooming techniques that will facilitate the physical efforts necessary for the task. At the same time, we can teach the wife how to engage her husband in an activity that she perceives to be respectful to his image and that is manageable and meaningful to him as well. We can help her plan a weekly schedule and include in it times in which a paid helper or her children will handle the caregiving responsibilities to give her some relief and to enable her to engage in activities that are necessary to run her household and other activities that are important to her.

The four steps occur in a dynamic and cyclical order and serve mainly as principles to understand the inner meanings of caregiving to different caregivers so that we can design individualized intervention programs.

Caregiver Stress and Burnout

Throughout this chapter, we discuss the various ways in which caregiving can be stressful both for informal family caregivers and for formal caregivers, including occupational therapy practitioners. A certain amount of stress is inherent in the caregiving situation, and the caregiver should expect that. However, prolonged or inordinately high levels of stress can lead to burnout, a condition in which the negative aspects of the situation totally overwhelm the caregiver to the point that he or she is unable to continue without incurring serious physical or psychological damage. Support groups for caregivers, for clients and family members, and for professionals are generally an important protective action (Cohen, 1996; Peiffer & Crooker, 1990).

Occupational therapy practitioners may need to provide training to caregivers in effective ways to accomplish their caregiving activities so that they are less likely to become exhausted and discouraged. Practitioners can advise persons already experiencing burnout about strategies to overcome it and about coping techniques to help them continue to function despite their tremendous amount of stress. Occupational therapy practitioners can refer family members to appropriate support groups and provide information and appropriate referrals to other care alternatives when family members reach the end of their ability to provide total care.

Engaging Clients in Caregiving

Many persons who have chronic physical, mental, cognitive, or developmental disabilities do not have the opportunity to engage in caregiving. Similarly, others often deny young persons with physical and developmental disabilities initial access to any caregiving responsibility. In addition, persons who are injured may suddenly lose their caregiving abilities and unexpectedly lose their customary caregiving roles. Finally, older persons often renounce their role as caregivers, even though the role may have been central to their lives. Moreover, if a caregiver's health deteriorates as a result of illness, stroke, a mental condition, or cognitive deterioration, they generally lose their remaining activities and responsibilities for caregiving.

In this way, caregiving seems to be incompatible with receiving care because often clients with disabilities do not have the right to care for others. For some of these persons, especially women, taking care of the welfare of their family members and neighbors had been a central part of their existence. With others, especially younger persons with developmental, cognitive, or physical disabilities, although we recognize the importance of helping them move from receiving care to caring for themselves, we often fail to consider the advantages and consequences of moving them further along that continuum to giving care to others. To help all of these persons, therefore, we must be aware of the importance of caregiving as a developmental and empowering experience to many persons and give them opportunities to engage in the tasks involved in caregiving.

Another potential benefit of clients engaging in caregiving exists. Because caregiving is such a complex activity that requires multilevel skills, through involvement in the required tasks, clients can possibly improve their level of functioning in other areas. Moreover, involvement in caregiving activities usually has enhanced meaning because, in the past, caregiving has usually been important in most persons' lives. Nevertheless, we should always remember that caregiving does have different meanings for different persons. Therefore, although we should make caregiving available to clients, we must always give them the choice of whether and how to become involved.

Occupational Therapy Interventions

The following examples illustrate how caregiving is useful in the treatment of different groups of clients. Much of the emphasis in this chapter thus far has been on the caregiver, both informal (family members) and formal (paid nonprofessional or professional) and on the caregivers' needs for skills specifically used in the caregiving process and for strategies to deal with stress and to prevent possible burnout. We have already discussed how occupational therapy practitioners provide information and activities as interventions for both of these groups of caregivers as clients. We have shown how occupational therapy practitioners, as professional caregivers themselves, can develop ways to guide themselves and other professionals in methods of delivering care in difficult situations and can develop strategies to deal with their own stress and possible burnout as caregivers.

This section of the chapter deals with the perhaps more obvious, but often unserved, population of clients who because of age, impairment, or lack of opportunity have themselves reduced or eliminated the element of caregiving in their own lives or whom others have forced to relinquish caregiving. As we have demonstrated, whether the occupation of caregiving to others was an important part of their previous life roles or in situations in which they never fully developed this occupation, we now know that having the opportunity to give care to others is a fundamental and important part of being human and living a meaningful life. Therefore, we, as occupational therapy practitioners, must provide such opportunities for caregiving to our clients. We can provide education or reeducation in caring as an occupation when necessary and in the supportive environment in which this caregiving occurs by structuring appropriate activities in which our clients can participate. Accordingly, below are some examples of the kinds of activities that will accomplish this objective.

Case Scenario 11

Young children can become involved in being sensitive to and providing care for the needs of others in many ways. When children see their teachers or their therapists being sensitive to the feelings of others and doing small caring actions such as making sure that persons are comfortable in their wheelchairs, that persons can reach all of the supplies they need while doing a project, or that persons are not left out of a conversation in a social situation, the children learn appropriate attitudes and behaviors. Children can participate in a toy or book drive by selecting one of their own toys or books or holiday gifts to give away, or they can make gifts during the holidays to donate to less fortunate children. Children can "adopt" an elderly nursing home resident and send drawings, photographs, or small gifts to their adopted grandparent; they can then be encouraged to visit the nursing home in a group to sing songs or to bring their pets or a favorite object to talk about with the elderly person.

Case Scenario 12

We can work with adolescents with cognitive, physical, or mental disabilities and help them become involved in taking care of others. Frequently, no one in the family will consider involving these adolescents in family caregiving tasks, which denies them the opportunity to develop a caring attitude, to acquire the skills that are within their capability, and to experience the satisfaction and social recognition connected to the role. We can teach adolescents the skills necessary for feeding or cleaning their pet and taking the responsibility for its well-being. To do so, we must prepare family members to change their attitudes toward these adolescents. We may need to alter the social environment if necessary. With the support of the human and nonhuman environment, we can create opportunities for these young persons to practice some caregiving tasks and to change their self-perception and that of their parents from being solely care receivers to being caregivers.

Case Scenario 13

An occupational therapy program for a group of young male clients with traumatic brain injury addressed caregiving to others as an area of deficit and a lost role that would, if regained, help these men to feel as if they are able to pursue male roles in society once again. Intervention involved identifying with each man the kinds of roles he had formerly occupied and the ways in which he had cared for or provided for others before his brain injury. After that, the therapist developed specific strategies with each man to take advantage of opportunities within his current environment to either resume some of the caregiving activities or to substitute other caregiving activities that would offer the same kinds of fulfillment. The men who engaged in satisfying activities by volunteering at a nursing home or by contributing to others through resuming community member and extended family roles indicated that doing these activities helped them to feel more like men (Gutman, 1999).

Case Scenario 14

Persons who are injured or who have illnesses that force them to relinquish caregiving roles at the height of their responsibilities may feel a double loss in being unable to fulfill a role of great value to them when they realize that their inability to do so causes hardship for loved ones. This situation may arise when a parent with young children is injured or when the caregiving spouse of an elderly person suddenly has a stroke. In such situations, the occupational therapist can help the person evaluate the extent of the injury and the likelihood of their being able to resume their caregiving responsibilities with appropriate training, assistance, or assistive devices. If the person is not going to be able to resume these activities, then helping to make appropriate alternative caregiving arrangements would solve the immediate situation and may alleviate worry and guilt. Finally, clients should find alternative ways of expressing caregiving, for example, by talking to and reading to their children if performing physical caregiving activities is no longer possible.

Case Scenario 15

We can involve elderly persons in community projects or help them to improve the skills necessary for taking care of their spouse, their children, or their grand-children at home. For example, we can establish a cooking group in a community-based center for elderly persons. The group can engage in cooking food and giving it to the needy members of the community. Moreover, during holiday periods, the group can have special projects by preparing different meals and bringing them to charity dinners in churches, hospitals, or assisted living facilities. The group can focus on preparing traditional holiday dinners, such as Italian or German Christmas dinners, a Jewish Passover Seder, a Chinese New Year meal, or a Ramadan nightly dinner, and distribute these to needy persons in their community. In this way, the group members can connect to their own traditions and history while engaging in giving care to persons from their own community at spiritually important times of the year. Cooking can help by combining old skills and knowledge with exercising new or relearning impaired skills. Cooking can help to improve executive functions such as reading, counting, following a sequence of steps, and decision making as well as improve physical skills. Cooking requires planning, following directions and sequencing, recalling old knowledge and memorizing new directions, identifying mistakes, problem solving, fine and gross motor function, mobility, and more. The group activity requires social and interpersonal skills such as sharing responsibility, tasks, appliances, and working together in a shared space toward a common goal. At the same time, the therapist can plan the activity in such a way that each member of the group will contribute according to his or her ability. The opportunity to provide caring for others through feeding them, literally and symbolically, can be extremely satisfying to those whose life experience involved receiving satisfaction from fulfilling the needs of others in their families or social circles.

Case Scenario 16

Hasselkus (1993) movingly described the caregiving role of the occupational therapy practitioner during the dying process in her description of her own experience in caring for her dying mother. Her situation involved a very elderly person who was physically frail but cognitively alert in a hospital in which other hospital staff members performed her physical care. Not all deaths take place in this manner, of course. In this situation, Hasselkus described the stages of care that she went through and suggested that, whatever the actual time sequence, caregiving for the dying may start out as what she terms "caregiving from a distance," which involves watching, monitoring, and offering suggestions. She then progressed to more frequent caregiving in which she began taking responsibility for household matters. Then, during the dying phase, her caregiving tasks changed to listening, talking, helping her mother conduct life reviews, funeral planning, and helping her mother face dying and the death process.

Summary

In this chapter, we explored the meaning of caring, caregiving, and care receiving. We discussed the importance of maintaining our opportunities to be caregivers throughout our lifetimes, and we gave examples of the ways in which persons can care. Finally, we presented some ways in which occupational therapy practitioners can encourage caregiving for persons of all ages and with all kinds of disabilities through the use of purposeful activities. ■

Appendix

Exercise 3 Discussion

1. For the mother, although caregiving to her children and parents is satisfying for her and is part of her self-perception, she mainly associates caregiving with burden and stress. She may have difficulty dividing her time between the needs of her parents and the needs of her children (the "sandwich generation" phenomenon), which could cause her guilt. She may use the situation to teach her children about the importance of caring for their elderly grandparents by role modeling such caring behaviors. In addition, the mother may focus on teaching her children independence and transferring to them some of the caregiving responsibilities for their younger siblings.

2. For the grandmother, although caregiving for her grandchild will involve some physical and emotional burdens, caregiving may be mainly a satisfying activity related to her occupational history that is deeply connected to her self-definition. Although the grandmother will be involved in the one-to-one relationship with her grandchild, she may need to be somewhat careful and use good ergonomic techniques with tasks requiring physical effort to avoid injuring herself.

3. The paid aide may focus mainly on the hands-on tasks of caregiving while being cautiously emotionally involved. Her job satisfaction is connected to salary and to her personal and cultural perception of caring. She may or may not try to help ease the frustration and loneliness of her client, and she may have difficulty with her own hostility toward him.

4. The son can be more involved in organizing help for his mother, in talking with her, in giving her guidance on how to manage her difficulties, and in being emotionally involved and deeply concerned about her well-being. His caregiving may have financial implications as well, if by his doing so she can avoid having to hire a personal attendant or moving into a nursing home. At some point, however, he may have to relinquish some caring activities to a paid caregiver or help his mother find and make the transition to an assisted living or long-term care facility.

5. The child care worker or babysitter may enjoy interacting with the child and establish a relationship with her but may focus on the hands-on tasks of playing with her and keeping the child safe until her mother returns. In addition, her rewards are connected to the salary earned for the job.

6. The wife may be frustrated about the drudgery of taking care of her husband, who is getting progressively weaker. She may be sad about the loss of their lifestyle in earlier years when he was healthy, and their lives were easier. She may still, however, love him enough to do all of the tasks that are necessary without overwhelming stress. She may need to consider the effect of his illness and her caregiving on other family members, including their children. After a while, she may become physically and emotionally exhausted and may need the help of a support group for well spouses. At some point, she may need to consider alternative caregiving settings.

7. The elderly man may be in failing health himself or may not be used to performing the domestic household tasks that his wife formerly handled, or he may be uncomfortable with caring for his wife's personal needs. Still, because of their lifelong relationship, this may be a labor of love and respect that he refuses to relinquish to a professional caregiver. He may be fearful of losing his companion and of what may happen to him if she dies or must move to a nursing home if he can no longer care for her.

8. The daughter may find spiritual comfort in taking care of her dying mother, and at the same time, she may be overwhelmed with grief at the prospect of her mother's death. The daughter may be relieved at not having to care for her mother's routine daily physical needs and may thus be able to concentrate on helping her mother through life review and other preparatory activities to have a peaceful dying experience. This experience could be extremely meaningful for both of them.

9. The religious leader can advise his or her congregation about how to improve the quality of their lives, organize projects to help the needy members of the community, and establish a moral commitment to helping others. He or she receives continual feedback from the congregation in the form of demands for attention, complaints, compliments, thanks, love, and respect. The religious

leader may feel a special calling and may receive spiritual rewards for religious activities. At the same time, he or she receives a salary for the work, which may be the leader's livelihood.

References

American Association of Retired Persons. (1999). News excerpt. *AARP Bulletin, 40*, 20.

Abel, E. K. (1991). *Who cares for the elderly? Public policy and experiences of adult daughters.* Philadelphia: Temple University.

Abbot, N. (1990). The caregiving alliance. *Occupational Therapy Practice, 2*, 60–65.

Beach, D. L. (1997). Family caregiving: The positive impact on adolescent relationships. *The Gerontologist, 37*, 233–238.

Bowden, P. (1997). *Caring: Gender-sensitive ethics.* New York: Routledge.

Brody, E. M., & Lang, A. (1982). They can't do it all: Aging daughters with aged mothers. *Generations, 7*, 18–20.

Cahn, A. (1975). *Women in the U.S. labor force.* New York: Praeger.

Chang, C. F., & White-Means, S. I. (1991). The men who care: An analysis of male primary caregivers who care for frail elderly at home. *Journal for Applied Gerontology, 10*, 343–358.

Christiansen, C., & Baum, C. (1997). Person–environment occupational performance: A conceptual model for practice. In C. H. Christiansen, & C. M. Baum (Eds.), *Enabling function and well-being* (pp. 46–70). Thorofare, NJ: Slack.

Clark, C. A., Corcoran, M., & Gitlin, L. N. (1995). An exploratory study of how occupational therapists develop therapeutic relationships with family caregivers. *American Journal of Occupational Therapy, 49*, 587–594.

Clement, G. (1996). *Care, autonomy, and justice: Feminism and an ethic of care.* Boulder, CO: Westview Press.

Cohen, M. D. (1996). *Dirty details: The days and nights of a well spouse.* Philadelphia: Temple University Press.

Corcoran, M., & Gitlin, L. N. (1992). Dementia management: An occupational therapy home-based intervention for caregivers. *American Journal of Occupational Therapy, 46*, 801–808.

Dear Abby. (1999, February 16). *The Intelligencer Record*, p. D4.

Diemut Bubeck, E. (1995). *Care, gender and justice.* Oxford: Clarendon Press.

Dougherty, P. M., & Radomski, M. V. (Eds.). (1990). The caregiving alliance (Special issue). *Occupational Therapy Practice, 2.*

Dwyer, J. W., & Coward, R. T. (1991). A multivariate comparison of the involvement of adult sons versus adult daughters in the care of impaired parents. *Journal of Gerontology, 46*, 258–269.

Fisher, B., & Tronto, J. (1990). Toward a feminist theory of caring. In E. K. Abel & M. K. Nelson (Eds.), *Circles of care: Work and identity in women's life* (pp. 35–62). Albany, NY: State University of New York.

Fogelman, E. (1994). *Conscience and courage: Rescuers of Jews during the holocaust.* New York: Anchor Books.

Gilligan, C. (1982). *In a different voice.* Cambridge, MA: Harvard University.

Gitlin, L. N., & Corcoran, M. (1993). Expanding caregiver ability to use environmental solutions for problems of bathing and incontinence in the elderly with dementia. *Technology and Disability, 2,* 12–21.

Gitlin, L. N., Corcoran, M., & Leinmiller-Eckhardt, S. (1995). Understanding the family perspective: An ethnographic framework for providing occupational therapy in the home. *American Journal of Occupational Therapy, 49,* 802–809.

Graham, H. (1983). Caring: A labour of love. In J. Finch & D. Groves (Eds.), *A labour of love: Women, work and caring.* Boston: Routledge & Kegan Paul.

Greif, J. (1994). *AIDS care at home: A guide for caregivers, loved ones, and people with AIDS.* New York: Wiley.

Grott, G. (1998, March 16). The caregiving therapist. *Advance for Occupational Therapists,* 19.

Gutman, S. A. (1999). Alleviating gender role strain in adult men with traumatic brain injury: An evaluation of a set of guidelines for occupational therapy. *American Journal of Occupational Therapy, 53,* 101–110.

Harris, P. B. (1998). Listening to caregiving sons: Misunderstood realities. *Gerontologist, 38,* 342–352.

Harris, P. B., & Bichler, J. (1997). *Men giving care: Reflections of husbands and sons.* New York: Garland.

Hasselkus, B. R. (1988). Meaning in family caregiving: Perspectives on caregiver/professional relationships. *Gerontologist, 28,* 686–691.

Hasselkus, B. R. (1990). Ethnographic interviewing: A tool for practice with family caregivers for the elderly. *Occupational Therapy Practice, 2,* 9–16.

Hasselkus, B. R. (1991). Ethical dilemmas in family caregiving for the elderly: Implication for occupational therapy. *American Journal of Occupational Therapy, 45,* 206–212.

Hasselkus, B. R. (1993). Death in very old age: A personal journey of caregiving. *American Journal of Occupational Therapy, 47,* 717–723.

Hasselkus, B. R. (1998). Occupation and well-being in dementia: The experience of day-care staff. *American Journal of Occupational Therapy, 52,* 423–434.

Hochschild, A. R. (1983). Emotion work, feeling rules, and social structure. *American Journal of Sociology, 85,* 551–575.

Horowitz, A. (1985). Family caregiving to the frail elderly. *Annual Review of Gerontology and Geriatrics, 5,* 194–246.

Humphry, R., & Case-Smith, J. (1996). Working with families. In J. Case-Smith, A. S. Allen, & P. N. Clark (Eds.), *Occupational therapy for children* (3rd ed., pp. 67–98). St. Louis: Mosby.

Mason, R. (1999, March). Foreign assistance. *Hadassah Magazine,* 80.

McRae, H. (1998). Managing feelings: Caregiving as emotion work. *Research on Aging, 20,* 137–160.

Moroney, R. M., Dokecki, P. R., Gated, J. J., Noser Haynes, K., Newbrough, J. R., & Nottingham, J. A. (1998). *Caring and competent caregivers.* Athens, GA: University of Georgia.

National Family Caregivers Association. (1997). *NCFA/Fortis report: Caregiving across the life cycle.* Kensington, MD: Author.

Nieva, V. F., & Gutek, B. A. (1981). *Women and work: A psychological perspective.* New York: Praeger.

Oliner, S., & Oliner, P. (1988). *The altruistic personality: Rescuers of Jews in Nazi Europe.* New York: Free Press.

Peiffer, M., & Crooker, B. M. (1990). Our story: Two perspectives of family caregiving. *Occupational Therapy Practice, 2,* 45–52.

Piercy, K. W. (1998). Theorizing about family caregiving: The role of responsibility. *Journal of Marriage and the Family, 60,* 109–118.

Rudick, S. (1989). *Maternal thinking toward a politics of peace.* Boston: Beacon Press.

Sachs, D. (1988). *The perception of caring held by female occupational therapists: Implications for professional role and identity.* Unpublished doctoral dissertation, New York University.

Sachs, D., & Labovitz, D. R. (1994). The caring occupational therapist: Scope of professional roles and boundaries. *American Journal of Occupational Therapy, 48,* 997–1005.

Scharlach, A., Low, B., & Schneider, E. (1991). *Elder care and the work force: Blueprint for action.* Lexington, MA: Lexington Books.

Smalley, S. (1990). Chronic illness and codependence: The caring role. *Occupational Therapy Practice, 2,* 1–8.

Vergara, E. R., & Angley, J. C. (1990). Preparing families to take home a high-risk infant. *Occupational Therapy Practice, 2,* 66–83.

Williams, J. H. (1983). *Psychology of women: Behavior in the biosocial context* (2nd ed.). New York: Norton.

Wuthnow, R. (1995). *Learning to care: Elementary kindness in an age of indifference.* London: Oxford University Press.

16

Activities, the Empowerment Process, and Client-Motivated Change

Sharon A. Gutman, PhD, OTR
Paula McCreedy, MEd, OT/L
Prudence Heisler, MA, OT/L

Since the profession's inception in the early 1900s, occupational therapists have observed that engagement in meaningful activity facilitates a sense of competence or empowerment (Clark et al., 1991; Dunton, 1919; Kielhofner, 1995; Meyer, 1922; Mosey, 1986; Reilly, 1974). Therapists have not, however, been able to articulate as thoroughly the process by which activity is able to facilitate empowerment. This chapter explores the use of activity to empower persons with disabilities, delineates the principal elements involved in the empowerment process, and illustrates the role of client-motivated change by using case examples.

The Empowerment Process

Empowerment is the process through which persons obtain the competence necessary to exert a positive influence on the social systems, groups, persons, and personal behaviors that affect their quality of life (Wilson, 1996). Quality of life is the extent to which persons believe that life is meaningful, manageable and comprehensible and provides opportunities for personal growth and goal attainment (Hood, Beaudet, & Catlin, 1996). Persons often measure quality of life by the degree to which they have been able to establish satisfying interpersonal relationships (and the internalization of acceptance by family members or friends), the presence of a supportive social network for needed resources and guidance, and participation in activity that provides a sense of meaning and personal gratification (Antonovsky, 1992).

Empowerment often involves the presence of five fundamental elements (Gutierrez, 1995).

1. A repertoire of skills. Persons must establish a repertoire of skills that will help them to meet environmental challenges and demands.

2. A sense of competence. A sense of competence involves the belief that one's skills are sufficient to achieve desired goals.

3. Feelings of self-determination. Self-determination is the belief that one can exert volitional control or personal will over life circumstances to enhance one's quality of life.

4. A sense of belonging. A sense of belonging involves the recognition that one deserves acceptance as a member of the community (or larger society) versus having others ostracize him or her because of disability. Recognizing that one deserves acceptance as a member of the community involves the corollary beliefs that one is entitled to participate in and contribute to the community as any other group member would and that one's contributions are valuable to the community.

5. A sense of equality. A sense of equality is the belief that one has the same rights as all others to strive for and achieve a personally satisfying quality of life.

These five fundamental elements underlie the empowerment process and are present when persons believe that they can exert a positive influence on their life circumstances to enhance their quality of life. The empowerment process additionally requires the person to make four attitudinal and behavioral changes (Wilson, 1996).

1. The belief in personal change. The first change necessitates that persons accept the belief that they have choices and that they can act on them. Recognizing that one has choices is the first step in the empowerment process and is necessary for persons to replace stagnation with action.

2. Internal motivation. A second change requires that persons mobilize their internal resources to take action. To mobilize one's internal resources, persons must be internally motivated to engage in the change process. Such internal motivation results from the belief in both personal choice and in one's ability to implement desired change.

3. The belief in self-effectiveness. A third change mandates that persons obtain a repertoire of skills necessary to meet environmental challenges and demands. Self-effectiveness requires the initial belief that one can learn and master the skills necessary to implement desired change.

4. The establishment of external support. A fourth change requires persons to develop a supportive social network consisting of family members, peers, and health care providers to rely on during the natural setbacks and gains that occur in every change process. Persons must internalize such external support to use

effectively the material and emotional resources of the support system when members of the support network are not present.

Disempowerment as a Result of Disability

To understand fully the components of the empowerment process, one must explore the factors that precipitate disempowerment. Disability is often disempowering because it limits a person's capacity to perform the skills needed to function competently in family systems, at school and work sites, and in communities. Disability disrupts long-established roles and relationships among persons and their family members, friends, and coworkers, which causes role strain and role loss (Goffman, 1963; Mosey, 1986; Pearlin & Schooler, 1978). As a result of such role strain, persons often lose their predisability identity and must recreate and renegotiate roles and relationships that were once familiar and stable.

For example, a change in one family member's roles, abilities, and identity affects and alters the family system as an entity. Other family members may need to adopt new roles to maintain the family system's functioning. Therapists must gain an understanding of the effects of change on all family roles and relationships to help the family system adapt to and survive the disruptions that result from a loved one's disability. Practitioners should encourage family members to collaborate with and participate in their loved one's treatment planning and therapy.

Practitioners must recognize that an unwanted disability has forced such change processes on persons and their family members. All change processes are difficult and frequently require protracted periods of time. Change processes that a disability thrusts on the person are disempowering, particularly because these changes disrupt one's sense of control and volition.

Practitioners must additionally recognize that the traditional medical model often disempowers persons with disability because the patient assumes a passive "sick" role, and the medical authority assumes a position of dominance and control. The traditional medical model often encourages persons who become patients to believe in their ineffectiveness and powerlessness, which, in turn, produces feelings of alienation, loss of self-esteem, and loss of dignity (Mattingly & Fleming, 1994).

We can measure disempowerment by the presence of six principle elements.

1. Loss of self-determination. Loss of self-determination occurs when the person believes that the disability has taken away volitional control and personal choice.

2. Loss of competence. Loss of competence and the concomitant feeling of inadequacy occur when the person loses the skills necessary to meet the demands of the environment and consequently feels a lack of proficiency regarding previously mastered daily life activities.

3.   The experience of stigmatization. Stigmatization occurs when the person believes that the larger community has ostracized or set apart him or her because of disability, appearance, or a difference in functional abilities.

4.   Feelings of devaluation. One feels devalued by the larger society when one perceives that the community, work site, or family system neither accepts nor respects his or her contributions.

5.   Feelings of inequality. Feeling unequal to other community members occurs when the person believes that the community, work site, and family system no longer consider the person to have the same rights as all others to strive for and to achieve a personally satisfying quality of life as a result of the disability.

6.   Loss of self-identity. Loss of one's predisability identity occurs when the person no longer understands himself or herself in relation to familiar persons and objects in the environment. Loss of self-identity occurs as a result of the disruption in predisability activities, roles, and relationships. Practitioners must understand that persons experience even the loss of dysfunctional activities, roles, and relationships as a disempowering loss of identity and should acknowledge this loss as such.

Therapeutic Facilitation of Client-Motivated Change

Understanding how to address therapeutically the components of disempowerment is a critical skill that often differentiates the experienced clinician from the novice (Benner, 1984; Benner & Tanner, 1987; Mattingly & Fleming, 1994). The ability to assist persons who feel disempowered to mobilize their internal resources requires the practitioner both to instill hope and to confront the defense mechanisms that enable the person to remain in a disempowered state. Denial, rationalization, and attachment to dysfunctional activities, roles, and relationships are defense mechanisms that may hinder a person from mobilizing the internal resources necessary to alter one's quality of life positively (Horney, 1950). Practitioners must be aware of a client's use of defense mechanisms and understand how to confront their operation in a client's life therapeutically.

The concept of ambivalence is critical for practitioners to understand when helping clients through a change process resulting from a disability. Ambivalence occurs when persons hold opposing or contradicting affective orientations toward a specific person, object, or event (Smelser, 1998). Clients commonly experience ambivalent emotions toward their disability, their practitioners, and their treatment process. Practitioners must understand that, although ambivalence hinders motivation, ambivalence is a normal experience in the range of human responses to disability. Practitioners must learn to tolerate a client's ambivalence to help that client to use his or her ambivalent feelings to bring about positive change. Helping a client both to recognize and accept ambivalence consciously is a critical step in the facilitation of motivation.

The instillation of hope (or the ability to persuade persons to believe that they either possess or can develop the skills necessary to enhance their life satisfaction) can often be more difficult than confronting defense mechanisms and ambivalence, and the degree of resilience, tenacity, and perseverance persons possess can greatly influence their level of hope. Why some clients experience successful rehabilitation courses whereas others lose motivation likely depends on both genetic traits and life experience, among other factors. Regardless of whether a person possesses high or low levels of resilience and perseverance, however, practitioners can use specific techniques to facilitate motivation when persons feel disempowered. Bandura (1977) described motivation as coming from four principal sources.

1.   Performance accomplishments

2.   Vicarious experience

3.   Verbal persuasion

4.   Optimal emotional states

First, performance accomplishments are the success experiences that clients must encounter to develop the motivation to change. When clients who participate in new activities experience a series of successes, they are more likely to develop the confidence and skills necessary to accomplish feared but desired life goals eventually (Bandura, 1977). Occupational therapy practitioners grade activities in accordance with a client's skill level to facilitate success experiences. Practitioners choose activities that allow the client to practice needed skills in a safe, nonthreatening environment. The participation in activities should begin in simulated settings (e.g., the occupational therapy clinic) and move to the natural environment (e.g., a community shopping center, the work site) as the client gains competence. The therapist continually grades the activity higher until the client is practicing the actual set of skills necessary to enhance his or her quality of life.

For example, a client may need to obtain the skills necessary for a job interview. The practitioner and client may role-play the job interview scenario, first in the safety of the occupational therapy clinic and then in a simulated office setting. The practitioner may ask the client initially to practice one skill, such as maintaining eye contact while answering interview questions. When the client masters this skill, the practitioner grades the activity higher so that the client may then need to maintain eye contact while answering questions, dress appropriately for an employment interview, and shake hands with the employer both before and after the interview. Later in the sequence of therapy, the client may practice interviewing skills in a series of real-life employment interviews for jobs that he or she does not want. The practitioner provides continual feedback so that the client can continue to make improvements in skill level. In this way, the practitioner sets up the optimal conditions through which a client can gradually experience success until the client masters the highest level of desired skill.

Second, vicarious experience involves learning from observing others or modeling (Bandura, 1977). Providing opportunities for clients to observe similar others who have successfully gained the skills the client desires can encourage motivation. Opportunities for clients to observe how others engage in specific skill behaviors should occur in both simulated (e.g., television, film) and natural environments (e.g., the community shopping center) to provide optimal learning experiences in graded settings.

Practitioners can grade vicarious experience by providing the opportunity for clients to receive mentorship from a peer who has experienced a successful rehabilitation course. Alcoholics Anonymous and many consumer service organizations have effectively used the peer mentorship or buddy system to provide persons with a mentor who, through vicarious experience, can model appropriate behaviors that the client must adopt to enhance his or her quality of life (Caron & Bergeron, 1995; Hutchison, Osborne-Way, & Lord, 1986). For example, Gutman and Swarbrick (1998) described a woman, Eli, who sustained a head injury as a result of abuse perpetrated by a male partner. As part of her participation in an occupational therapy group, the therapist paired Eli with a woman who had successfully extricated herself from prior abusive relationships and had learned the skills necessary to lead a more healthful lifestyle and have a positive self-regard. Through peer mentorship, this woman was able to both challenge Eli's risk-taking behaviors and model the positive skills Eli needed to end her pattern of participation in abusive relationships.

Vicarious experience is often a powerful method of learning because it offers the client an opportunity to observe that others sharing similar life circumstances were able to make the positive life changes that the client wants to make. Such an observation can be highly motivating because persons often find more credibility in peer mentors who have lived similar experiences than in practitioners who may not share the same gender, race, socioeconomic class, or cultural belief systems as the client (Krefting, 1991; Mattingly & Fleming, 1994). The use of peer mentors to facilitate learning specific life skills is an important therapeutic tool that all occupational therapy practitioners should use when treating clients who may not be able to relate to the practitioner's own cultural background and life experience.

Vicarious experience is an effective motivator because it allows clients to observe the accomplishments of similar others and inspires the belief that clients, too, can achieve desired positive outcomes. Vicarious experience becomes most effective when the client is able to transform the modeled behaviors into an internal resource guide that the client can refer to when the peer mentor is not present.

Third, verbal persuasion is a form of motivation in which others persuade the person to believe that he or she possesses the ability to master difficult skills (Bandura, 1977). In the initial use of verbal persuasion, the practitioner (or peer mentor) seeks to build confidence in the client by verbally coaxing him or her to attempt the performance of new and often feared activities. As the client begins to practice desired skills on a consistent basis, verbal persuasion takes the form of a set of instructions regarding the performance of specific behaviors. Such instructions act as a guide for the client to follow independently when the practitioner is not present. Later, when the client has internalized the verbal instructions, he or she can use verbal persuasion to talk himself or herself through a particular activity requiring the newly learned skills.

For example, a client who wants to learn assertiveness training skills to deal more effectively with demanding employers and coworkers may initially need the verbal coaxing of a practitioner or peer mentor to believe that he or she can indeed learn and use desired assertive behaviors. The practitioner and client may role-play the use of assertiveness techniques in specific scenarios that the client is likely to encounter, and other group members may verbally encourage the client as he or she practices the use of new assertive behaviors. Additionally, the practitioner may talk the client through a specific scenario that requires assertive behaviors as the client engages in role-playing activities with another client. In either case, the verbal persuasion becomes a set of instructions to help the client to learn and master assertiveness techniques in specific situations. A goal of therapy is that the client will later internalize such verbal persuasion and that the persuasion will serve as a guide in social situations when the practitioner and group members are not present. For such internalization to occur, the practitioner must provide the opportunity for a sufficient amount of role-playing and real-life practice until the client demonstrates comfort and independent mastery of desired skills.

Finally, Bandura (1977) described optimal emotional arousal as a fourth form of motivation. Because high degrees of arousal often reduce one's performance level, practitioners must help clients to achieve optimal emotional states through stress reduction techniques. Persons rely in part on their anxiety level and physiological arousal when evaluating their ability to perform feared or novel activities. When clients experience high degrees of anxiety in response to specific feared or novel activities, they are likely to believe that they are unable to learn the skills necessary to perform those activities effectively. Until a client's physiological state reaches a comfortable level (i.e., a level in which the client can comfortably engage in the practice of feared activities), new learning will not take place. The practitioner has the responsibility to address reducing anxiety before all other desired therapeutic activities. Stress reduction techniques may take the form of breathing exercises, meditation, guided imagery, and biofeedback. If such therapeutic techniques are not effective, then the client may need a referral for pharmacological intervention to reduce anxiety (American Psychiatric Association, 1994). The therapist has the responsibility to determine when pharmacological intervention is necessary.

One of the most effective forms of stress reduction is desensitization therapy (Wolpe, 1958, 1981). Before actually practicing the skills necessary for a specific feared or novel activity, the client engages in a series of visualization techniques in which he or she visually imagines participating in the feared activity while in the safety of the therapy setting. The client practices desensitization therapy until he or she is able visually to imagine himself or herself participating in the feared activity without concomitant feelings of anxiety. At this time, the practitioner can direct therapeutic activities toward role-playing and, later, real-life practice. For example, John, a client with a history of depression, panic disorder, and substance abuse, reported that he experienced anxiety in response to various job stressors, including the need to make presentations for his job. John's attempt to alleviate his performance anxiety through alcohol intake resulted in a temporary suspension from his employment, and his employer required that John participate in a compulsory drug and alcohol abuse program before returning to work. As part of his rehabilitation, John participated in an occupational therapy group in which he learned stress reduction techniques such as meditation and biofeedback. John received one-to-one desensitization therapy with an occupational therapist that enabled him to practice public speaking in his mind in the safety of the therapeutic setting. When John reported that he could imagine himself engaged in the activity of public speaking without experiencing debilitating levels of anxiety, John then began to practice making short presentations aloud in front of the occupational therapist. Shortly thereafter, John attempted to present in front of his five-member occupational therapy group. At this time, because John reexperienced high degrees of anxiety that rendered his presentation skills non-functional, the facility's psychiatrist prescribed an antianxiety medication for John. The medication enabled John to continue his practice of public speaking in front of the occupational therapy group without feelings of extreme apprehension. As a result of continued practice without anxiety, John was able to learn the skills of public speaking necessary to maintain his current employment.

Knowing when to use performance accomplishments, vicarious experience, verbal persuasion, and stress reduction techniques to motivate clients is a skill that develops with clinical experience. A clinician who initiates such techniques too quickly in the therapeutic process without respecting the client's need to grieve over losses may unwittingly dissolve a client's trust and further inhibit motivation. Before initiating motivation techniques, practitioners must understand that a period of grieving about lost roles and relationships (even dysfunctional ones) must occur before clients can mobilize their internal resources to recreate meaningful lives.

Practitioners must recognize that change processes are difficult and that each client will require varying lengths of time to grow more comfortable with changes resulting from disability or illness. Practitioners must help their clients to understand that rehabilitation often involves a series of gains and setbacks. Setbacks that occur in a rehabilitation course are not indications of failure but rather are a natural occurrence of all change processes. Practitioners who are able to convey an understanding of these ideas to their clients have made major strides in the initial stages of the motivation process.

Use of Activity in the Empowerment Process

One of the principle philosophical assumptions of occupational therapy is that participating in meaningful occupation is necessary for persons to gain a sense of mastery over their environment and life circumstances (Mosey, 1986; Reilly, 1974).

Occupational therapy practitioners assist persons with disabilities in performing desired activities that are necessary for them to function as members of a community and family system. Participation in activity is empowering because it provides the opportunity for humans to interact with the objects and persons in their surroundings. Activity is the primary medium through which persons seek a human experience (i.e., activity is the medium through which persons experience themselves in relation to the human and nonhuman environment). Persons know themselves through their engagement in activities that support their roles and relationships. Activity is innately empowering because it is almost always the medium through which humans communicate and socialize with each other. Thus, because humans are interdependent beings who know themselves through their interactions with the persons and objects in their environment, the engagement in activity is necessary to form a human identity.

The formation of human identity is a tiered process involving three primary steps (see Figure 1).

1.   In the first stage of identity formation, persons participate in specific chosen activities that can support the assumption of desired social roles.

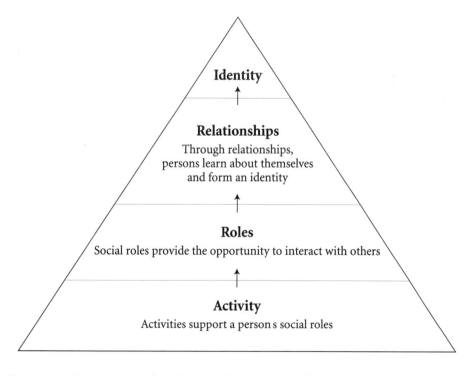

Figure 1. Activities support the roles and relationships that form a human identity.

2.   The assumption of specific social roles provides the opportunity for persons to engage in relationships with others.

3.   Through engagement in relationships and the activities and roles that support those relationships, humans come to know themselves as persons who are part of larger communities.

When disability causes the loss of meaningful activities, roles, and relationships, persons lose an understanding of who they are in relation to others in their environment. Consequently, one's sense of self or identity often becomes displaced as persons struggle to maintain familiar activities and roles that the onset of disability has jeopardized. For example, a woman 40 years of age with multiple sclerosis (MS) found that she could no longer participate in many of the caregiving activities required by her toddler, who was 4 years of age. As a result of the lost ability to participate in parenting activities, the client believed that she was losing her role as a mother and believed that her relationship with her husband was strained and uncomfortable. Because MS had disrupted the activities that supported her roles and relationships as a wife and mother, the client experienced a loss of the predisability identity that she had established before her diagnosis. Disability strips persons of familiar activities, roles, and relationships and forces them to surrender long-established and often comfortable identities.

Use of Activity To Empower Persons With Disabilities

By assisting persons with disabilities in engaging in the daily life activities that support their roles within communities, family systems, and work and school settings, occupational therapy practitioners provide one of the first opportunities for persons to feel empowered after the onset of disability. Practitioners address two primary categories of activity: activities of daily living (ADL), or basic self-care tasks, and instrumental ADL (IADL), or complex multistep activities that require the integration of higher-level cognitive skills (e.g., meal preparation, money management, community travel). In a broader sense, ADL and IADL are similar to Maslow's (1968) categorization of basic needs (or deficiency needs) and metaneeds (or growth needs; see Table 1). Basic needs include both physiological needs and safety needs and are akin to the basic self-care ADL that occupational therapy practitioners address (e.g., eating, bathing, dressing, home safety). Metaneeds involve the human need to experience a sense of belonging, self-esteem or personal competence, and self-actualization or feeling empowered in one's ability to accomplish life goals. The activities that support metaneeds mainly relate to the IADL that persons must perform to participate in complex social relationships and societal organizations. For example, the need to feel a sense of belonging requires a person to obtain the skills necessary to reintegrate into the community and to develop a supportive social network that provides needed resources and guidance. Self-esteem and competence needs require the person to develop a set of skills sufficient to meet specific environmental challenges

Table 1
A Comparison of ADL and Maslow's Need Hierarchy

ADL (Basic Needs)	*IADL (Metaneeds)*

Physiological needs
    The person can transfer from a bed to a toilet.
Safety needs
    The person is cognitively safe to live independently in his or her environment.
	Belongingness
	    The person has reintegrated into the community and become a participating group member whose contributions are valued. The person has developed a supportive network that provides resources and guidance.
	Self-esteem
	    The person is confident that his or her skills are sufficient to meet environmental challenges and demands.
	Self-actualization and empowerment
	    The person possesses the skills necessary to exert positive change to create a personally meaningful quality of life.

Note. ADL = activities of daily living, IADL = instrumental activities of daily living.

and demands (e.g., the ability to adhere to a monthly budget to maintain independent apartment living). Self-actualization needs require a person to develop the skills necessary to rebuild a personally satisfying quality of life in which he or she can accomplish desired life goals despite the presence of disability. For example, a person with quadriplegia may want to develop the skills necessary to return to school to embark on a more satisfying career postinjury.

Occupational therapy practitioners help clients to fulfill both basic and metaneeds through participation in activities that can support the roles and relationships that disability has disrupted. The process through which practitioners use activity to help clients to rebuild desired roles and relationships involves a sequence of five primary steps.

1. In the first therapeutic stage, the practitioner and client identify the specific roles and relationships that the client has lost as a result of disability or never gained as a result of developmental delay.

2. After identifying lost roles and relationships, the client and practitioner then indicate the specific activities that the client used to support lost roles and relationships. For persons who never obtained desired roles and relationships as a result of developmental delay, the practitioner must help the client to identify activities that could support desired but never obtained roles and relationships.

3.   The practitioner then encourages the client to determine which roles and relationships he or she wants to rebuild or build anew after the onset of disability or delay.

4.   The practitioner and client choose activities that will support the rebuilding of desired roles and relationships. The practitioner should assist the client in the adaptation of predisability activities in accordance with sequelae secondary to the client's disability. The practitioner should help the client to explore novel activities that could support the client's desired roles and relationships after the onset of disability or delay. In this way, the practitioner assists the client in accessing new resources (both internal and external).

5.   In the final therapeutic stages, the practitioner and client continue to practice the skills necessary to participate in the specific activities supporting desired roles and relationships. Through the engagement in such activities, the client is able to begin to rebuild an identity on the basis of satisfying interactions with the persons and objects in his or her environment.

To facilitate these steps, a practitioner can use the motivation techniques of Bandura (1977): performance accomplishments, vicarious experience, verbal persuasion, and stress reduction strategies. For example, a practitioner may set up the environmental conditions in which a client can experience graded performance accomplishments until he or she has attained a specific desired goal (e.g., perhaps regaining full-time employment in the community after experiencing drug and alcohol abuse problems). The practitioner may provide the opportunity for the client to observe, through vicarious experience, how others overcame their substance abuse and were able to regain full-time employment and personally satisfying friendships and family relationships. Stress reduction techniques may help the client to deal more effectively with work-related and social stressors that previously facilitated the client's substance abuse. The practitioner may use verbal persuasion to assist the client in creating an internal set of instructions that the client can use to talk himself or herself through specific stressful events.

Case Scenarios

The following case scenarios illustrate how occupational therapy practitioners can use activity to facilitate the resumption of desired roles and relationships. The five-step process outlined above serves as a guide for the reader to follow the therapeutic process.

Case Scenario 1

Tom was a white heterosexual man 40 years of age who at 24 years of age sustained a traumatic brain injury in an alcohol-related motor vehicle crash. As a result of his injury, Tom experienced severe short-term memory deficits and sexual disinhibition. Because of these deficits, Tom required supportive living services and spent the past 16 years in four different residential facilities for persons with brain injury. At his current residential placement, Tom was living in a community group home that housed four other men with traumatic brain injuries. Although Tom possessed the cognitive ability to perform most basic self-care activities with distant supervision (e.g., bathing, toileting, grooming, dressing, and household chores), he required close supervision for many IADL (e.g., meal preparation and money management). Although Tom additionally possessed the ability to remember the walking routes around his local community to access shopping, movies, recreational entertainment, and restaurants independently, Tom required the assistance of a staff member out in the larger community because of his impulsivity and sexual disinhibition.

Step 1: Identification of Roles and Relationships Disrupted by Injury

One of Tom's most disturbing role losses after injury concerned his inability to resume a dating or courtship role. Before his accident, Tom had enjoyed an active social life that included a series of monogamous sexual relationships with women. Tom's injury occurred to the dorsolateral frontal cortex and hypothalamic neural regions of the brain, areas that play a role in regulating sexual desire and response (Miller, 1993). As a result of neurological insult to these structures, Tom became sexually disinhibited and began to exhibit socially inappropriate behaviors with women in public settings. Because of his sexual disinhibition, Tom's placement in traumatic brain injury residential programs became problematic, and, consequently, Tom experienced a series of admissions and discharges from various residential facilities. Discharges were often in response to a specific event in which the facility could no longer tolerate Tom's sexually inappropriate behaviors.

During the first year that Tom resided in his current community group home, a similar situation occurred in which he became sexually and physically aggressive with a female client whom he wanted to date. Rather than discharge Tom from the facility, however, his treatment team physically separated him from female clients by moving him to an all-male group home and restricting his community access. When Tom began to receive occupational therapy services in his current residential placement, he identified his desire to engage in dating roles and relationships as his foremost priority.

Step 2: Identification of Lost Activities That Supported Predisability Roles and Relationships

Tom was able to list the activities that supported his dating role before his injury. Such activities included dinner, dancing, and attending films, shows, and concerts. However, although Tom was able to identify appropriate dating activities, he was not able to articulate or demonstrate the social skills necessary to interact appropriately with women. Initially, Tom needed to obtain a repertoire of social skills that would enable him to address a woman appropriately, introduce himself, and conduct a conversation without exhibiting sexually disinhibited behaviors. Tom and his therapist compiled a list of the socially inappropriate behaviors that he displayed in public, including prolonged staring, violating social norms of personal space, frequently touching others' shoulders and arms, and verbalizing sexual propositions. Tom was aware that he exhibited these behaviors and that they are inappropriate. The therapist and Tom then discussed how to replace these behaviors with more socially acceptable ones. To identify appropriate interaction skills with women, Tom and his therapist observed men and women interacting in the larger community environment (e.g., at shopping centers and malls, in restaurants, and at the bank). During these observation sessions, Tom and the therapist noted appropriate eye contact, respect for another's personal space, and appropriate conversational topics. Tom and the therapist began to role-play the use of appropriate interaction skills, first in the safety of the clinic and then in the actual community setting.

Step 3: Determination of Which Roles and Relationships the Client Wants To Rebuild and Build Anew

Although Tom indicated that he wanted to have a monogamous sexual relationship with a woman, he recognized that he would be unable to do so without first developing the interaction skills necessary to engage in informal social contact with women. Tom decided that a casual social role with women whom he considered friends would provide the opportunity for him to practice the interaction skills he needed to develop and maintain a more intimate relationship with a woman.

Step 4: Specification of Activities That Can Support Desired Roles and Relationships

Tom chose to practice social skills with a female friend who resided at the traumatic brain injury residential facility. Activities in which Tom chose to participate included shopping at a local mall with his female companion, walking in a community park, and dining at a nearby restaurant. On these occasions, Tom's therapist was present to cue him when his behaviors deviated from those he had learned in his role-playing sessions. When Tom began to demonstrate consistently socially appropriate behaviors with his female friend, the therapist's level of supervision changed from close to distant observation. For example, as Tom continued to accompany his female friend to dinner at a local restaurant, the therapist began to sit at a nearby table rather than joining the couple.

After one month in which Tom consistently demonstrated socially appropriate behaviors with his female friend, Tom and his therapist were confident that he was ready to engage in dating activities with women with whom he wanted to establish a greater degree of intimacy. Tom began dating a woman he was attracted to who resided in a nearby community group home. Again, Tom's therapist initially provided close supervision to cue him if his behaviors differed from socially appropriate ones and eventually used distant supervision as Tom demonstrated consistency in the use of acceptable behaviors.

As Tom's relationship with his dating partner became more intimate, the occupational therapist and nursing staff members reinforced safe-sex practices so that the couple could engage in the activities of a sexual relationship in the same way that adult couples in the larger society often do.

Step 5: Development of a Satisfactory Postinjury Identity on the Basis of Desired Roles and Relationships

Through the above activities, Tom was able to rebuild an identity as a dating partner, a role inherently related to his concept of himself as an adult male that enabled him to experience greater satisfaction with male gender roles. Tom's treatment team members had not attempted to offer him social skill training in the context of dating relationships; rather, they attempted to deal with his inappropriate behaviors by restricting his access to women. By allowing Tom to practice interaction skills with women in progressively less supervised settings, Tom was able to demonstrate that he could assume more socially acceptable behaviors.

Tom's therapist used three of the four motivation techniques that Bandura described (1977): performance accomplishments, vicarious experience, and verbal persuasion. Tom achieved a series of performance accomplishments by having the opportunity to use appropriate social skills in graded situations successfully, first in role-playing scenarios with the therapist, then with a female friend, and finally with a woman with whom Tom wanted to establish a more intimate relationship. The therapist used vicarious experience as a form of learning when she provided the opportunity for Tom to observe the social skills of men and women interacting in the natural community setting. Verbal persuasion in the initial role-playing sessions helped Tom to internalize a repertoire of appropriate social skills that he could use when the therapist was not present.

Through these activities, Tom obtained the skills necessary to engage in dating relationships. Such skills enabled Tom to feel empowered in his ability to make personal changes to achieve a more satisfactory quality of life.

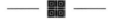

Exercise 1

1. In what other ways could Tom's therapist have used vicarious experience as a learning tool?

2.   What other performance accomplishments could Tom have experienced to enhance his social interaction skills with women? How would a therapist set up the environment so that Tom could experience such performance accomplishments?

3.   How did the participation in activity help Tom to reobtain his role as a dating partner?

4.   What other activities could Tom have participated in to enhance his social skills with women?

5.   Describe the process of empowerment that enabled Tom to learn the skills necessary to make positive changes in his quality of life.

<hr>

Case Scenario 2

Archie is a white male child 4 years of age who lives with his mother, father, and younger brother. Archie's mother reported having an uncomplicated pregnancy and a normal delivery. According to his mother, Archie achieved common developmental milestones by his second year (e.g., walking, talking) but began to lose his language skills shortly thereafter and received a referral for occupational therapy as part of an early-intervention, home-based program. Although Archie's parents identified his language delay, they were less concerned about other apparent behavioral issues that were evident in clinical evaluations. Archie demonstrated outbursts of temper when shifting from the performance of one activity to another. He displayed great difficulty with sustained eye contact and could neither tolerate physical touch nor initiate interaction with others in his environment. Archie's play was perseverative, rigid, and limited to two or three specific, favored toys. Additionally, Archie demonstrated notable sensitivity to visual, tactile, and auditory stimulation.

On his first occupational therapy home visit, Archie ran randomly around his house and avoided any visual, tactile, or auditory contact. Even when seated in his bedroom with his own selected, preferred toys, Archie continued to resist the therapist's overtures. The therapist attempted to initiate interaction and build rapport by playing with toys on the floor at Archie's own level. Archie fleetingly joined the therapist in a game of peekaboo but screamed inconsolably when the therapist attempted to alter the rules of his play.

<hr>

Step 1: Identification of Roles and Relationships Disrupted by Developmental Dysfunction

One of his most apparent role impairments was Archie's difficulty in establishing play and social roles typical of a preschooler his age. Archie demonstrated great difficulty in interacting with others and in initiating free play. Instead, he often only engaged in solitary play and would typically roll one of his toy cars back and forth until he remained standing still, fixed and motionless with his hand on the car, staring off into space. Archie would remain in this position for minutes at a time and would show signs of distress if disturbed.

Step 2: Identification of Lost Activities That Supported Predisability Roles and Relationships

Archie's parents were able to identify words and language activities (e.g., singing toddler songs and rhymes) that Archie had previously engaged in and now appeared to be losing. His parents strongly maintained that, as a young infant, Archie tolerated holding, eye contact, and sounds and played similarly to most other babies. After the birth of their second child, Archie's mother was more able to identify behavioral differences between her sons.

Archie's family system required time to adjust to the presence of therapists in their home. Similarly, the occupational therapist needed to provide time not only for the child but also for Archie's parents. Thus, Archie's parents and babysitter were frequently involved in the weekly therapy sessions for the first year of therapy. Archie's parents received information about the types of activities that could help remediate Archie's developmentally delayed behaviors. The therapist suggested that the parents exclude complicated and rule-bound activities from the games they played with Archie. Instead, they used games that allowed Archie to exercise his own control and independence. For example, the therapist and Archie built furniture and cubby houses that allowed him to initiate his own entrance and exit. Providing Archie with multiple safe spaces in which he could relate and interact with the therapist was important. Although language was his parents' primary concern, the therapist would not demand syntactically correct speech. Instead, the therapist would engage in Archie's own language if the theme of his communication was clear. Archie brought one or two of his toys into the cubby house, and the therapist used them to initiate interactive play. Archie's parents extended this type of therapeutic activity and purchased a small tent in which one of the parents would often sit with Archie and play. Both parents were consistently able to demonstrate pride in Archie's accomplishments. Despite advice from other therapists and a service coordinator, Archie's parents refused to seek any evaluation or treatment from a traditional medical model approach. They did not want anyone to assign Archie to a diagnostic category, even if that meant a consequential lack of funding.

Step 3: Determination of Which Roles and Relationships the Client Wants To Rebuild and Build Anew

Although Archie learned to function more adaptively in his own home, he was overwhelmed and frightened when he ventured into larger, unpredictable environments, such as the local playground. Therefore, therapy sessions more frequently took place in a playground setting to expand Archie's opportunities to interact with other children and build relationships. Initially, Archie would passively allow others to place him in a swing and push him back and forth until his stimulation level was so diminished that he appeared to be in a trance. He could not initiate play on novel playground equipment. The therapist used singing and counting activities to help Archie assume greater control over his arousal level. Games included more active motor planning such as expanded games of peekaboo and hide-and-seek. Again, the therapist maintained the theme of creating smaller, more manageable spaces within larger settings by climbing into tunnels and playground equipment to rest and talk for rapport building and relationship development.

Step 4: Specification of Activities That Can Support Desired Roles and Relationships

Archie wanted to learn how to use preschool toys and equipment (e.g., scissors, Playdough®, puzzles, bats and balls) within the context of his own rules. The therapist began having sessions with Archie at his preschool with small groups of children. Archie's peers quickly included him as a center of games because he had become a willing participant in preschool activities by this stage of therapy. His social behavior had advanced from the random running movement and aversion to any close contact with others that the therapist had first observed in the initial home visits. Archie now could initiate social greetings to the therapist, a behavior that carried over to his teachers. In fact, Archie became quite attached to his teachers and therapist. He was able to put his hands on his therapist's chin if he believed the therapist was ignoring him, move the therapist's face into his eye contact, and say, "I'm talking to you." This normalization of social responsiveness and adoption of appropriate social roles provided great comfort to Archie's parents, who all along fought the medical categorization of his potential. Archie's ability to move from one activity to another and his capacity to use language syntactically and communicatively had begun to approach his actual age as his social network expanded.

Step 5: Development of a Satisfactory Identity on the Basis of Desired Roles and Relationships

Archie has moved into an integrated school setting, travels by public transportation to an urban occupational therapy practice, and participates in more challenging activities in which he is required to adapt to, rather than adapt, his environment. In occupational therapy, Archie sometimes complains, "These are not my toys," but he is able to accept the novel toys and can interact and play appropriately with other children (in a therapy group) whom he does not see on a regular basis. He currently exercises autonomy with the typical willfulness of a developing preschooler. During one session, a friend from his preschool came to the occupational therapy practice at the same time as Archie's session and enthusiastically embraced Archie and covered him with hugs and kisses. Archie not only tolerated such physical contact but tentatively reciprocated.

Archie's therapist used the four motivation techniques that Bandura (1977) described: performance accomplishments, vicarious experience, verbal persuasion, and stress reduction techniques. Archie achieved a series of performance accomplishments by having the opportunity to interact successfully with others in graded situations, first with the occupational therapist in newly created safe spaces within the home (cubby houses), then with the therapist in the larger setting of a local playground, and finally in a preschool setting with other children. The therapist used vicarious experience as a form of learning when she provided the opportunity for Archie to observe the play and social skills of other preschoolers in the playground setting, in Archie's preschool classroom, and in therapy group sessions with other children at the occupational therapy practice. The therapist used verbal persuasion to help Archie attempt interactive play with her and with others in his environment. Stress reduction techniques focused on helping Archie to have a greater sense of control in what he perceived to be unpredictable environments. For example, the therapist created cubby spaces in which Archie was freely allowed to enter and exit as he wanted, Archie and the therapist played games in which others' rules did not restrict Archie's behaviors, and the therapist encouraged communication that allowed Archie to speak freely without demanding syntactically correct speech.

Through these activities, Archie was able to learn interactive play styles and began to build relationships with others in which he was able to demonstrate appropriate eye contact, tolerate physical touching, and initiate verbal communication. Such social and play skills enabled Archie to feel empowered and in control of his environment and allowed him to build relationships that enriched his emotional life and facilitated greater social and cognitive development.

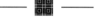

Exercise 2

1. In what other ways could Archie's therapist have used vicarious experience as a learning tool?

2. What other performance accomplishments could Archie have experienced to enhance his social interaction skills with others? How would a therapist set up the environment so that Archie could experience such performance accomplishments?

3. How did participation in activity help Archie to reobtain his role as a member in give-and-take family and school systems?

4. What other activities could Archie have participated in to enhance his social skills with others?

5. Describe the process of empowerment that enabled Archie to learn the skills necessary to make positive changes in his quality of life.

Summary

This chapter primarily concerns issues related to empowerment and how empowerment interacts with activity. The fundamental goal of this chapter is to demonstrate how this quest for personal empowerment leads to a better quality of life.

Empowerment is a combination of skills, competence, self-determination, belonging, and equality. In addition, persons who are empowered have personal qualities and attitudes that allow them to make changes in their life situations.

Occupational therapy practitioners apply knowledge of empowerment as a process in the relationship between disability and disempowerment. When persons lose the skills and qualities that are crucial to their sense of self, when the "sick" role forces them to accept dependence, and when the stigma associated with disability influences how others perceive them, a therapeutic process is available that can restore the experience of empowerment.

The role of the occupational therapy practitioner is to assist persons who have lost the ability to assert themselves with a disability to learn how to facilitate change by developing new skills, by learning from others, and by seeing the accomplishments thus produced. Bringing clients to this empowerment process involves powers of persuasion and learning how to deal with added stress. Occupational therapy practitioners can help clients accomplish empowerment by offering many levels of activity as the means, from ADL to countless activities of leisure and work. ■

References

American Psychiatric Association. (1994). *Diagnostic and statistical manual of mental disorders* (4th ed.). Washington, DC: Author.

Antonovsky, A. (1992). Can attitudes contribute to health? *Advances: The Journal of Mind–Body Health, 8*(4), 33–49.

Bandura, A. (1977). Self-efficacy: Toward a unifying theory of behavioral change. *Psychological Review, 84*(2), 191–215.

Benner, P. (1984). *From novice to expert: Excellence and power in clinical nursing practice.* Reading, MA: Addison-Wesley.

Benner, P., & Tanner, C. (1987). Clinical judgment: How expert nurses use intuition. *American Journal of Nursing, 87,* 23–31.

Caron, J., & Bergeron, N. (1995). A self-help partnership group for people who have experienced psychiatric hospitalization: An exploratory study. *Canada's Mental Health, 43*(2), 19–28.

Clark, F. A., Parham, D., Carlson, M. E., Frank, G., Jackson, J., Pierce, D., Wolfe, R. J., & Zemke, R. (1991). Occupational science: Academic innovation in the service of occupational therapy's future. *American Journal of Occupational Therapy, 45,* 300–310.

Dunton, W. R., Jr. (1919). *Reconstruction therapy.* Philadelphia: Saunders.

Goffman, E. (1963). *Stigma: Notes on the management of spoiled identity.* New York: Simon & Schuster.

Gutierrez, L. M. (1995). Understanding the empowerment process: Does consciousness make a difference? *Social Work Research, 19*(4), 229–237.

Gutman, S. A., & Swarbrick, M. (1998). The multiple linkages between women, head injury, alcoholism, and sexual abuse. *Occupational Therapy in Mental Health, 14,* 33–65.

Hood, S., Beaudet, M., & Catlin, G. (1996). A healthy outlook. *Health Reports: Statistics Canada, 7*(4), 25–32.

Horney, K. (1950). *Neurosis and human growth: The struggle toward self-realization.* New York: Norton.

Hutchison, P., Osborne-Way, L., & Lord, J. (1986). *Participating with people who have directly experienced the mental health system.* Toronto: Canadian Mental Health Association.

Kielhofner, G. (Ed.). (1995). *A model of human occupation: Theory and application* (2nd ed.). Baltimore: Williams & Wilkins.

Krefting, L. (1991). The culture concept in the everyday practice of occupational and physical therapy. *Physical and Occupational Therapy in Pediatrics, 11,* 1–6.

Maslow, A. H. (1968). *Toward a psychology of being* (2nd ed.). New York: Van Nostrand Reinhold.

Mattingly, C., & Fleming, M. H. (1994). *Clinical reasoning: Forms of inquiry in a therapeutic practice.* Philadelphia: F. A. Davis.

Meyer, A. (1922). The philosophy of occupational therapy. *Archives of Occupational Therapy, 1,* 2–3.

Miller, L. (1993). *Psychotherapy of the brain-injured patient: Reclaiming the shattered self.* New York: Norton.

Mosey, A. C. (1986). *Psychosocial components of occupational therapy.* New York: Raven Press.

Pearlin, L. I., & Schooler, C. (1978). The structure of coping. *Journal of Health and Social Behavior, 19,* 2–21.

Reilly, M. (1974). *Play as exploratory learning.* Beverly Hills, CA: Sage.

Smelser, N. J. (1998). The rational and the ambivalent in the social sciences: 1997 presidential address. *American Sociological Review, 63,* 1–16.

Wilson, S. (1996). Consumer empowerment in the mental health field. *Canadian Journal of Community Mental Health, 15*(2), 69–85.

Wolpe, J. (1958). *Psychotherapy by reciprocal inhibition.* Stanford, CA: Stanford University Press.

Wolpe, J. (1981). *Our useless fears.* Boston: Houghton Mifflin.

17

Moving Toward a Scientific Base for One of the Oldest and Most Important Ideas in Occupational Therapy

Julie Jepsen Thomas, PhD, OTR/L, FAOTA
David L. Nelson, PhD, OTR/L, FAOTA

Occupational therapists have been creating therapeutic occupational forms (e.g., purposeful activities, situations, conditions, environments, contexts) to facilitate occupational performance since the inception of the profession. Some of the earliest writings in the field refer to the importance of occupation in the process of recovering from illness and injury and promoting well-being (Dunton, 1931; National Society for the Promotion of Occupational Therapy, 1917). In fact, as discussed in chapter 1 of this book, the use of occupation (purposeful activity and sometimes occupations themselves) as the method of therapy is what makes the profession of occupational therapy unique from other helping professions.

One would imagine, given the central place of occupation in the delivery of occupational therapy services, that research on the effects of occupation would be longstanding and abundant. Indeed, early in the profession, Bird T. Baldwin (1919) strongly recommended that occupational therapists develop an experimental science of how common, everyday occupations may help restore movement abilities. He even developed quantitative measurements of movement. The first published empirical test on the effects of differing occupational forms on performance was as recent as 1984 (Kircher, 1984). Since then, numerous studies have used scientific methods to

---

Editors' Note. The authors of this chapter use David Nelson's terminology as described in chapter 2. Their work presents valuable information about research related to activities and occupation. Therefore, we have included their terminology, even though it is not congruent with our terminology and definitions as discussed in chapter 1.

investigate the effects of occupational forms on performance, and these studies are the focus of this chapter.

This chapter will introduce the reader to a conceptual framework for studying therapeutic occupation. Authors whose research we cite in this chapter use various terms to describe essential variables. For example, among the terms are *occupationally embedded movement, occupational form, purposeful activity, added-purpose activity, task constraints*, and *materials-based occupation*. Table 1 and an accompanying discussion summarize what we have derived from research to date. This chapter then identifies and discusses some of the issues that are inherent in conducting research in this area. Finally, we describe ideas for future research on occupation that can expand our knowledge of important principles of occupational therapy and inform practice. We invite readers to deepen their understanding of the empirical support for an important principle of our profession by reading the original articles that we cite in this chapter. Only by reading the original works can one truly develop a full appreciation of the nature and nuances of each study.

Figure 1 shows a conceptual framework for therapeutic occupation. Briefly, *occupation* is the relationship between an occupational form and an occupational performance. Occupational therapists synthesize or create occupational forms (objective circumstances with sociocultural and physical dimensions) that will guide or elicit a person's occupational performance (doing, behaving). The person, through his or her unique developmental structure, finds varying degrees of meaning in the occupational form that lead to purposes for engaging in an occupational performance. This framework provides a "road map" for the investigation of occupation. An *independent variable* consists of two or more occupational forms that we compare with each other. For example, the independent variable may involve a comparison between a therapist asking a client to reach for a glass of water and having the client reach out without a specific target. A *dependent variable* is some observable measure of occupational performance or effect. To use the same example of reaching, the dependent variable may be the speed of the reach.

We must study important principles of occupational therapy in a systematic way. For example, occupational therapists believe that engaging a person in an occupational form with enhanced meaning and purpose will result in better performance compared with an occupational form that provides less meaning and purpose. To study this important principle, a researcher would begin by identifying the independent variables. For a sound study, researchers must choose variables carefully to control for extraneous factors that could provide an alternative explanation of the findings. Next, the researcher must decide on a dependent variable. The framework identifies several possibilities. One could measure range of motion (ROM), number of repetitions completed, reported meaning or purpose, effect on subsequent occupational form, or adaptations of the participants' developmental structure (e.g., cardiovascular conditioning, learning, self-esteem). Choosing dependent variables may seem simple, but it involves careful planning to avoid threats to internal and external

Table 1

Summary of Research Studies on Occupational Forms

Study	Participants	Independent Variables (Occupational Forms)	Dependent Variables	Results
Bakshi, Bhambhani, and Madill (1991)	20 female students	Two crafts (one preferred and one not) vs. two rote exercises	Frequency of repetitions Blood pressure change Rate of perceived exertion Heart rate change	NS NS NS Rote > crafts
Beauregard, Thomas, and Nelson (1998)	2 female children with cerebral palsy (single-subject design)	Reaching for a doll as part of a game vs. reaching for a cylinder	Movement units Movement time Displacement Peak velocity % of reach to peak velocity	Doll < cylinder Doll < cylinder NS Doll > cylinder Doll > cylinder for one child and NS for the other
Bloch, Smith, and Nelson (1989)	30 female students	Jumping with vs. jumping without a rope	Heart rate increase Duration Affective meanings Preference	With rope > without rope NS NS NS
DeKuiper, Nelson, and White (1993)	24 women and 4 men residing in a nursing home	Kicking a balloon vs. imagining kicking a balloon vs. rote kicking	Vertical distance Speed Frequency of kicks	NS NS ■ Kicking balloon > imagining ■ Kicking balloon > rote ■ NS imagining vs. rote

			Dependent variable	Results
Hall and Nelson (1998)	47 female students	Eating with a spoon (materials) vs. imagining eating with a spoon (partial imagery) vs. imagining eating without a spoon (imagery)	Movement time	■ Materials > partial imagery/imagery ■ Partial imagery > imagery
			Movement units	■ Materials > partial imagery/imagery ■ Partial imagery > imagery ■ NS materials vs. partial imagery/imagery
			Displacement	■ Partial imagery < imagery
			Peak velocity	■ Materials < partial imagery/imagery ■ Partial imagery < imagery
			% of reach for peak velocity	■ Materials < partial imagery ■ Materials < imagery ■ NS partial imagery vs. imagery
Heck (1988)	5 female and 15 male students	Duplicating a pattern vs. repeatedly tracing an X in the center of the paper while experiencing electrical stimulation into painful range	Duration of pain tolerance	Pattern > tracing
Hoppes (1997)	6 women and 4 men residing in a nursing home	Game playing vs. nonplayful forms while standing	Duration of standing tolerance	Game playing > nonplayful forms

(continued)

Table 1 (*continued*)

Study	Participants	Independent Variables (Occupational Forms)	Dependent Variables	Results
Hsieh, Nelson, Smith, and Peterson (1996)	9 women and 12 men with hemiplegia	Picking up balls from the floor and tossing them at a target vs. imagining picking up balls and tossing them at a target vs. rote movement	Frequency of repetitions	■ Balls > rote ■ Imagining > rote
King (1993)	84 male and 62 female patients in a hand clinic	Gripping vs. pinching devices with computer program vs. rote exercise using gripping and pinching devices	Frequency of gripping Frequency of pinching	With computer program > without program With computer program > without program
Kircher (1984)	26 females	Jumping with vs. jumping without a rope	Heart rate increase Duration	With rope > without rope NS
Lang, Nelson, and Bush (1992)	12 women and 3 men residing in a nursing home	Kicking a balloon vs. imagining kicking a balloon vs. rote kicking	Frequency of kicks	■ Kicking balloon > imagining ■ Kicking balloon > rote ■ NS imagining vs. rote
Licht and Nelson (1990)	22 women and 8 men residing in a nursing home	Copying familiar vs. nonfamiliar objects	Accuracy of drawing	Familiar > nonfamiliar

Study	Sample	Comparison	Measure	Results
Mathiowetz and Wade (1995)	14 women and 6 men without multiple sclerosis and 17 women and 3 men with multiple sclerosis	Eating with a spoon (materials) vs. imagining eating while using a spoon (partial imagery) vs. imagining eating without a spoon (imagery)	Movement time	■ Materials > partial imagery ■ Materials > imagery ■ NS partial imagery and imagery
			Displacement	■ Materials < partial imagery ■ Materials < imagery ■ Partial imagery < imagery
			Velocity variability	■ Materials < partial imagery ■ Materials < imagery ■ Partial imagery < imagery
		Drinking from a glass (materials) vs. imagining drinking while using a glass (partial imagery) vs. imagining drinking without a glass (imagery)	Movement time	■ Materials > partial imagery ■ Materials > imagery ■ Partial imagery > imagery
			Displacement	■ Materials < partial imagery ■ Materials < imagery ■ NS partial imagery and imagery
			Velocity variability	■ Materials < partial imagery ■ Materials < imagery ■ Partial imagery < imagery

(continued)

Table 17.1 (*continued*)

Study	Participants	Independent Variables (Occupational Forms)	Dependent Variables	Results
		Turning pages of a book (materials) vs. imagining turning pages while using a book (partial imagery) vs. imagining turning pages without a book (imagery)	Movement time	■ Materials > partial imagery ■ Materials > imagery ■ NS partial imagery and imagery
			Displacement	■ Materials < partial imagery ■ Materials < imagery ■ NS partial imagery and imagery
			Velocity variability	■ Materials < partial imagery ■ Materials < imagery ■ NS partial imagery and imagery
Maurer, Smith, & Armetta (1989)	14 men and 4 women with chronic schizophrenia	Arm movement with vs. without a ribbon stick	Frequency of rotations Duration	Ribbon stick > without Ribbon stick > without
Miller and Nelson (1987)	30 female students	Stirring cookie dough vs. rote movement	Frequency Duration OSD evaluation OSD power OSD action	Cookie dough > rote NS Cookie dough > rote NS NS

Morton, Barnett, and Hale (1992)	15 women and 15 men	Moving a weighted box to ring a bell vs. rote moving a box without using a bell	Frequency of repetitions Duration Heart rate	NS NS NS
Moyer and Nelson (1998)	21 female and 7 male rehabilitation patients	Squeezing a bulb in a hockey game against another player vs. rote squeezing alone vs. rote squeezing in presence of another person	Frequency of repetitions Cumulative air pressure dispersed from bulb	NS NS
Mullins, Nelson, and Smith (1987)	18 women and 10 men residing in a nursing home	Stenciling vs. rote movement	Preference for stenciling or rote movement for exercise	NS ($p = .06$)
Nelson et al. (1996)	12 women and 14 men after cerebro-vascular accident	Bilaterally assisted supination game vs. bilaterally assisted rote supination	Degrees of handle rotation	Game > rote exercise
Paul and Ramsey (1998)	9 women and 11 men with hemiplegia	Making music with drums vs. exercise group	Degrees of active shoulder flexion	NS
			Degrees of active elbow extension	NS

(continued)

Table 1 (*continued*)

Study	Participants	Independent Variables (Occupational Forms)	Dependent Variables	Results
Riccio, Nelson, and Bush (1990)	27 elderly women residing in a nursing home	Imagining picking apples vs. rote reaching up imagining picking coins vs. rote reaching down	Frequency of reaching up Frequency of reaching down	Imagining > rote NS; order effect
Rice (1998)	24 women and 12 men	Turning wing nuts in or out vs. rote supination pronation movement vs. control group	Movement time	■ Turning wing nuts < control ■ NS turning wing nuts and rote ■ NS rote and control ■ Untrained limb-opposite movement practice < control ■ NS untrained limb-same movement practice and control ■ NS opposite limb practice (rote) and control
		Right or left turn in and right or left turn out vs. right or left rote vs. control	Movement time of cross-transfer effects in untrained limb	
Ross and Nelson (in press)	60 female students	Reaching for a pencil (materials) vs. imagining reaching for a pencil (imagery) vs. rote reaching	Reaction time Movement time	■ Materials < imagery/rote ■ NS rote vs. imagery ■ Materials < imagery/rote ■ Rote < imagery

		Measures	Results
		Movement units	■ Materials < imagery/rote ■ Rote < imagery
		Displacement	■ Materials < imagery/rote ■ NS rote vs. imagery
		Peak velocity	■ Materials < imagery/rote ■ Imagery < rote
		% of reach to peak velocity	■ Imagery < materials ■ Imagery < rote
		End velocity	■ Materials < rote ■ Materials < rote ■ Imagery < rote ■ NS materials vs. imagery
Sakemiller and Nelson (1998)	2 female children with cerebral palsy (single-subject design)	Game playing vs. verbal directions to encourage prone extension	Neck extension Game > verbal Back extension Game > verbal Total extension Game > verbal
Schmidt and Nelson (1996)	10 female and 9 male rehabilitation patients	Sanding a board for a child's rocking horse (altruistic occupation) *vs.* sanding a board for a shelf *vs.* sanding a board for rote exercise	Distance of movement NS Frequency of movement NS
Sietsema, Nelson, Mulder, Mervau-Scheidel, and White (1993)	3 women and 17 men with traumatic brain injury	Reaching forward to play game vs. rote reaching forward without a game	Range of motion during reach Game > rote

(continued)

Table 1 (*continued*)

Study	Participants	Independent Variables (Occupational Forms)	Dependent Variables	Results
Steinbeck (1986)	15 female and 15 male students	Lower extremity drill press with project vs. exercise cycle; Squeezing bulb for game vs. rote squeezing bulb	Frequency of repetitions	■ Drill press > exercise cycle ■ Game > rote
Thibodeaux and Ludwig (1988)	15 female students	Sanding a cutting board to keep vs. sanding a piece of wood not to keep	Duration of sanding Heart rate standing	NS NS
Thomas (1996)	45 elderly women residing in the community	Kicking a balloon vs. imagining kicking a balloon vs. rote kicking	Frequency of kicks Rest period required before another set of kicks Heart rate change	■ Kicking balloon > imagining ■ Kicking balloon > rote ■ NS imagining vs. rote ■ Kicking balloon > imagining ■ Kicking balloon > rote ■ NS imagining vs. rote NS
Thomas, Vander Wyk, and Boyer (1999)	15 patients in cardiac rehabilitation	Soccer kicking game vs. imagining game vs. rote kicking	Frequency of kicks	■ Game > imagining game ■ Game > rote kicking ■ NS imagining vs. rote

Study	Sample	Task	Measure	Results
			Rest period required before another set of kicks	NS
			Heart rate change	NS
			Affective meanings	NS
van der Weel, van der Meer, and Lee (1991)	2 girls and 7 boys with cerebral palsy and 7 girls and 5 boys without cerebral palsy	Bang drums using pronation/supination movements vs. rote pronation/supination	Pronation/supination amplitude	▪ Drums > rote for children with cerebral palsy ▪ NS for children without cerebral palsy
Wagner, Krauss, and Horowitz (1995)	45 male students	Squeezing a bulb in a hockey game against another player vs. rote squeezing alone vs. rote squeezing in the presence of another person	Frequency of repetitions	▪ Rote alone > game ▪ Rote with another > game
Wu, Trombly, and Lin (1994)	37 female students	Picking up a pencil and preparing to write (materials) vs. imagining picking up a pencil (imagery) vs. rote exercise	Reaction time	▪ Materials < imagery/rote ▪ NS rote vs. imagery
			Movement time	▪ Materials < imagery/rote ▪ Rote < imagery
			Movement units	▪ Materials < imagery/rote ▪ Rote < imagery
			Displacement	▪ Materials < imagery/rote ▪ Rote < imagery
			Peak velocity	▪ Materials < imagery/rote ▪ NS rote vs. imagery
			% of reach to peak velocit	▪ Materials < imagery/rote ▪ Rote < imager

(continued)

Table 1 (*continued*)

Study	Participants	Independent Variables (Occupational Forms)	Dependent Variables	Results
Yoder, Nelson, and Smith (1989)	30 elderly women	Stirring cookie dough vs. rote movement	Frequency of rotations	Cookie dough > rote
Yuen, Nelson, Peterson, and Dickinson (1994)	52 male students	Prosthetic training connecting dots with pen light vs. training without light or dots	Accuracy of maze tracing with a pen	Dots and pen light > without dots and pen light
Zimmerer-Branum and Nelson (1995)	37 women and 15 men residing in nursing home	Dunking a basketball vs. rote movement	Preference for exercise method	Basketball > rote

Note. NS = no significant differences found for variables; OSD = Osgood Semantic Differential.

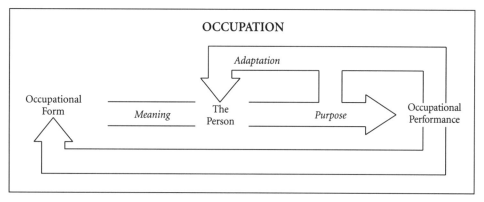

Figure 1. Conceptual framework for therapeutic occupation. *Note.* From "Why the Profession of Occupational Therapy Will Flourish in the 21st Century, 1996 Eleanor Clarke Slagle Lecture" by D. L. Nelson, 1997, *American Journal of Occupational Therapy, 51,* p. 13. Copyright 1997 by the American Occupational Therapy Association. Reprinted with permission.

validity. Careful selection of reliable and valid instruments is necessary to measure the chosen dependent variables.

What Do We Know From the Research to Date?

Kircher (1984) published the first experimental study to examine whether persons would behave differently in response to contrasting occupational forms. We review this study in some detail as an example of how researchers have constructed studies of this type. The goal of Kircher's study was to determine whether occupationally embedded exercise (purposeful activity) provided enhanced meaning (intrinsic motivation) and purpose that could result in different performance compared with an occupational form that was more rote. Kircher compared the independent variables of jumping while using a rope with jumping without using a rope by using a counterbalanced design. The participants were 26 healthy women who reported that they liked to jump rope when they were younger and had no conditions that would prevent full participation in a jumping occupation. The researcher randomly assigned participants to one of two jumping orders (jumping with the rope first and then without or jumping without the rope first and then with the rope). This design allowed the researcher to determine whether the order of experiencing the independent variables influenced the dependent variables. The participants wore electrocardiogram (ECG) monitors, and the evaluator instructed the participants to jump until they believed they were working "very hard" on the Borg Rate of Perceived Exertion scale (Borg & Linderholm, 1973).

The dependent variables for the study were heart rate increases (measured by counting the heart rate on the ECG rhythm strips) and duration of participation in the two jumping conditions (measured by a stopwatch). Kircher (1984) found that heart rate increases at a given level of perceived exertion (working very hard) were significantly higher for the condition involving jumping with a rope than for the condition involving jumping without a rope. She did not find any significant differences in terms of duration of jumping.

What do these results mean? Kircher related the results to the occupational therapy and cardiophysiology literature. Other researchers have shown that heart rate has a high positive correlation with rate of perceived exertion. She concluded that something else must have intervened with these participants because they perceived the same level of exertion when jumping with a rope, even though their hearts were actually working more rapidly than in the rote condition. Kircher believed that the occupational form of jumping with a rope provided enhanced motivation and resulted in "persons not perceiving fatigue as readily when his or her attention is focused on an appropriately selected activity" (Kircher, 1984, p. 168). The implication for practice is that, when clients are engaged in an occupationally enhanced exercise, they may work harder (generate a higher heart rate) before they perceive themselves to be at the same level of exertion as when they are engaged in a rote exercise.

Every study has limitations, and Kircher's is no exception. Identifying possible limitations is important so that subsequent research can address these issues and improve our understanding of important concepts. Kircher believed that the participants possibly perceived the two conditions differently by responding to local factors (peripheral muscle fatigue) in one condition and central factors (cardiopulmonary fatigue) in the other. Perhaps the rhythm of jumping or the preference for condition were mitigating factors. Kircher argued that, even if these factors did play a role, they were all part of the defined package of purposefulness. Another possible limitation was the relatively small sample size. Whenever a study fails to find significant differences, as this one did in duration of participation, one must be concerned about the possibility of missing true differences that would be more detectable with a larger sample size. This is referred to as a *Type II error*, and we discuss this phenomenon in more detail later in this chapter.

The importance of Kircher's study is twofold. She showed that, with an occupationally embedded exercise (jumping with a rope), participants behaved differently than when they were engaged in a rote exercise (one in which the focus is on the movement as directed by the evaluator). This was the first study to lend empirical support to this basic occupational therapy principle. Second, Kircher's study provided an example for future studies and as such spawned additional studies that have continued this important line of inquiry concerning occupationally embedded versus rote exercise movement. Table 1 provides a synopsis of many of these studies. From the table, the reader will be able to quickly determine the populations studied to date. For each study, we briefly identify the independent variables and the dependent variables. Finally, the table shows the results of the study for each of the dependent variables.

A perusal of the dependent variables in Table 1 reveals that researchers have studied various aspects of occupational performance. For example, several researchers measured the number of repetitions of various movements when participants were engaged in contrasting occupational forms. Researchers contrasted movement elicited from occupationally enhanced forms and imagery and rote exercise forms. The independent variables involved the upper extremities, lower extremities, or both. Most of these studies demonstrated that occupationally enhanced forms resulted in notably more repetitions of movement than rote exercise or imagery forms (DeKuiper, Nelson, & White, 1993; Hsieh, Nelson, Smith, & Peterson, 1996; King, 1993; Lang, Nelson, & Bush, 1992; Maurer, Smith, & Armetta, 1989; Miller & Nelson, 1987; Riccio, Nelson, & Bush, 1990; Steinbeck, 1986; Thomas, 1996; Thomas, Vander Wyk, & Boyer, 1999; Yoder, Nelson, & Smith, 1989). Subjects for these studies have included men and women, elderly residents of nursing homes, community-dwelling elderly persons, persons with hemiplegia, clients with hand injuries, clients with schizophrenia, clients in cardiac rehabilitation, and college-age students.

Not every study has found notable differences when contrasting occupational forms in terms of number of repetitions (Bakshi, Bhambhani, & Madill, 1991; Morton, Barnett, & Hale, 1992; Moyer & Nelson, 1998; Schmidt & Nelson, 1996), and one study found that rote exercise forms elicited more repetitions than occupationally enhanced forms (Wagner, Krauss, & Horowitz, 1995). What could explain this discrepancy in results? One possibility is the degree of contrast present in the occupational forms. For example, Morton and associates (1992) contrasted moving a weighted box up an incline to ring a bell (an occupationally embedded task) with moving the same box up the incline without ringing the bell. Insufficient contrast may possibly have existed between these similar occupational forms. Perhaps participants found the tasks so close in terms of meaning that they elicited no differences in purpose, and, therefore, subsequent occupational performance was virtually the same. Another possibility could be small sample size. For example, Schmidt and Nelson (1996) found no difference in the number of repetitions in 19 persons involved in a rehabilitation program. This number may have been too small to detect true differences. As scientists, we must be open to the possibility that rote exercise may be as valuable as occupationally embedded exercise for certain populations under certain conditions. For example, Schmidt and Nelson (1996) suggested that clients in rehabilitation hospitals who do not have cognitive impairments may be highly motivated to carry out certain types of rote exercise, especially those of short duration and those in which the possible benefits of the exercise are clear.

Other studies investigated the amount of motion or ROM elicited by contrasting occupational forms. Most of these studies found that occupationally enhanced forms resulted in more or further movement of designated body parts than rote exercise forms (Nelson et al., 1996; Sakemiller & Nelson, 1998; Sietsema, Nelson, Mulder, Mervau-Scheidel, & White, 1993; van der Weel, van der Meer, & Lee, 1991). Others have not found such differences in amount of movement elicited (DeKuiper et al., 1993; Paul & Ramsey, 1998; Schmidt & Nelson, 1996). Possible explanations for these results may rest in the requirements of the independent variables or in the approach to data analysis. The occupationally enhanced form in DeKuiper and colleagues' (1993) study did not require full ROM to engage successfully in the occupation, which would have a direct effect on the ROM dependent variable. Paul and Ramsey (1998) compared the actual number of degrees of ROM achieved at posttest instead of comparing the change in number of degrees from pretest to posttest, which may have revealed significant differences.

Studies have shown that using enhancing occupational forms resulted in greater duration of pain tolerance (Heck, 1988), greater accuracy of drawing (Licht & Nelson, 1990), greater duration of standing tolerance (Hoppes, 1997), greater subjective preference for occupationally embedded exercise (Zimmerer-Branum & Nelson, 1995), and greater accuracy in tracing a maze while using an upper-extremity prosthesis (Yuen, Nelson, Peterson, & Dickinson, 1994). Research has been less definitive when investigating physiological responses to contrasting occupational forms in terms of heart rate and blood pressure changes or psychological response in terms of eliciting affective meaning.

A recent application of technology designed to quantify aspects of movement has allowed researchers to examine not only the product of movement (e.g., number of repetitions, pain tolerance, degrees of movement, accuracy of drawing) but also the process of moving. Technology now permits investigation of qualities of movement such as movement units (smoothness), movement time (speed), displacement (directness), peak velocity during movement, and the percentage of reach in which peak velocity occurs. This technology involves the simultaneous recording of movement in three planes by using high-speed cameras. Analysis of velocity profiles results in quantification of the dependent variables mentioned above. Taken together, these dependent variables provide a picture of the quality of reach. The motor control literature has described patterns of reaching that reflect greater efficiency, maturity, and higher levels of skill development.

Occupational therapy researchers have used this technology to demonstrate that reaching dynamics during an occupationally embedded movement are different from those in a matched rote exercise or imagery movement. Researchers have found that occupationally embedded movement results in a better quality of reach than when a person is engaged in an imagery or rote exercise occupational form. Subjects have included children with cerebral palsy (Beauregard, Thomas, & Nelson, 1998), adults with and without multiple sclerosis (Mathiowetz & Wade, 1995), and female college students (Hall & Nelson, 1998; Wu, Trombly, & Lin, 1994).

The studies summarized in Table 1 are noteworthy because they help inform practice and support important principles of occupational therapy. Taken as a whole, the preponderance of evidence supports the use of an occupational approach to elicit desired aspects of occupational performance. One way of analyzing the results of a group of studies is to conduct a meta-analysis (Glass, 1976). This technique involves combining the results of related studies by calculating and comparing effect sizes.

Effect sizes indicate the degree to which the null hypothesis is false, in this case, that the occupational forms or independent variables had no effect on performance or the dependent variables (Cohen, 1988). The results of a meta-analysis conducted on 17 occupational therapy research studies concerning motor performance dependent variables found effect sizes ranging from (–0.07 to 0.92 with a mean effect size of 0.50 (Lin, Wu, Tickle-Degnen, & Coster, 1997). The authors contrasted the studies on the basis of other relevant factors such as whether the participants had a deficit, the type of dependent variable, the age of subjects, and so forth. The authors concluded that their findings "support the concept that naturalistic occupations involving objects may serve as effective means to promote motor performance" (Lin et al., 1997, p. 40).

These results are good news for occupational therapists, who have long advocated that engagement in meaningful occupations results in benefits to clients but did not have empirical support for such assertions. Occupational therapists can now point to a growing body of literature that documents these ideas in an objective manner.

Issues in Conducting Research on Occupation

Designing and conducting research studies in any area of inquiry demands careful planning and, depending on one's skill, consultation with more experienced researchers. These precautions help the researcher to avoid pitfalls that would invalidate one's research results and thus waste valuable time, energy, and resources. Several issues are relevant when one conducts research on the effects of occupational form on performance. We identify these issues to alert the reader to some of the requirements and conventions of the research process.

Experimental research requires careful control of the independent variables. Controlling for as many aspects of the occupational forms selected as possible is necessary, except for the elements that one is testing. For example, Miller and Nelson (1987) compared the occupationally embedded exercise condition of stirring cookie dough with the rote exercise condition of merely stirring. To be a fair comparison, all aspects of the two forms were the same (e.g., the resistance provided by the substance stirred, the container and spoon used to stir, the position of the participants), except for the aspects that make one condition occupational in nature and the other rote in nature. The container for stirring was the same in both conditions and had a cover to prevent participants from seeing the substance stirred. Both conditions used the same ingredients for the dough, except that the researchers added vanilla to simulate the smell of cookie dough in the occupationally embedded condition, and they added water in the rote condition. The researchers further enhanced the form for the occupationally embedded condition by having the aroma of baking cookies and the sight of freshly baked cookies in the room. These procedures allowed for careful matching of physical effort and specific movements required while still contrasting elements that make one condition occupational and the other rote.

This careful matching of conditions often requires specially constructed equipment to provide the same movement requirements to participants in all conditions, which can limit the types of movements and occupations that one can investigate. For example, a complex occupation such as building a birdhouse requires multiple patterns of movement. Converting this occupation into a rote movement to contrast the two would be difficult. This need for control may result in a rather artificial environment and one that is necessarily contrived.

Another problem is that the researcher must use the same occupational form with all subjects assigned to the condition. Of course, the same form will not be equally meaningful and purposeful to everyone. The researcher must make an educated guess (on the basis of a pilot study if possible) that the form will be meaningful and purposeful enough for the entire cohort of subjects to show an overall difference versus the rote condition.

In everyday practice, the requirements of research do not constrain occupational therapists. The therapist can use unlimited creativity to synthesize therapeutic occupational forms and can individualize them for each person. In fact, if the benefits of enhanced occupational forms are evident in even contrived research conditions, imagine what occurs when the therapist is free to use his or her full talents to create meaningful, purposeful forms in active collaboration with the recipient of services.

Another concern in research is the possibility of Type II errors. Type II errors can occur when the study fails to find significant differences in the dependent variables when those differences truly exist. Whenever a researcher finds no difference in the independent variables, one should consider the possibility of a Type II error. This phenomenon can occur for several reasons. One is sample size. Sample size directly relates to the power of a study to detect subtle but real differences that exist in the dependent variables. The smaller the sample size, the more difficult detecting those differences is. Investigators often conduct occupational therapy research with a relatively small number of participants. This is especially true when we study persons with disabilities. Finding sufficient numbers of persons with disabilities who meet the study's selection criteria is often quite difficult. If one uses a small sample size, one must be concerned about the possibility of Type II error.

Another factor that will contribute to Type II errors is large variances in the dependent variables. The power to detect differences increases as variance decreases. Researchers can reduce variance by carefully considering who to include in the study. For example, large age ranges or greatly differing ability levels in participants will potentially increase the variance in the data and make finding true differences difficult. Research designs such as a counterbalanced approach or a repeated-measures design will reduce variance by having participants experience all conditions and therefore act as their own control subjects. In addition, the lack of sensitivity and reliability of the instruments that measure the dependent variables can create random measurement error. This can increase variance and contribute to a Type II error.

Finally, the effect size of the independent variables relates to the power to detect true differences. If the effect of the occupationally embedded form is great, then detecting differences will be easier. For example, in Morton and colleagues' (1992) study, the small difference in the independent variables (ringing a bell versus not ringing the bell) may not have created enough of a difference between the conditions. With more contrast, the conditions will result in more power to detect true differences.

As the number of studies comparing different occupational forms grows, we can learn from the experience of the researchers who have published before us. A careful critique of the methods and results of studies when considering these issues will help us design studies that can discern differences and thus have a better chance of finding those that do exist when using enhanced, occupationally embedded forms.

Ideas for Future Research

The future is bright for occupational therapists who accept the challenge of including research in their professional goals. An unlimited need certainly exists for more studies that will inform practice and add to our understanding of the underpinnings of occupational therapy. We offer the reader the following ideas to build on previous work and to expand the research of the future into new areas.

One study in and of itself is not sufficient to support a principle or to change the way one practices. We accumulate knowledge slowly, with studies building on previous work to create a consensus of empirical support. Generally, consensus occurs through studies that replicate the results of previous studies. We need more replication studies in occupational therapy (Ross, Hall, & Heater, 1998) to verify results and to increase our confidence in them. For example, Bloch, Smith, and Nelson (1989) replicated Kircher's (1984) original work and had similar results. This verification adds to our confidence that the results of Kircher's study were not the result of chance alone.

We must conduct related studies that extend our ability to apply results to other independent variables, dependent variables, and populations. For example, Lang and colleagues (1992) originally studied residents in nursing homes and contrasted the independent variables of kicking a balloon versus kicking an imaginary balloon versus the rote exercise of kicking. They found that the frequency of kicks was greatest for the more occupationally embedded condition and was no different between the imagined and rote condition. DeKuiper and associates (1993) repeated the experiment and included speed of kicking and vertical distance traveled. They found the same results as Lang and associates (1992) for frequency of kicking but no difference among the conditions for the new variables included. Thomas (1996) repeated the Lang study but studied well elderly women who lived in the community. In addition to the variable for frequency of kicks, she included heart rate change and the length of rest period that the seniors wanted before completing another round of kicks. She found the same results for the frequency of kicking that the two previous studies did and found no differences among the participants in terms of heart rate changes. In addition, Thomas (1996) found that participants required a longer period of rest before continuing in the occupationally embedded condition than during the other conditions, with no differences evident between the imagined and rote conditions. This process of replicating and extending studies builds the body of knowledge in occupational therapy.

Many studies listed in Table 1 involved college-age students and well elderly persons. These studies are helpful, especially in relatively new areas of investigation. They give us a baseline of results for healthy populations. Some studies likewise involve persons with disabilities; however, these studies are fewer in number and do not address the gamut of possible disabling conditions. These studies are particularly important because they explore important variables with persons who are similar to clients with whom occupational therapists work. Even though studies with populations of persons with disabilities pose challenges, we must persist in this effort. One approach to studying persons with disabilities is to use a single-subject research design (Ottenbacher, 1986). For example, Beauregard and colleagues (1998) used a single-subject ABA design to study the quality of reach in two young girls with cerebral palsy. Additional single-subject studies with persons with disabilities can add to our understanding of the effect of contrasting occupations for these important persons.

Careful study of the existing research reveals that researchers measured many dependent variables after one exposure to and immediately after experiencing the independent variables. In other words, researchers measured the immediate effects of the independent variables. In practice, we are particularly interested in the longer-term effects of the treatments we provide. More research is necessary to document the longer-term effects of these important independent variables. This goal can add to the complexity of a study and is certainly a logical next step for further linking research to practice.

The use of sophisticated technology to measure process variables such as quality of movement in addition to outcome variables such as amount or frequency of movement has great potential. This technology enhances our ability to understand the extent to which occupationally enhanced approaches can benefit the person. These technologies may allow us to study more complex occupational forms that are closer to those that practitioners use in everyday practice. This is an exciting area for future research and one that occupational therapy has just begun to apply to important questions for our discipline.

So far, researchers have studied the effects of individual occupational forms on the occupational performance of the person. A future direction for research is to study important principles at the program level. For example, occupational therapists are interested in research that contrasts a naturalistic or occupationally oriented program for a particular population with a program that is more reductionistic in nature. For example, Clark and colleagues (1997) contrasted programming that was occupational in nature with that of a social activities programming approach and a nontreatment control group. The researchers found notable benefits with the occupational therapy approach on several functional and quality-of-life measures. Another study contrasted an occupationally enhanced educational approach with a lecture approach for clients undergoing phase I cardiac rehabilitation. The results showed that clients in the occupationally enhanced cohort group had more self-efficacy (confidence) in their skills (Thomas, 1993) and less anxiety at discharge (Thomas, 1995) than clients in the lecture-based group. This type of research can be quite complex but is extremely important to demonstrate the value of occupational therapy programs that use an occupational approach.

To date, we have a lack of qualitatively designed research in this line of inquiry. Qualitative studies may enhance our understanding of some of the complex aspects of contrasting occupational forms that do not lend themselves well to quantitative measurement. Qualitative studies may likewise be important in the study of questions at the program level mentioned above. Of particular interest are phenomena such as the meaning that particular occupational forms hold for the person. Because meaning is an internal process unique to each person, meaning has eluded direct measurement. Qualitative methods may explore personal meaning and broaden our understanding of it. Other studies could investigate the purposes generated by contrasting occupational forms. We make assumptions about a person's purposes from his or her actions, but purpose is another concept that is internal and that we cannot directly measure. Qualitative methods are appropriate for studying these and other important questions in future studies.

As the body of research grows to include several studies investigating a particular set of variables, conducting additional meta-analyses is helpful. This approach synthesizes the research in a systematic way and clearly communicates the size of the effect of occupationally enhanced forms on important performance variables. Meta-analyses have the advantage of increased power because they combine multiple studies. This technique can produce a valuable contribution to the occupational therapy literature.

We hope you have a better understanding of the research literature as it relates to the study of occupational forms or purposeful activities. Without research, we must base our practice decisions on tradition, hunches, or observations. These methods will not provide us with the systematically tested knowledge that we need to meet society's needs. Research is necessary to help define our scope of practice and is necessary for occupational therapy to handle the scrutiny of external forces such as third-party payers. Research allows us to take our rightful place among other disciplines who treat the same persons with whom we work and likewise claim function to be their outcome. We challenge you to learn more about research, to read and develop skill in analyzing research published in the literature, to "get your research feet wet," to collaborate with others who want to engage in research, and to value this important role as crucial in advancing the profession of occupational therapy in the future. ∎

Exercise

1. Start a research support group and meet once a month to discuss an interesting occupational therapy research article. Analyze the article individually and then as a group. Ask faculty members to serve as mentors to check your understanding of the research article.

2. Ask fieldwork supervisors for questions they would like to see research answer. As you observe occupational therapy during Level I fieldwork, keep a list of questions you would like research to answer. At the end of these experiences, share your list with those of your classmates. Sort the questions in terms of complexity. Do the more simple questions have potential for investigation through student projects? Use this information in your research courses.

3. Check the "future research" section of published research studies. Do any of these ideas have potential for your student project?

4. As you study occupations to use therapeutically, try to devise a matching rote exercise condition that you could use in a study as a contrasting occupational form.

References

Bakshi, R., Bhambhani, Y., & Madill, H. (1991). The effects of task preference on performance during purposeful and nonpurposeful activities. *American Journal of Occupational Therapy, 45,* 912–916.

Baldwin, B. T. (1919). *Occupational therapy applied to restoration of movement.* Washington, DC: Commanding Officer and Surgeon General of the Army, Walter Reed General Hospital.

Beauregard, R., Thomas, J. J., & Nelson, D. L. (1998). Quality of reach during a game and during a rote movement in children with cerebral palsy. *Physical and Occupational Therapy in Pediatrics, 18*(3/4), 67–84.

Bloch, M. W., Smith, D. A., & Nelson, D. L. (1989). Heart rate, activity and affect in added-purpose versus single-purpose jumping activities. *American Journal of Occupational Therapy, 43,* 25–30.

Borg, G., & Linderholm, H. (1973). Exercise performance and perceived exertion in patients with coronary insufficiency, arterial hyperextension and vasoregulatory asthenia. *Acta Medica Scandinavica, 187,* 1–26.

Clark, F., Azen, S. P., Zemke, R., Jackson, J., Carlson, M., Mandel, D., Hay, J., Josephson, K., Cherry, B., Hessel, C., Palmer, J., & Lipson, L. (1997). Occupational therapy for independent-living older adults: A randomized controlled trial. *JAMA, 278,* 1321–1326.

Cohen, J. (1988). *Statistical power analysis for the behavioral sciences.* Hillsdale, NJ: Lawrence Erlbaum.

DeKuiper, W. P., Nelson, D. L., & White, B. E. (1993). Materials-based occupation versus imagery-based occupation versus rote exercise: A replication and extension. *Occupational Therapy Journal of Research, 13,* 183–197.

Dunton, W. R. (1931). Occupational therapy. *Occupational Therapy and Rehabilitation, 10,* 113–121.

Glass, G. V. (1976). Primary, secondary, and meta-analysis of research. *Educational Researcher, 5,* 3–8.

Hall, B. A., & Nelson, D. L. (1998). The effect of materials on performance: A kinematic analysis of eating. *Scandinavian Journal of Occupational Therapy, 5,* 69–81.

Heck, S. A. (1988). The effect of purposeful activity on pain tolerance. *American Journal of Occupational Therapy, 42,* 577–581.

Hoppes, S. (1997). Can play increase standing tolerance? A pilot-study. *Physical and Occupational Therapy in Geriatrics, 15,* 65–73.

Hsieh, C. L., Nelson, D. L., Smith, D. A., & Peterson, C. Q. (1996). A comparison of performance in added-purpose occupations and rote exercise for dynamic standing balance in persons with hemiplegia. *American Journal of Occupational Therapy, 50,* 10–16.

King, T. I. (1993). Hand strengthening with a computer for purposeful activity. *American Journal of Occupational Therapy, 47,* 635–637.

Kircher, M. A. (1984). Motivation as a factor of perceived exertion in purposeful versus non-purposeful activity. *American Journal of Occupational Therapy, 38,* 165–170.

Lang, E. M., Nelson, D. L., & Bush, M. A. (1992). Comparison of performance in materials-based occupation, imagery-based occupation, and rote exercise in nursing home residents. *American Journal of Occupational Therapy, 46,* 607–611.

Licht, B. C., & Nelson, D. L. (1990). Adding meaning to a design copy task through representational stimuli. *American Journal of Occupational Therapy, 44,* 408–413.

Lin, K., Wu, C., Tickle-Degnen, L., & Coster, W. (1997). Enhancing occupational performance through occupationally embedded exercise: A meta-analytic review. *Occupational Therapy Journal of Research, 17,* 25–47.

Mathiowetz, V., & Wade, M. G. (1995). Task constraints and functional motor performance of individuals with and without multiple sclerosis. *Ecological Psychology, 7,* 99–123.

Maurer, T. L., Smith, D. A., & Armetta, C. L. (1989). Single purpose vs. added purpose activity: Performance comparisons with chronic schizophrenics. *Occupational Therapy in Mental Health, 9,* 9–20.

Miller, L., & Nelson, D. L. (1987). Dual-purpose activity versus single-purpose activity in terms of duration on task, exertion level, and affect. *Occupational Therapy in Mental Health, 7,* 55–67.

Morton, G. G., Barnett, D. W., & Hale, L. S. (1992). A comparison of performance measures of an added-purpose task versus a single purpose task for upper extremities. *American Journal of Occupational Therapy, 46,* 128–133.

Moyer, J. A., & Nelson, D. L. (1998). Replication and resynthesis of an occupationally embedded exercise with adult rehabilitation patients. *Israel Journal of Occupational Therapy, 7,* E57–E75.

Mullins, C. S., Nelson, D. L., & Smith, D. A. (1987). Exercise through dual-purpose activity in the institutionalized elderly. *Physical and Occupational Therapy in Geriatrics, 5,* 29–39.

National Society for the Promotion of Occupational Therapy. (1917). *Constitution.* Baltimore: Sheppard Hospital.

Nelson, D. L. (1997). Why the profession of occupational therapy will flourish in the 21st century, 1996 Eleanor Clarke Slagle lecture. *American Journal of Occupational Therapy, 51,* 11–24.

Nelson, D. L., Konosky, K., Fleharty, K., Webb, R., Newer, K., Hazboun, V. P., Fontaine, C., & Licht, B. (1996). The effects of an occupationally embedded exercise on bilaterally assisted supination in persons with hemiplgaia. *American journal of Occupational Therapy, 50,* 639–646.

Ottenbacher, K. J. (1986). *Evaluating clinical change: Strategies for occupational and physical therapists.* Baltimore: Williams & Wilkins.

Paul, S., & Ramsey, D. (1998). The effects of electronic music-making as a therapeutic activity for improving active range of motion. *Occupational Therapy International, 5,* 223–237.

Riccio, C. M., Nelson, D. L., & Bush, M. A. (1990). Adding purpose to the repetitive exercise of elderly women through imagery. *American Journal of Occupational Therapy, 44,* 714–719.

Rice, M. S. (1998). Purposefulness and cross transfer in a forearm supination and pronation task. *Scandinavian Journal of Occupational Therapy, 5,* 31–37.

Ross, L. M., Hall, B. A., & Heater, S. L. (1998). The Issue Is—Why are occupational therapists not doing more replication research? *American Journal of Occupational Therapy, 52,* 234–235.

Ross, L. M., & Nelson, D. L. (in press). Comparing materials-based occupation, imagery-based occupation, and rote movement through kinematic analysis of reach. *Occupational Therapy Journal of Research.*

Sakemiller, L. M., & Nelson, D. L. (1998). Eliciting functional extension in prone through the use of a game. *American Journal of Occupational Therapy, 52,* 150–157.

Schmidt, C. L., & Nelson, D. L. (1996). A comparison of three occupational forms in rehabilitation inpatients receiving upper extremity strengthening. *Occupational Therapy Journal of Research, 16,* 200–215.

Sietsema, J. M., Nelson, D. L., Mulder, R. M., Mervau-Scheidel, D., & White, B. E. (1993). The use of a game to promote arm reach in persons with traumatic brain injury. *American Journal of Occupational Therapy, 47,* 19–24.

Steinbeck, T. M. (1986). Purposeful activity and performance. *American Journal of Occupational Therapy, 40,* 529–534.

Thibodeaux, C. S., & Ludwig, F. M. (1988). Intrinsic motivation in product oriented and non-product oriented activities. *American Journal of Occupational Therapy, 42,* 169–175.

Thomas, J. J. (1993). Self-efficacy and patient education: A comparison of two programs. *Journal of Cardiopulmonary Rehabilitation, 13,* 398–405.

Thomas, J. J. (1995). Reducing anxiety during phase I cardiac rehabilitation. *Journal of Psychosomatic Research, 39,* 295–304.

Thomas, J. J. (1996). Materials-based, imagery-based, and rote exercise occupational forms: Effect on repetitions, heart rate, duration of performance, and self-perceived rest period in well elderly women. *American Journal of Occupational Therapy, 50,* 783–789.

Thomas, J. J., Vander Wyk, S. A., & Boyer, J. (1999). Contrasting occupational forms: Effects on performance and affect in patients undergoing phase II cardiac rehabilitation. *Occupational Therapy Journal of Research, 19,* 187–202.

van der Weel, F. R., van der Meer, A. L. H., & Lee, D. N. (1991). Effect of task on movement control in cerebral palsy: Implications for assessment and therapy. *Developmental Medicine and Child Neurology, 33,* 419–426.

Wagner, M. R., Krauss, A., & Horowitz, B. (1995). Occupationally embedded exercise, rote exercise, and the presence of another person in the exercise context. *Israel Journal of Occupational Therapy, 4,* E87–E101.

Wu, C., Trombly, C. A., & Lin, K. (1994). The relationship between occupational form and occupational performance: A kinematic perspective. *American Journal of Occupational Therapy, 48,* 679–687.

Yoder, R. M., Nelson, D. L., & Smith, D. A. (1989). Added-purpose versus rote exercise in female nursing home residents. *American Journal of Occupational Therapy, 43,* 581–586.

Yuen, H. K., Nelson, D. L., Peterson, C. Q., & Dickinson, A. (1994). Prosthesis training as a context for studying occupational forms and motoric adaptation. *American Journal of Occupational Therapy, 48,* 55–61.

Zimmerer-Branum, S., & Nelson, D. L. (1995). Occupationally embedded exercise versus rote exercise: A choice between forms by elderly nursing home residents. *American Journal of Occupational Therapy, 49,* 394–402.

18

Preparing for Activity
in the Future

Marie-Louise Blount, AM, OT, FAOTA
Paula Kramer, PhD, OTR, FAOTA
Jim Hinojosa, PhD, OT, FAOTA

Many of us are interested in predicting and understanding what the future will hold. The life course itself leads us to speculate about what the future holds for us, and, in a larger sense, we would like to know the shape of the future for those close to us, for our professions, for our nation's interests, and for the people on our planet. Some project these interests into the universe and, with more or less information, tie our course to long-term celestial change. For that matter, considerations about the future lead many to speculate about matters of religion and ultimate fate.

This chapter has a more mundane intent: to examine the future of human activity and how it may affect occupational therapy. We begin, however, with some notions about change at the societal level to put these thoughts into some context and to provide them with some shape.

The future as an area of unknown terrain may seem as inviting as the persons, places, and events that may inhabit it, and we may anticipate it with joy, or the future may seem fearsome, inhabited by unwanted changes, anticipated losses, and debility. Clearly, our view of future events will vary by age, circumstances, health, and belief systems. We sometimes seek knowledge and understanding in a vain effort to control the future or at least to make it less uncertain.

Media depictions of the future have long included sleek young persons wearing bodysuits (never winter coats or umbrellas) standing near glossily curved spaceships or missilelike automobiles with ultramodern, uncluttered homes and soaring highways or transit flyovers hurtling through the background. We can see some of these elements every day in our world. But the world we inhabit is very different from space-age fantasies. We live with the juxtaposition of startlingly new and strikingly innovative changes with familiar, expected, tried-and-true, everyday experiences.

—— ▦ ——

Exercise 1

Answer each of the following questions in three sentences or less: Who am I? Who would I like to be? What are the similarities between the person you perceive yourself to be and the person you would like to be? What are the differences? What conclusions can you draw from this assignment? (Insel & Roth, 1985, p. 74)

We have no way to actually predict what will happen tomorrow, next week, next year, or in the year 2100. We do, of course, live with certain indicators of direction and possibility, which include knowledge of the past and the present in human affairs, the acceleration of technological change, information about population trends, and calculations about acid rain and global warming. On the basis of some of these indicators, we can therefore discuss some of the areas of most notable change and how they affect human activity but only as we can perceive them now. Sudden, transforming change may be less likely than incremental change, but it too can occur and can make all careful study of trends futile.

Media and Modes of Communication

Some of the most rapidly changing aspects of our environment in the mid-to-late 20th century have been in our modes and means of communication as well as the content of what we communicate. A recent report (Standage, 1998) suggested that the introduction of telegraphy was, in its day, as societally transforming as computer technology is today. Since the introduction of the telegraph, however, we have seen the development of all sorts of radio and wireless communication (including wireless telephones), global print media delivered via wireless communication and rapid transportation systems, television and videorecordings in rapidly proliferating forms, and computer technology that has spawned new applications, wonders, and intrusions every day. The Information Age indeed is here, and it has already had some interesting effects on the way in which we incorporate activity into our lives.

Persons now commonly have access to television with many channels, a wide range of radio stations of varying types, and on-line news with chat room options. These sources of information and entertainment have transformed persons' lives in a short time. Yet, persons still say that they are bored or that "there is nothing on" television or radio. Changes in media and modes of communication have likewise transformed our activity lives, including the following results: many persons spend a good part of their workday sitting at a monitor and keyboard; television watching but not much physical activity fills the leisure hours of many (perhaps the same) persons; and knowing which buttons to push and when not only operates the stereo and videocassette recorder but also many household appliances, cars, and jet aircraft. The use of exercise equipment is one mode of balancing human activity. Contemporary lives have overall become much more sedentary.

In addition, the ways in which we use our hands to accomplish tasks have radically changed. Technology has freed us from many manual tasks. Instead of writing letters and going to the post office to mail them, we send e-mail. Yet in some cases, technological changes have created the need for more complex fine motor skills. Programs exist that allow persons to talk into the computer rather than typing. These trends are likely to continue in coming decades.

Technological Change

Although communication technology has a primary effect on our lives, technological change likewise affects many aspects of our existence. These changes primarily affect the lives of persons in the so-called "developed" world. Some places exist in which finding a telephone is difficult, in which many persons cannot read, and in which hand tools are the principal means of activity in the home, leisure, and work environments. How technological changes will move to new populations in the future is a challenging topic to consider.

With rapidly developing and available technological devices and equipment, persons have developed new ways of interacting with devices and with each other. Today, many persons must have special skills to operate a stereo and videocassette recorder, a digital satellite television, and many household appliances. Special skills and knowledge are necessary to operate modern cars. Even more expertise and experience are necessary to control the advanced equipment that is an essential aspect of flying a jet or information processing.

For most of us, now and in the future, changing technology will affect every aspect of our lives, from high-powered toothbrushes, to food processors (Hafner, 1999), to color photocopiers, to magnetic resonance imaging, to robotics, to mood- and activity-enhancing drugs. Technological change and new products will affect not only our knowledge and interaction but also our bodies, how and why we move, and what we think and desire "we have always been empowered—yet oddly constrained—by the vocabulary of the moment" (Hall, 1999, p. 128). All of this will lead to some transformations in our daily activities, including, for occupational therapists, the need to analyze these changes and new activity patterns and to explore them with our clients, whose own lives will have altered activity patterns, emerging interests, and restructured circumstances. This will be true even before considering the influence of disability and possible new limitations on the lives of these clients.

Technological change will add to the resources available in the rehabilitation process and may, like other societal changes, affect the necessity for and method of delivering our services. These changes affect the way in which we carry out our daily activities, the way we feel about the activities that we do, and the tools we use.

Changing Resources

Recent history indicates that the way in which we generate, trade, and expend money, goods, and other resources has changed. We can be sure that such change will continue. We can be fairly sure that economic troughs and booms and consequent adjustments in all quarters of society will occur. This chapter discusses how some recent economic changes influence the delivery of health care. Fluctuating resources and, in the United States, the lack of guaranteed health care coverage for all suggest that any type of health care may not be available to some portion of society. Any economic uncertainty and resulting shortages of services will lead to segments of society being unable to fulfill their personal goals for well-being, to consequent social unrest, and to anomie. In good times, more possibilities exist for addressing social ills and shortages, but the choices that we make will never address all of the social inequities that exist. Persons seeking to improve their life chances and to find solutions for their own personal dilemmas will have difficulty doing so when the economy is faltering and will have more opportunities to meet their goals in prosperous times.

In the future, occupational therapists must consider issues of resources and their effects on persons' lives when planning intervention, perhaps even more so than we do now. Creativity and ingenuity will be particularly necessary for persons who have fewer resources and pressing needs, whereas knowledge of how to access on-line investing and the latest sophisticated adaptive equipment may be necessary for other clients. Thus, because we must be prepared to work in a world in which types and knowledge of technology are ever changing and are continually more demanding, we must likewise give more attention to our own adaptive skills, our knowledge of the simplest and most rudimentary ways to solve problems of living and doing, and our willingness to offer our services pro bono when necessary to provide those services in a somewhat equitable fashion.

Tradition: The Pull of the Familiar

The *X-Files* world of sleek mystery and intellect is not the one we live in every day, and it may not be the one in which we will live in the future. Most of us would not be satisfied with form-fitting spacesuits and barren landscapes filled only with objects constructed by persons, objects that emphasize efficiency above other features.

Within most of us is a desire for the asymmetrical, the familiar, even the traditional. As one of the authors writes this, the surrounding landscape strongly influences her. The goldfinches and the wildflowers distract her as she sits outdoors while she writes. The natural beauty all around her reinforces the obverse of the electronic world that was at her fingertips. Yes, electricity, telephones, and a computer are nearby, but family, expected behaviors, familiar foods, joys of work, and beautiful objects likewise shape her world.

Most of us enjoy a world that combines the new and startling with the established and familiar (Friedman, 1999). Sociologists have termed the fireplaces in our homes, the oatmeal we eat for breakfast, and the flowers in our window boxes *rural survivals*. We have every reason to believe that the good and bad in our past and present activity lives will follow us in some form into the future. Occupational therapy practitioners who emphasize the importance of arts and crafts in purposeful activities remind us that our knowledge of how to make things with our hands, of how to shape beauty, is a human impulse that will not be lost to us or to our clients in the future.

Consequences of Change

When examining our daily activities and even those activities that are special or unusual, clearly adaptation to change is a requirement of the human condition. This is true for each of us just as it is true for the small child who is trying to overcome difficulties of movement, the young adult who is trying to cope with a devastating injury, or the elderly person who is dealing with even modest physical and mental changes resulting from aging.

Human beings hold some aspects of their futures in their heads and hands. As stated earlier, past actions and circumstances have determined some aspects of the future. We can foresee some of these developments by carefully examining current trends. Most persons make choices that shape their futures. Nations, too, plan educational, transportation, and communication systems as well as relationships with other nations that influence the future, the environment, and the ability to deal with one another.

Human beings do not plan much of what occurs in our lives and in the larger world, and indeed much is unplannable. Furthermore, all of our actions have unintended consequences. At one time, we had no knowledge of a link between tobacco smoking and lung cancer. We now see discernible but unintended connections among World Wars I and II and developments in the Balkan republics. Our efforts to lead healthy lives do not invariably lead us to the outcomes that we anticipated. Serendipity and tragedy are always available to surprise and shock us. These observations only serve to remind us that a good future is always uncharted and that the best treatment plans need reconsideration.

The Life Course

One scientific genre that provides us with reports from time to time is the approach to human development that promotes the extension of the healthy human life span, a world that, during the past several centuries, has become cleaner for many of us and has provided better nutrition, safer childbirth, fewer children per family, and the eradication or decreased incidence of some diseases. A conscious plan and intent by some to move further in that direction holds tantalizing notions of even longer, more successful lives.

Nonetheless, as occupational therapists, a major concern of our emphasis on normal and therapeutic activity must currently and in the future be on enhancing and fulfilling an already extended life course. We must continue to attend to all the issues of human development, both healthy and deleterious, that we have made our focus. In the future, the promises and consequences of human development and aging and how they interact with purposeful activities and occupation will continue to be a central theme for us. In doing so, we should not over- or underemphasize either end of the life cycle nor should we neglect adolescence, young adulthood, or middle adulthood, no matter what chronological ages these periods encompass. The transitions of life and aging as a usual and inexorable process will always influence our activities and interests and therefore the way in which we apply activities therapeutically.

Belief Systems and Human Actions

Predictions of the future and generalizations about outcomes cannot fail to consider how ideology, convictions, and political actions affect human behavior. Neat plans not only become messy because of unintended consequences but also because the choices we make are outcomes of our interpretations of the world, sometimes resulting from fervently held beliefs, religious traditions, political leanings, or ideological conditioning. Part of what makes the future unpredictable are these very belief systems that lead persons to make war, demand conformity with the tenets of their religion, promote new educational systems, fear change, and engage in new individual or shared activities. Therefore, we truly cannot know what the future will hold for occupational therapy, even though we have a responsibility as occupational therapists to stand for, promulgate, and adapt the tenets of our profession in the climate of the belief systems that develop. Furthermore, those of us who have been engaged in this process must pave the way for you, the occupational therapists of the future, to draw from the knowledge and achievements of the past, to avoid the pitfalls that experience has shown us, to learn from the indicators that others provided in which purposeful activities are moving and changing, and to apply their positive attributes to assist persons who need such assistance to lead fuller and more satisfying lives.

Genetic Engineering

In efforts to evaluate the scope of the future and how it will affect human activity, one area of knowledge that is bound to influence us is the burgeoning science of genetics and efforts to understand how the genetic map works. Work to increase knowledge in this area has been and will continue to be wildly successful. Alterations in the gene pool, in how we treat illnesses and disabilities, and in how to promote fertility or to vary heritability are highly likely to affect the practice of our profession and even who our clients will be. For example, future practice will no doubt embrace more twins and triplets. In some cases, low birth weights and more complex multiple pregnancies will produce children requiring intervention. Even more likely, however, will be a changing human landscape resulting from increased knowledge of and success with various methods of enhancing fertility.

Changes in the field of fertility intervention are already coming to our attention, but some commentators believe that these advances will affect a relatively small proportion of the population. Nonetheless, occupational therapists specializing in pediatrics will probably see many representatives from this population.

In the future, some will use cloning, efforts to modify genetic impairment, and even selective eugenics to control reproduction, reproductive choices, and heritable diseases. As with other predictions for the future, one can be sure that some of these creations will have unintended consequences. Possibilities for new and unimagined developments in the areas of genetics and reproductive technology are probably among the most revolutionary changes that will affect our notions about family, our definitions of human beings and relationships, and occupational therapy practice.

Future Practice

As the chapters in this book describe, occupational therapy practice is rooted in the use of purposeful activities with the ultimate goal that clients engage in occupations. As occupational therapy practitioners, we believe in the importance of activities and occupations. In the real world, however, many occupational therapy practitioners are often unable, unwilling, or reluctant to use purposeful activities as part of their daily interventions. Why do some occupational therapy practitioners not use purposeful activities? Frequently, when occupational therapy practitioners describe what they do in practice, they often discuss specific intervention strategies or techniques. Many describe specific hands-on manipulations or exercises that they perform during the treatment sessions. These kinds of answers reinforce the belief that the techniques for the treatments are more important than the performance of the specific activity itself, when the ability to perform the activity may be the goal that the client is trying to achieve. Occupational therapy practitioners are ultimately concerned with the client's ability to engage in occupations. Engagement in occupations requires that clients be able to perform the many purposeful activities that are the foundations of the specific occupations of their lives. Therefore, as occupational therapy practitioners, we should be comfortable explaining the outcomes of intervention in terms of the client's ability to engage in occupations. Activities are useful in treatment because they are the foundation for engaging in occupations. Thus, our measures of success are the client's abilities to perform the specific activities so that he or she can ultimately engage in occupations. As occupational therapy practitioners, we must reaffirm the importance of the person's ability to perform occupations.

The future of occupational therapy is rich because society focuses on function or the person's ability to engage in meaningful tasks. The challenge to occupational therapy practitioners is to move forward and yet be true to our roots. We must value personal needs and desires and what is meaningful to our clients. We must put aside our expectations of the client and focus on the client's expectations for himself or herself. We must learn about the cultures of our clients and work together with the clients to identify meaningful activities and occupations that are consistent with their values and their heritage. This is the art of our practice: focusing on the will of the client and not on the desires of the practitioner. Once we have mastered artful practice that is true to our profession, we must move forward in the world of science, which involves documenting what we do and explaining how valuable it is to the person. Once we recognize the importance of occupation to the person, the value of the occupation to society becomes immediately apparent. Through the effective use of occupational therapy, society can use persons who are willing and able to engage in meaningful occupation.

Occupational therapy's concern with a person's ability to do purposeful activities and occupations is grounded in functional outcomes. In the therapeutic process, the therapist first establishes functional goals that are meaningful to the client and will assist the client in performing activities and occupations successfully. To determine whether the intervention has been effective, occupational therapists must clearly identify functional outcomes. Inherent in functional outcomes is the client's ability to perform purposeful activities so that he or she can engage in occupations. Functional performance implies that a person is able to perform specific activities that allow him or her to perform occupations and, thus, be a more functional human being. What could be more functional than dressing oneself, feeding oneself, or being able to take care of one's children? In our view, occupational therapy involves a concern for developing optimal and independent function. The foci of future practice will be the measurement of the success of the intervention through the demonstration of functional outcomes and the refinement of our theoretical base through the determination of which frames of reference or types of interventions are most effective for our clients. Furthermore, by highlighting the importance of the person's ability to do something he or she values as a measure of the success of our interventions, we will demonstrate the value of occupational therapy to society.

Our concern for the person must additionally involve the context of his or her life. We can no longer focus solely on the person's needs and physical environment. Activities occur in a broader framework. Meaningful activities for a person often relate to others. Interventions must include family members and social and community contexts. Currently, we do this in a limited manner. We treat children with family-centered care. Inpatient units now focus on involving the family members of clients. In general, however, our focus is still the person without concern for the broader context of his or her life. This conceptual expansion will bring interventions out of the clinical setting and make the activity more meaningful to the client and other important persons in his or her life. Broadening our scope brings the practice of occupational therapy into contact with a larger population and demonstrates our value to a broader public.

Another possible change in our practice will involve attending to groups as well as persons. We use groups in intervention, but this is a broader conceptualization of groups as populations. Currently, we treat persons with repetitive motion injuries. In the future, however, we may direct more of our attention to the prevention of such injuries by intervening with groups who may be prone to such problems. We may change the environment, or we may try to change the way a person performs specific activities. Prevention is just a small part of our practice today, but it should become more prominent in the future. Our increasingly aging population will demand our attention to help them adapt their activities so that they can continue to be vitally involved in their chosen occupations. The adaptation of activities on a broader scale will become an essential component of practice.

In reflecting on future practice, we realize that the future is always unpredictable, sometimes exciting, and often threatening. Although we cannot predict what the future holds, we can reflect on whether we have a sound foundation on which the future can evolve. Today, occupational therapy has the potential of being a prominent profession in the 21st century. This will become a reality if occupational therapy practitioners continue to provide interventions that are responsive to societal change. Shifts in the sites of practice and service delivery models are evident in all areas of practice. Since the 1990s, occupational therapy services have shifted from clinic settings to more integrated community, classroom, and home settings.

The strength of occupational therapy has always been its practitioners' willingness and abilities to adapt and change in response to society. If occupational therapy is to continue to be viable, practitioners must continually examine their interventions in the light of a changing society. We must examine society to set our intervention priorities and to select the most appropriate tools for interventions. What activities do persons value? What are the activities that persons desire and in which they need to engage? How can occupational therapy practitioners use activities therapeutically if they do not know which activities in a society are foundational to its members' occupations? Additionally, occupational therapy practitioners must have an expanded appreciation of society that includes understanding the needs of minorities and persons who are poor, chronically ill, and elderly. Whether and how occupational therapy addresses these issues may determine how viable occupational therapy will be in the next decade. Occupational therapy practitioners must become familiar with changes in the health care and education systems as they evolve. Occupational therapy practitioners cannot afford to continue to watch passively and attempt to respond to changes; occupational therapy practitioners must become active in shaping newly emerging systems. To move beyond direct services, occupational therapy practitioners must advocate for the concerns of the individual client within managed services. Practitioners must begin to create new service delivery models that ensure quality care in natural environments.

Education: Purposeful Activities and Occupation

Many aspects of the world are cyclical. Ideas go in and out of fashion just as skirt lengths do. As professions grow and develop over time, they, too, experience a fluctuation of ideas. Professions either respond to societal changes, or they become obsolete. When occupational therapy began, its basis was occupation, and it stressed the importance of engaging in occupation for a healthy, productive life.

During the years, the centrality of the term *occupation* to occupational therapy changed. During the 1940s, occupation became much less crucial to the profession. We focused more on activities and activity analysis and moved away from the importance of occupation to the client. The intent was to match the activity with the client's condition. Our practice became somewhat mechanistic and focused on the goals of the therapist rather than the needs of the client. We worked within a medical model and followed many medical procedures and dictates. Therapeutic modalities became crafts, exercises, and the use of machinery. We attempted to move toward a concentration on science (or what we perceived at that time to be science). The profession wanted to closely align itself with medicine so that others would view occupational therapy more scientifically. At this time, the American Occupational Therapy Association (AOTA) and the American Medical Association jointly accredited educational programs. Educational programs became more science oriented as well and introduced more basic sciences into the curriculum and decreased the emphasis on crafts. The relationship of art and crafts to the profession became less clear, and many practitioners questioned the relevance of crafts to practice. The term *occupation* is almost nonexistent in the literature during that time. Other professions absorbed much of what we generally considered to be part of our domain of concern, some traditional and others that were just developing at this time. In retrospect, we were seemingly less aware of the value of what we do than others were.

War efforts changed the focus of life. During World War II, occupational therapists were an essential part of the rehabilitation team. The focus of intervention included activities of daily living, work, and exercise. Medicine devalued the active involvement of the patient in care, and occupational therapists' use of crafts and having the patient be actively involved in his or her own treatment did not fit well with this perspective. Although practitioners continued to use crafts, the use of crafts was questionable. From this period through the 1960s, therapeutic intervention minimally involved the positive aspects of activities and occupation and concentrated on function. Education during this time focused even more heavily on the sciences, with a strong emphasis on the motor system. Activities were still a part of curricula, but they were quite prescriptive. Practitioners matched activities to the person's deficit areas, not to the person's interests or values.

During the late 1970s, occupational therapy literature began exploring the importance of getting back to the roots of the profession, which resulted in an increase in theory building and a discussion of the importance of research. Some of the literature focused on promoting occupational therapy as a basic science with concepts that are easy to measure, whereas other writings focused on the concept of occupation. Researchers used the terms *activities*, *purposeful activities*, and *occupation* interchangeably and believed they were synonymous. In treatment, therapists moved away from using diversional activities, and interventions flowed from theoretical information. Frames of reference became more prominent in practice. The profession began to debate its philosophical base and finally adopted "The Philosophical Base of Occupational Therapy" (AOTA, 1979). The terms *occupation* and *purposeful activities* were synonymous.

Education made a dramatic change during the 1970s. Theories of occupational therapy became part of curricula. Several persons articulated models of practice for the profession. Various degree levels emerged, as did postprofessional education opportunities. Students learned to relate their activities for clients to theory. This evolution continued through the 1980s with the development of more theories and frames of reference. Researchers formulated clearer relationships between theory and practice.

During the past decade, our profession has learned that science is not necessarily synonymous with the basic sciences and may include the social and behavioral sciences and the concept of scientific inquiry. We have experienced a renewed emphasis on scholarship and research but from a broader perspective, including both quantitative and qualitative methodologies. A renewed focus on occupation has emerged.

The change in our perspective is evident in the changes in educational standards as well. The 1983 and 1991 *Essentials and Guidelines for an Accredited Educational Program for the Occupational Therapist* (AOTA, 1983a, 1991a) and *Essentials and Guidelines for an Accredited Educational Program for the Occupational Therapy Assistant* (AOTA, 1983b, 1991b) do not even use the word *occupation*. Instead, they use terms *activity* and *purposeful activities*. The most recent educational standards, *Standards for an Accredited Educational Program for the Occupational Therapist* (Accreditation Council for Occupational Therapy Education [ACOTE], 1998a), and *Standards for an Accredited Educational Program for the Occupational Therapy Assistant* (ACOTE, 1998b), use *occupation*, *activity*, and *purposeful activities* but focus most heavily on occupation.

Exercise 2

Review the *Standards for an Accredited Educational Program for the Occupational Therapist* and the *Standards for an Accredited Educational Program for the Occupational Therapy Assistant*. Answer each of the following questions: Do the definitions in the glossary of *activity, purposeful activity,* and *occupation* clearly describe the relationship between these terms? What is that relationship? Identify the relationship between purposeful activities and occupation in your own life. Think of three examples. Keeping these three examples in mind, closely examine Section B 2.0, "The Basic Tenets of Occupational Therapy." In your educational experience to this point, how have the differences between these terms been exemplified?

Although little agreement exists among scholars on the definitions of *occupation* and *purposeful activities*, most agree that these concepts are basic to occupational therapy. The profession adopted a hierarchy (AOTA, 1997) in which *occupation* is the umbrella term, and *purposeful activities* is an important component under that umbrella. The newest educational standards suggest a hierarchy that is somewhat different. Our profession must continue to explore these terms, define them, and debate their relationship to each other and to the practice of occupational therapy.

The challenge to education in the future is to encourage the exploration of these concepts, to debate their meanings, and to identify how they relate to practice. Students must learn to think about the relationships among activity, purposeful activity, and occupation and how these concepts apply to intervention and to the profession as a whole. These concepts are the cornerstone of our profession and require our attention. Although our profession has grown extensively, it has likewise come full circle by moving closer to its roots. We must clarify the meaning and importance of occupation and purposeful activities and through them explain and describe what we do and its importance to society.

Summary

In 1961, Mary Reilly claimed that "occupational therapy can be one of the greatest ideas of 20th century medicine" (Reilly, 1962, p. 1). As we move into the 21st century, despite changes in society and technology, occupational therapy continues to provide a valuable service to persons and society. We have changed and grown, just as society has changed and grown, and yet we still provide a fundamental and meaningful service to persons by helping them maintain control of their lives through participation in occupations and activities that are meaningful to them. The future will provide the practice of occupational therapy with many challenges, yet behind each challenge is an opportunity to promote the importance of human activity and occupation. ■

References

Accreditation Council for Occupational Therapy Education. (1998a). *Standards for an accredited educational program for the occupational therapist.* Bethesda, MD: American Occupational Therapy Association.

Accreditation Council for Occupational Therapy Education. (1998b). *Standards for an accredited educational program for the occupational therapy assistant.* Bethesda, MD: American Occupational Therapy Association.

American Occupational Therapy Association. (1979). The philosophical base of occupational therapy. *American Journal of Occupational Therapy, 33,* 785.

American Occupational Therapy Association. (1983a). Essentials of an accredited educational program for the occupational therapist. *American Journal of Occupational Therapy, 37,* 817–823.

American Occupational Therapy Association. (1983b). Essentials of an accredited educational program for the occupational therapy assistant. *American Journal of Occupational Therapy, 37,* 824–830.

American Occupational Therapy Association. (1991a). Essentials and guidelines for an accredited educational program for the occupational therapist. *American Journal of Occupational Therapy, 45,* 1077–1084.

American Occupational Therapy Association. (1991b). Essentials and guidelines for an accredited educational program for the occupational therapy assistant. *American Journal of Occupational Therapy, 45,* 1085–1092.

American Occupational Therapy Association. (1997). Statement—Fundamental concepts of occupational therapy: Occupation, purposeful activity, and function. *American Journal of Occupational Therapy, 51,* 864–866.

Friedman, T. L. (1999). *The Lexus and the olive tree: Understanding globalization.* New York: Farrar, Straus & Giroux.

Hafner, K. (1999, May 27). Honey, I programmed the blanket: The omnipresent chip has invaded everything from dishwashers to dogs. *New York Times,* p. G125.

Hall, S. S. (1999, June 6). Journey to the center of my mind. *New York Times Magazine,* 122–128.

Insel, G. M., & Roth W. T. (1985). *Core concepts in health* (4th ed.). Palo Alto, CA: Mayfield.

Reilly, M. (1962). Occupational therapy can be one of the greatest ideas of 20th century medicine. *American Journal of Occupational Therapy, 16,* 1–9.

Standage, T. (1998). *The Victorian Internet: The remarkable story of the telegraph and the nineteenth century's on-line pioneers.* New York: Walker.

Index